Goodheart's

Same-Site Differential Diagnosis

A RAPID METHOD OF DIAGNOSING AND TREATING COMMON SKIN DISORDERS

Goodheart's

Same-Site Differential Diagnosis

A RAPID METHOD OF DIAGNOSING AND TREATING COMMON SKIN DISORDERS

HERBERT P. GOODHEART, M.D.

Associate Clinical Professor
Department of Dermatology
Mount Sinai School of Medicine
New York, New York
Director of Dermatology
Elmhurst Hospital Center
Elmhurst, New York

Wolters Kluwer | Lippincott Williams & Wilkins
Health

Philadelphia • Baltimore • New York • London
Buenos Aires • Hong Kong • Sydney • Tokyo

Acquisitions Editor: Sonya Seigafuse
Product Manager: Kerry Barrett
Production Manager: Alicia Jackson
Senior Manufacturing Manager: Benjamin Rivera
Marketing Manager: Kim Schonberger
Design Coordinator: Doug Smock
Production Service: Aptara, Inc.

Printed in China

Library of Congress Cataloging-in-Publication Data

Goodheart, Herbert P.
    Goodheart's same-site differential diagnosis : a rapid method of diagnosing and treating common skin disorders /
Herbert P. Goodheart.
        p. ; cm.
    Other title: Same-site differential diagnosis
    Includes bibliographical references and index.
    Summary: "Goodheart's Same-Site Differential Diagnosis is an easy-to-use reference for primary care physicians who are often on the front line of diagnosing and treating skin disorders. Organized in a head-to-toe fashion, the book presents 400 full-color images of common skin disorders and places them side by side with their clinical look-alikes or other diagnostic possibilities that occur at the same anatomic site. Since many skin disorders tend to occur at specific sites, this organization by region is helpful in narrowing the number of diagnostic possibilities and reaching a specific diagnosis or differential diagnosis quickly and accurately. The book presents differential diagnoses by region, along with key physical findings, laboratory tests, and historical information to help make a definitive diagnosis. Once a diagnosis is made, the management of each condition is described in step-by-step fashion on a facing page. Recommended first-line, second-line, and alternative therapies are briefly listed. A companion website will offer the fully searchable text and many additional images"–Provided by publisher.
    ISBN-13: 978-1-60547-746-6 (alk. paper)
    ISBN-10: 1-60547-746-X (alk. paper)
    1. Skin–Diseases–Diagnosis–Handbooks, manuals, etc. 2. Diagnosis, Differential–Handbooks, manuals, etc.
I. Title.   II. Title: Same-site differential diagnosis.
    [DNLM: 1. Skin Diseases–diagnosis–Handbooks. 2. Diagnosis, Differential–Handbooks.
3. Skin Diseases–therapy—Handbooks. WR 39]
    RL105.G66 2011
    616.5–dc22

                                                                    2010027791

To purchase additional copies of this book, call our customer service department at (800)
638-3030 or fax orders to (301) 223-2320. International customers should call (301) 223-2300.

Visit Lippincott Williams & Wilkins on the Internet: at LWW.com. Lippincott Williams & Wilkins customer service representatives are available from 8:30 am to 6 pm, EST.

10 9 8 7 6 5 4 3 2 1

Dedicated to Karen, my wife, my love, for her support, encouragement, and patience

Foreword: *Same-Site Differential Diagnosis*

Herb Goodheart is an astute, seasoned clinician who brings years of experience to this extraordinarily useful textbook that should be on the shelf of every practicing dermatologist, family practitioner, and resident. *Same-Site Differential Diagnosis* is an invaluable tool to help clinicians navigate through the differential diagnoses of various dermatologic disorders based on the part of the body that is affected. This easy-to-read book starts with dermatologic disorders of the head and proceeds all the way down to the feet, covering every body part between the two. Disorders of the hair, nails, and mucous membranes are reviewed as well. The latter are covered in two separate chapters- one dealing with the oral cavity and tongue and the second dealing with the pubic and genital area. The closing chapter deals with generalized eruptions not covered in earlier chapters of the book. Specifically, it offers an organized approach to the differential diagnosis of exfoliated dermatitis versus toxic epidermal necrolysis versus staphylococcal scalded skin syndrome.

Every chapter in the book is illustrated beautifully with photographs showing characteristic lesions to help readers recognize the conditions discussed. There is a simple, organized approach to the diagnosis of each disease or condition. Sections entitled *"Distinguishing Features," "Diagnosis,"* and *"Management"* are followed by bulleted points that are very simple to read and incredibly helpful. For example, distinguishing features of perioral dermatitis that help differentiate it from rosacea include its appearance in women between 15 and 40 years of age; small erythematous papules or pustules resembling acne, without telangiectasias; and occasional concomitant seborrheic dermatitis-like scaling. The bulleted points under the *"Diagnosis"* section are brief and to the point: Is biopsy helpful or are clinical features sufficient? The *"Management"* sections for each disorder are loaded with useful pearls. For example, a single bullet in the *"Management"* section for rosacea reviews the order of all oral antibiotics used to treat this condition. Occasionally, there are conditions that are frustrating to manage because of a lack of therapies. True to Dr. Goodheart's approach to patients in the clinic, simple measurements like telling a patient that the condition is benign are often sufficient, and that point is appropriately made for some of the diagnoses covered.

For some conditions, there are also flagged items that again provide useful bulleted points in yellow boxes entitled *"Also Consider"* or *"Rarely."* In the discussion of diffuse alopecia, for example, telogen effluvium and anagen effluvium are reviewed, but in the separate box, readers are reminded to *"Also Consider"* conditions like hyperthyroidism and hypothyroidism, connective tissue disease, secondary syphilis, etc. In addition, readers should also think of conditions that *"Rarely"* cause diffuse alopecia like "loose anagen syndrome" in children, congenital hair shaft abnormalities, malnutrition, heavy metal poisoning, and others. *Same-Site Differential Diagnosis* is also highlighted with many tips and alerts that are clinically important pearls. One of my favorites involves the discussion of the use of topical corticosteroids in patients who have developed perioral dermatitis as a result of steroid use. As many clinicians know, in the short term, topical steroids may benefit steroid-induced perioral dermatitis, but in the long run they make it worse. Dr. Goodheart's tip that this is "one step forward, two steps backward" is truly appropriate.

The first chapter of *Same-Site Differential Diagnosis* is on hair and scalp. It begins with an overview of alopecia and an erudite discussion of the various causes of hair loss. The differential diagnosis is further broken down by age of the patient. For example, in infants and young children clinicians should think of atopic dermatitis, seborrheic dermatitis and tinea amiantacea, whereas in adults the dermatoses of the scalp are most likely to be seborrheic dermatitis, psoriasis, and atopic dermatitis. Differences between men and women and between patients of different races are also discussed.

One of the features I like most about the book is that it offers important clues pertinent not only to body sites but also to specific areas within those body sites. For example, in the chapter on hands and fingers, the precise part of the hand affected offers clues to the diagnosis. As an example, granuloma annulare affects the dorsum of the hand, not the palm. It is also appropriate that there is a separate chapter for the arms, and there is yet another chapter on fingernails. The latter chapter offers a beautifully written, comprehensive discussion of the differential diagnosis of nail disorders and nail lesions with stunning photographs illustrating the differences between the various diagnoses. In that chapter alone, there are photographs illustrating onycholysis, onycholysis and green nail syndrome, onychomycosis, psoriasis nail pitting, psoriasis oil spots, psoriasis subungual hyperkeratosis, psoriatic onycholysis, eczematous dermatitis with nail dystrophy, subungual warts, subungual squamous cell carcinoma, subungual hematoma, longitudinal melanonychia, and acral lentiginous melanoma involving the nail.

Before opening this book, I wondered how the author would deal with areas of the body like the face and trunk that are prone to so many different dermatoses. I was delighted to see that he divided the face into many different sections in a very appropriate way. There are separate sections on the forehead and temples; eyelids and periorbital area; ears; nose and perinasal area; cheeks; lips and perioral area; oral cavity and tongue; and chin and mandibular area. The wisdom in dividing the face is very evident in the chapter on eyelids and periorbital area. In fact, many of the conditions discussed in this section are unique to the eyelids and periorbital area and don't affect the remainder of the face. Conditions such as hordeolum, chalazion, syringomas, xanthelasma, hydrocystoma, ocular rosacea and blepharitis are appropriately discussed in a separate chapter on the eyelids and periorbital area rather than included in what would have been a much larger and more awkward chapter including all dermatoses of the face. For the trunk, there are separate chapters on the axillae; buttocks and perineal area; breasts and inframammary area; umbilical area and trunk. Itching is a common symptom on the trunk and the differential diagnosis of itching is often challenging. One of my favorite sections of this book is the discussion of that differential diagnosis: pruritus and necrotic excoriations versus notalgia paresthetica versus macular amyloid. There is a useful tip here pointing out that angiotensin converting enzyme inhibitors used for hypertension are frequent causes of pruritus; and there is also an important alert that the pruritus of Hodgkin's disease often precedes the diagnosis of that disease by up to five years. That chapter also contains a helpful table on the differential diagnosis of viral exanthems.

There are so many rare and common dermatoses in our specialty that it would be a real challenge for a book of differential diagnosis based on body site to cover all of them. Pseudoxanthoma elasticum is a rare inherited disease that is a major focus of my research interests. It most commonly presents with yellow papules on the neck, and in starting that chapter, I wondered if the diagnosis would be mentioned. Of course, I would expect a chapter reviewing dermatologic conditions of the neck to mention skin tags and atopic dermatitis, but would a disease as rare as pseudoxanthoma elasticum be mentioned? Sure enough, pseudoxanthoma elasticum is one of the bulleted points highlighted under "*Rarely*" at the end of the solar elastosis discussion.

In the short time I've had access to the proofs of this book, they have become a valuable tool for me and will be very useful for every practicing dermatologist and family practitioner. I'm not sure how I survived the incessant questions about differential diagnosis at our weekly Grand Rounds when I was a resident without access to this book. But I know that my residents will fare much better since they'll undoubtedly look at this book every week before they present their Grand Rounds cases. I am equally certain that I'll use this book on a regular basis when I am challenged by difficult to diagnose conditions in the office. *Same-Site Differential Diagnosis* is a wonderful resource for anyone taking care of patients with skin disorders.

Mark Lebwohl, M.D.
Sol and Clara Kest Professor and Chairman
Department of Dermatology
The Mount Sinai School of Medicine

Preface

Formulating a differential diagnosis by region is based on the fact that many skin disorders have a predilection to occur at specific sites. This book's objective is to lead the health care provider who sees patients with skin problems to a specific diagnosis or to quickly reach a differential diagnosis between disorders that are often confused with one another.

Instead of the customary, potentially bewildering, method of illustrating skin disorders alphabetically or by clinical characteristics, this book is organized anatomically, progressing down the body from head to toe. Thus, a lesion is matched to the body part, and those conditions that present in a similar fashion are shown on the same page with their clinical "look alikes" that occur at the same site for easy comparison.

Characteristic historical information, physical findings, and laboratory tests that help distinguish the different conditions are pointed out. Less common and rare disorders are included in the differential diagnosis. Once a diagnosis is made, the management of each condition is described in a step-by-step fashion. Recommended and alternative therapies are briefly listed. Extensive cross referencing is used to direct the reader to other body sites that describe the same disorder.

Finally, in Appendix A, many of the generic medications are listed along with their brand names. In Appendix B, diagnostic and therapeutic techniques are illustrated. In Appendix C, the management of acne and rosacea are described.

Herbert P. Goodheart, M.D.
Associate Clinical Professor
Department of Dermatology
Mount Sinai School of Medicine
New York, New York
Director of Dermatology
Elmhurst Hospital Center
Elmhurst, New York

Acknowledgments

I thank the following people who helped to create this book:

Sonya Seigafuse, once again, my acquisition editor had the foresight to envision its potential value. The other major player is Kerry Barrett. Kerry has shown amazing attention to detail and her availability and patience to answer my ongoing multitude of questions and complications has brought this project to the finish line. Martha Cushman's editing kept track of a stream of material. She found many things awry (not unusual) and corrected a multitude of loose ends. Indu Jawwad, my New Delhi Aptara connection, has been right on top of every modification thrown her way. Many thanks go to you, Indu.

Thanks also go to my colleagues at Derm-Chat/Derm-Rx, who keep me up-to-date on the latest diagnostic and therapeutic issues in dermatology: Art Huntley, who founded and maintains this valuable online resource, as well as the "heavy posters"—Steve Emmet, Joe Eastern, Haines Ely, Ben Barankin, Diane Thaler, Ashit Mahwar, Otto Bastos, Bob Rudolph, Sahar Ghannam, Keith Vaughan, Kim Frederickson, Larry Finkel, Bill Danby, Sate Hamza, Noah Scheinfeld, Steve Feldman, Barry Ginsberg, Bill Smith, Steve Comite, Pierre Jaffe, Omid Zargari, Becky Bushong, Ed Zabawski, Jerry Litt, Jo Bohannon-Grant, Ben Treen, Chuck Fishman, Kendra Bergstrom, Toni Notaro, Lennie Rosmarin, Barry Ginsburg, Susan Bushelman, Robin Berger, Maida Burow, Stu Kittay, Diane Davidson, Chuck Miller (x2), Norm Guzick, Pat Condry, Kevin Smith, Steve Stone, Gail Drayton, Linda Spencer, and many others who are too numerous to mention, have been my "online class-mates." This book is also dedicated to the memory of one of our truly great dermatologists, Skee Smith, an educator, a great clinician, and role model for all of us.

Contents

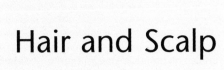

Hair and Scalp

Androgenetic alopecia, physiologic hair loss, is often viewed as an indication of diminished physical attractiveness, particularly in Western societies. Other types of alopecia may be due to temporary disease or medication reactions (e.g., cytotoxic drugs, birth control pills, anticoagulants). Androgenetic alopecia in men and women, diffuse alopecia in white women, and traumatic alopecia in women of African descent are the most common causes of hair loss in adults.

Various inflammatory scalp disorders such as extensive alopecia areata and folliculitis decalvans are also causes of alopecia that may lead to profound psychological problems. Chronic inflammatory scalp disorders such as dandruff (seborrheic dermatitis), atopic dermatitis, lichen simplex chronicus, and psoriasis are frequent causes of discomfort and embarrassment, but they generally do not result in permanent alopecia.

Scarring alopecia (permanent loss of hair follicles), also known as *cicatricial alopecia*, comprises a diverse group of disorders that may be due to infections, trauma (often self-induced), discoid lupus erythematosus, or lichen planopilaris. Scarring alopecia is seen in all ethnic groups and races; however, African American and African Caribbean black women and men are most often affected.

In young children, alopecia areata and tinea capitis account for most cases of alopecia. Seborrheic dermatitis ("cradle cap") and atopic dermatitis are the scalp disorders most often noted in infants.

The scalp is a common location for benign neoplastic lesions such as seborrheic keratoses, various nevi, pilar cysts, and premalignant solar keratoses. Squamous cell carcinoma, less commonly, basal cell carcinoma, and melanoma, may occur on the scalp.

IN THIS CHAPTER

- Androgenetic alopecia *vs* diffuse alopecia
- Alopecia areata *vs* tinea capitis
- Traction alopecia *vs* trichotillomania *vs* chemically induced alopecia
- Discoid lupus erythematosus *vs* lichen planopilaris *vs* folliculitis decalvans

Infants and Young Children
- Atopic dermatitis *vs* seborrheic dermatitis *vs* tinea amiantacea

Older Children and Adults
- Seborrheic dermatitis *vs* psoriasis *vs* atopic dermatitis
- Seborrheic keratosis *vs* solar keratosis *vs* squamous cell carcinoma

Androgenic Alopecia *vs* Diffuse Alopecia

Androgenic Alopecia

Androgenic alopecia (AGA), which manifests as male- or female-pattern common baldness, is not a disease but a normal consequence of aging. Seen more frequently in men, AGA tends to be less apparent in women because hair loss in women is generally incomplete and begins at a later age.

Androgenic alopecia is genetically influenced (autosomal dominant with variable penetrance); it is more common in whites than in Asians or blacks. It is caused by an androgenic action (dihydrotestosterone) on hair follicles that shortens the anagen (growth) phase of the hair cycle and thus produces thinner, shorter hairs in a process known as *miniaturization*.

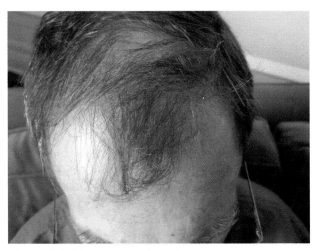

Figure 1-1 Male-pattern alopecia.

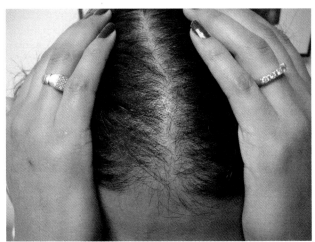

Figure 1-2 Female-pattern alopecia.

DISTINGUISHING FEATURES
- Males: *M-shaped* pattern, which subsequently may involve the vertex (Fig. 1-1)
- Females: *Christmas tree* pattern (widening of the part) on crown of scalp; more subtle and tends to begin later in life than in males (Fig. 1-2)

DIAGNOSIS
- Clinical pattern and absence specific disease that may cause hair loss
- Blood tests and other laboratory studies only when the diagnosis is in doubt

MANAGEMENT
- Females
  - Minoxidil 2% foam or solution **(Rogaine)**
  - Systemic antiandrogen therapy (e.g., spironolactone or oral contraceptives)
- Males
  - Minoxidil 5% solution **(Rogaine),** finasteride **(Propecia)**
- Males and females
  - Hair transplantation
  - Wigs/hairpieces

Diffuse Alopecia

Diffuse alopecia (Fig. 1-3) is seen almost exclusively in females. Causes include **telogen effluvium,** a diffuse, *non-patterned* shedding of resting hairs that may be due to a history of an acute event, such as an illness, childbirth (*post-partum effluvium*), drug reactions, iron deficiency, or low serum ferritin. Also, it may be the result of chronic illnesses and, rarely, inadequate protein in diet. When telogen effluvium results from an acute event, the hair usually regrows in a few months without treatment. **Anagen effluvium** results from the shedding of growing hairs and is most often due to cancer chemotherapeutic drugs.

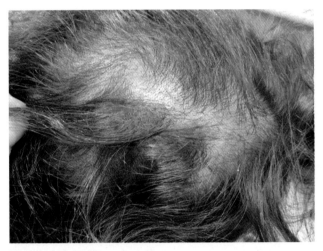

Figure 1-3 Diffuse alopecia.

DISTINGUISHING FEATURES
- Diffuse, nonpatterned alopecia due to loss of resting (telogen) or growing (anagen) hairs
- Frontal margin spared
- Usually without obvious bald patches

DIAGNOSIS
- Clinical presentation
- Comprehensive history
- Appropriate blood tests (e.g., thyroid-stimulating hormone, complete blood count, ferritin, total iron-binding capacity)
- Punch biopsy of scalp, if necessary (see Appendix B)

MANAGEMENT
- Correction of underlying medical or nutritional problem(s)
- Discontinuance of chemotherapeutic agent

☞ ALSO CONSIDER
- Senescent thinning
- Hyperthyroidism or hypothyroidism
- Sex hormone abnormality in women
- Acute connective tissue disease (e.g., systemic lupus erythematosus)
- Secondary syphilis

RARELY
- Diffuse alopecia areata
- Anagen hair loss in a child due to "loose anagen syndrome"
- Chronic telogen effluvium
- Congenital hair shaft abnormalities
- Insufficient calories, protein, vitamins, and heavy metal poisoning in the appropriate clinical context

Alopecia Areata *vs* Tinea Capitis

Alopecia Areata

Alopecia areata (AA), an idiopathic disorder, is characterized by nonscarring hair loss. Alopecia areata most commonly affects young adults and children. Persons with AA may also have a higher risk of atopy. The origin of AA is generally considered autoimmune because biopsy findings demonstrate T-cell infiltrates surrounding hair follicles and, albeit infrequently, may be associated with other autoimmune disorders, such as vitiligo, thyroid disease (Hashimoto disease), diabetes, Down syndrome, and pernicious anemia. Alopecia areata is most often found on the scalp, eyebrows, eyelashes, and other hair-bearing areas of the face, such as the beard or mustache.

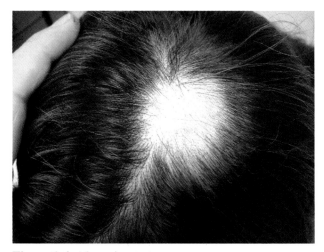

Figure 1-4 Alopecia areata.

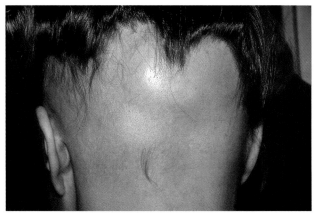

Figure 1-5 Alopecia areata (ophiasis pattern).

DISTINGUISHING FEATURES
- One or many smooth oval, round, or geometric patches of alopecia (Fig. 1-4)
- Bandlike at scalp margins (ophiasis) (Fig. 1-5)
- "Exclamation point hairs" at the periphery of bald spots
- Completely normal-appearing skin (i.e., no scale or erythema)
- Possible involvement of entire scalp (alopecia totalis) or entire body (alopecia universalis)

DIAGNOSIS
- Clinical appearance
- Rarely, a scalp biopsy is necessary if diagnosis in doubt (see Appendix B)

MANAGEMENT
- Observation and reassurance, because mild cases of AA often show spontaneous regrowth
- Superpotent (class 1) topical steroids with or without occlusion (see Appendix A)
- Intralesional triamcinolone injections administered every 6 to 8 weeks (see Appendix B)
- Systemic steroids (e.g., prednisone) in rapidly advancing alopecia
- Emotional support, the use of a wig, if necessary
- Possible workup for other diseases (e.g., thyroid disease) that may be suggested by history and/or physical examination
- Alternative treatments: topical minoxidil **(Rogaine),** scalp massage, heat, aloe vera, vitamins, hypnotherapy, oral psoralens combined with exposure to ultraviolet light in the A range (PUVA), topical cyclosporine, irritant contact dermatitis with anthralin, and immunotherapy by induction of contact dermatitis with various chemical compounds

Tinea Capitis

Tinea capitis, or "ringworm," is a fungal infection that most commonly occurs in prepubertal African American children. *Trichophyton tonsurans* is, by far, the most common etiologic agent (>90% of cases). Other species, such as *Microsporum audouinii*, which is spread from human to human, and *Microsporum canis*, which is spread from animals (cats and dogs), are more often seen in white children.

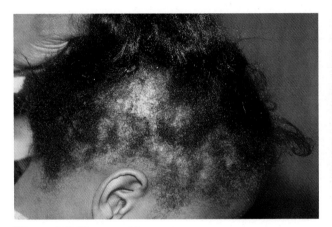

Figure 1-6 Tinea capitis.

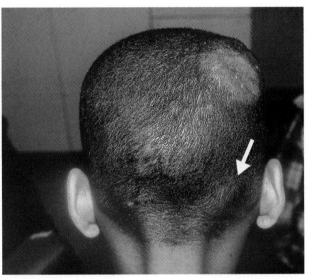

Figure 1-7 Tinea capitis (kerion). Note: Occipital lymph node (arrow). (From Goodheart HP. *Goodheart's Photoguide to Common Skin Disorders: Diagnosis and Management.* 3rd ed. Philadelphia, PA: Lippincott Williams & Wilkins; 2009, with permission.)

DISTINGUISHING FEATURES
- Focal or diffuse bald patches; often scaly, itchy, and inflamed (Fig. 1-6)
- Broken hair shafts, leaving residual black stumps ("black dot" ringworm)
- "Gray patch" ringworm, which consists of round, scaly plaques of alopecia in which hairs are broken off close to the surface of the scalp
- Possible inflammatory pustular nodules or plaques called *kerions*. A kerion is a boggy, pustular, indurated, tumorlike mass, which represents an inflammatory hypersensitivity reaction to the fungus (Fig. 1-7)
- Regional nontender adenopathy

DIAGNOSIS
- A potassium hydroxide (KOH) preparation or fungal culture confirms the diagnosis (see Appendix B)

MANAGEMENT
- Griseofulvin, terbinafine (**Lamisil**), itraconazole (**Sporanox**) (see Appendix A)
- Low-dose/short-term prednisone for kerion
- ☑ **TIP: Topical antifungal agents are of limited value.**

ALSO CONSIDER
- Tinea amiantacea
- Seborrheic dermatitis ("cradle cap")
- Atopic dermatitis
- Pediculosis capitis
- Traction alopecia
- Trichotillomania
- Folliculitis
- Secondary syphilis
- Bacterial pyoderma
- Psoriasis

Traction Alopecia *vs* Trichotillomania *vs* Chemically Induced Alopecia

Traction Alopecia

Traction alopecia is caused by the persistent physical stress of gripping injury from tight hair braiding (e.g., corn-rows), tight curlers, and other mechanical hair-styling techniques that have become very popular for many African American and African Caribbean people.

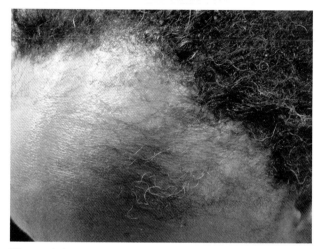

Figure 1-8 Traction alopecia.

DISTINGUISHING FEATURES
- Symmetric pattern of hair loss with broken hairs (Fig. 1-8)
- Alopecia at the temples and along the frontal hairline
- Characteristic border of residual hairs at the distal margin of alopecia
- Can lead to permanent alopecia

DIAGNOSIS
- Clinical appearance and a history of mechanical hair-straightening techniques

MANAGEMENT
- Discontinuance of responsible styling practices. If the patient decides to continue with her styling practices, she or he (rarely) should:
  - Have looser wrapping to produce less tension on hair roots
  - Have braids that are larger and looser
  - Unbraid every 2 weeks

Trichotillomania

Trichotillomania describes a repetitive, compulsive hair pulling, twirling, plucking, or twisting that results in alopecia. Manipulation of hair from the scalp, eyebrows, and eyelashes by the patient's own hand can reach the point of baldness. Often due to an underlying emotional problem, it becomes habitual once the behavior is established. Trichotillomania is seen most often in young white females. Like many other compulsive behaviors, it is thought to arise from an imbalance of levels of serotonin and glutamate in the brain.

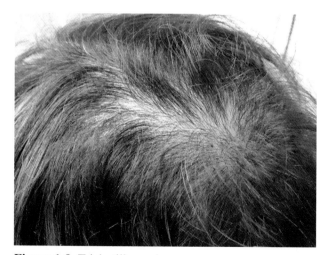

Figure 1-9 Trichotillomania.

DISTINGUISHING FEATURES
- Hairs that tend to be broken at different lengths (Fig. 1-9)
- Asymmetric hair loss
- Alopecia patches that tend to have irregular, angulated borders
- May involve eyebrows and eyelashes

DIAGNOSIS
- History and physical examination

MANAGEMENT
- Psychotherapy, behavior modification, hypnotherapy
- Selective serotonin uptake inhibitors and pimozide (**Orap**)

✔ **TIP: Alternative treatment—in a recent study, the nutritional supplement *N*-acetylcysteine, 1200 to 2400 mig, available in health food stores, has been shown to benefit more than 50% of people who took it.**

Chemically Induced Alopecia

Chemically induced alopecia and **central centrifugal cicatricial alopecia (CCCA)** are the current terms to describe this type of scarring alopecia that is mostly seen in African American women. The alopecia is most often caused by the use of various chemicals and/or heat to straighten hair (e.g., relaxers, hot combs, and permanent wave products); however, some cases also arise idiopathically. *Hot comb alopecia* and *follicular degeneration syndrome* are the traditional terms coined to describe this condition.

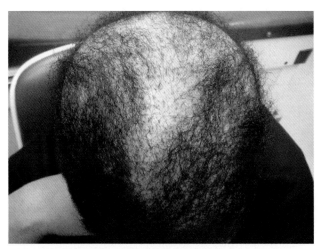

Figure 1-10 Chemically induced alopecia.

DISTINGUISHING FEATURES
- Most often seen on the crown and vertex in irregular pattern (less symmetric than traction alopecia) and reflects the areas where the chemicals or hot comb have been applied
- Possible scaling, pustules, and itching
- May result in permanent alopecia and scarring (Fig. 1-10)

MANAGEMENT
- Discontinuance of styling practices responsible for the condition. If the patient decides to continue with his or her styling practices, he or she should use chemicals only on the hair and not directly on the scalp
- Scalp biopsy if diagnosis is in doubt (see Appendix B)
- No effective therapy for CCCA

ALSO CONSIDER
- Systemic lupus erythematosus
- Alopecia areata
- Tinea capitis
- Cutaneous sarcoidosis
- Infectious or primary inflammatory scarring alopecia

Discoid Lupus Erythematosus *vs* Lichen Planopilaris *vs* Folliculitis Decalvans

Discoid Lupus Erythematosus

Discoid lupus erythematosus (DLE), also referred to as *chronic cutaneous lupus erythematosus*, consists of atrophic scarring plaques that commonly arise on the scalp, face, and ears. Discoid lesions affect 10% to 15% of patients with systemic lupus erythematosus. From 1% to 5% of cases of DLE progress to systemic lupus erythematosus (SLE), and serologic abnormalities suggestive of SLE are uncommon.

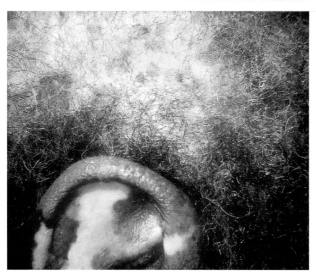

Figure 1-11 Discoid lupus erythematosus (chronic cutaneous lupus erythematosus).

DISTINGUISHING FEATURES
- More common in women
- Lesions begin as focal erythematous areas that evolve into atrophic disc-shaped plaques, characterized by scale, accentuated hair follicles ("follicular plugging"), and a permanent loss of hair
- Scarring alopecia ultimately results in a combination of hypopigmentation and hyperpigmentation (Fig. 1-11)
- Relatively asymptomatic, but skin may itch or be tender

DIAGNOSIS
- Clinical appearance and punch biopsy, if necessary (see Appendix B)

MANAGEMENT
- Avoidance of excessive sun exposure and use of broad-spectrum sunscreens
- Class 1 and 2 topical steroids (see Appendix A)
- Intralesional steroid injections (see Appendix B)
- Systemic antimalarials hydroxychloroquine **(Plaquenil)** and chloroquine **(Aralen),** systemic steroids, dapsone, oral retinoids, gold, clofazimine, methotrexate, thalidomide, tetracycline or erythromycin combined with niacinamide, and mycophenolate mofetil **(CellCept)**

Lichen Planopilaris

Lichen planopilaris (LPP) is considered to be a form of **lichen planus (LP)** that involves the scalp (Fig. 1-12). Lichen planus is an eruption with characteristic papules on the skin, nails, and mucous membranes (see Chapter 8, Oral Cavity and Tongue; Chapter 12, Arms; Chapter 21, Legs). Lichen planus infrequently affects the scalp; however, when it does, the inflammation results in a scarring alopecia, which is then referred to as LPP to highlight the hair follicle involvement. Lichen planopilaris and LP are considered to result from a cell-mediated immune response of unknown origin. In most cases of LPP, the inflammation is limited to the scalp, and typical LP lesions are not seen elsewhere on the skin.

 Frontal fibrosing alopecia (which affects the frontal area of the scalp) has recently been described and is believed to be a subtype of LPP (Fig. 1-13).

DISTINGUISHING FEATURES
- Erythema that progresses to the development of patchy, scarring alopecia most commonly noted on the vertex
- Tufting or polytrichia—clumped hairs due to surrounding scarring may be seen
- LPP tends to be progressive but often "burns out" after several years

DIAGNOSIS
- Clinical appearance and punch biopsy, if necessary (see Appendix B)

- Fungal cultures or periodic acid–Schiff staining should be done to rule out tinea capitis (see Appendix B)

MANAGEMENT
- First line of therapy: topical superpotent steroids or intralesional steroid injections
- Doxycycline or minocycline (100 to 200 mg/day) is often effective in mild cases of LPP
- Other therapies: cyclosporin, hydroxychloroquine, dapsone, and oral isotretinoin (see Appendix A)

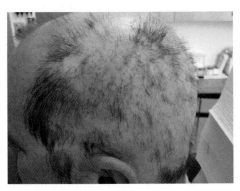

Figure 1-12 Lichen planopilaris.

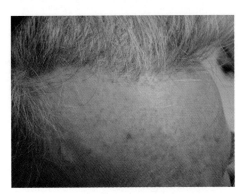

Figure 1-13 Frontal fibrosing alopecia. (Courtesy of Hendrik Uyttendaele, MD.)

Folliculitis Decalvans

Folliculitis decalvans, also referred to as *tufted folliculitis,* is a suppurative scalp disease of unknown etiology. It occurs mainly in black males in their second to fourth decades of life. The clinical course is chronic and unpredictable with relapses, although spontaneous resolution may occur. Bacterial infection appears to be a secondary event, not an etiologic factor. In many cases, *Staphylococcus aureus* can be isolated from the pustules, but its role is not clear.

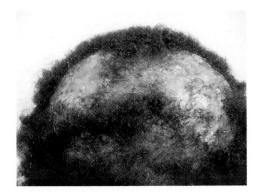

Figure 1-14 Folliculitis decalvans.

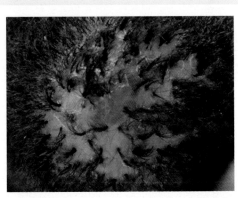

Figure 1-15 "Doll's head" sign. (Courtesy of Robert Rudolph, MD.)

DISTINGUISHING FEATURES
- Erythema and pustules (most often sterile) appear around the hair follicle (Fig. 1-14)
- May be itchy or tender
- Usually round or oval patches of hair loss with perifollicular pustules
- Characteristically, several or many hairs can be seen coming out of a single follicle, so the scalp looks tufted like a toothbrush ("doll's head" sign) (Fig. 1-15)
- Eventually the follicle is destroyed and leaves behind a scar

DIAGNOSIS (see Appendix B)
- Clinical appearance, bacterial culture, and punch biopsy, if necessary

MANAGEMENT (see Appendix A)
- Oral antibiotics: minocycline, tetracycline, rifampicin, clindamycin, ciprofloxacin, and dicloxacillin
- Oral and or intralesional corticosteroids
- Oral isotretinoin

ALSO CONSIDER
- Staphylococcal folliculitis
- Cutaneous sarcoidosis
- Acne keloidalis nuchae
- Scarring hair loss of unknown cause (pseudopelade)

RARELY
- Alopecia mucinosa
- Porphyria cutanea tarda
- Scleroderma
- Dissecting cellulitis (perifolliculitis capitis abscedens et suffodiens)
- Necrobiosis lipoidica
- Epidermolysis bullosa
- Cicatricial pemphigoid

Atopic Dermatitis *vs* Infantile Seborrheic Dermatitis *vs* Tinea Amiantacea

Atopic Dermatitis

Atopic dermatitis (AD), or atopic eczema (see also Chapter 3, Eyelids and Periorbital Area; Chapter 12, Arms; Chapter 21, Legs), is by far the most common cause of scalp rashes in prepubescent children. Atopic dermatitis is a chronic, inflammatory, itchy skin condition. It is also the most frequently seen skin disorder in people of Asian and African descent.

Atopic dermatitis occurs in association with a personal or family history of hay fever, asthma, allergic rhinitis, sinusitis, or AD itself. Also, a history of allergies to pollen, dust, house dust mites, ragweed, dogs, or cats may be uncovered. In many cases, AD first manifests as a severe "cradle cap."

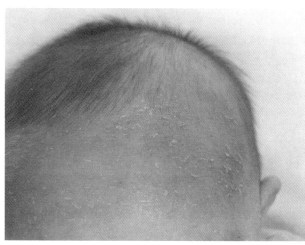

Figure 1-16 Atopic dermatitis.

DISTINGUISHING FEATURES
- Pruritus, scale, and erythema anywhere on the scalp (Fig. 1-16)
- Eczematous lesions are often present elsewhere on the body

DIAGNOSIS
- History of atopy and physical examination
- Depends on exclusion of tinea capitis, pediculosis capitis, and scabies

MANAGEMENT
- Intermittent application of low to mid potency topical steroids (see Appendix A)
- Minimal shampooing

Infantile Seborrheic Dermatitis ("Cradle Cap")

Infantile seborrheic dermatitis is a self-limited eruption that usually appears within the first 6 weeks of life. Most often, it presents on the scalp as "cradle cap"; less commonly, it affects other areas of the body: behind the ears, in the creases of the neck, armpits, and diaper area (diaper rash). The cause is unknown, but it possibly it has to do with over-active sebaceous glands in the skin of newborn infants due to maternal hormones. There also may be a relationship with the skin yeast, *Pityrosporum ovale*. Infantile seborrheic dermatitis may ultimately prove to be an early manifestation of AD, and rarely, psoriasis.

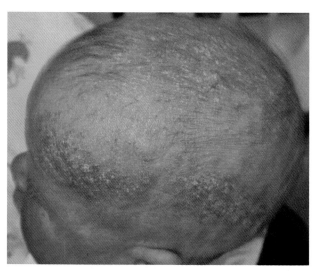

Figure 1-17 Seborrheic dermatitis ("cradle cap").

DISTINGUISHING FEATURES
- Varies from mild, patchy scaling resembling dandruff, to an oily, yellowish or brown crusting (Fig. 1-17)
- May become widespread
- Usually not pruritic

DIAGNOSIS
- Clinical

MANAGEMENT
- Mild baby shampoos, mineral or olive oil, and soft brushing to remove the scales; scale can also be removed with mild antiseborrheic shampoos that contain sulfur and salicylic acid, such as **Sebulex**
- A medicated shampoo containing ketoconazole, or a very mild class 5 or 6 topical steroid may be applied to any symptomatic (pruritic), inflamed, or reddened areas (see Appendix A)
- Stronger keratolytic agents such as **Salex cream** or **lotion**, or **Keralyt gel 6%**, or salicylic acid in petrolatum to remove thick, dense, adherent scale (see Appendix B)

Tinea Amiantacea

Tinea amiantacea (pityriasis amiantacea) is characterized by focal areas of thick adherent scale on the scalp and in the hair. This condition may be due to underlying seborrheic dermatitis, psoriasis, or AD; however, most often it appears without any evident cause.

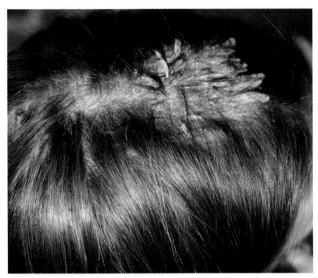

Figure 1-18 Tinea amiantacea.

DISTINGUISHING FEATURES
- One or more focal areas of yellow, silvery, or white scaly concretions arranged in an overlapping manner like tiles on a roof
- Scales surround hair shafts and are tightly adherent to them (Fig. 1-18)
- The underlying scalp may be erythematous and some hair loss may be evident in areas of severe scaling

DIAGNOSIS
- Clinical

MANAGEMENT
- Scale-removing keratolytic agents such as **Salex cream** or **lotion, Keralyt gel 6%,** or salicylic acid in petrolatum (see Appendix B)
- Mineral oil or olive oil also help remove scale. After scale is removed, topical steroids may be applied to underlying scalp to reduce inflammation

ALSO CONSIDER
- Tinea capitis
- Pediculosis capitis
- Scabies

RARELY
- Psoriasis
- Langerhans cell histiocytosis (histiocytosis X)
- Leiner disease

Seborrheic Dermatitis *vs* Psoriasis *vs* Atopic Dermatitis

In adults, seborrheic dermatitis, psoriasis, and AD of the scalp are very common inflammatory scalp disorders. All three are often clinically indistinguishable from one another; however, for therapeutic and prognostic reasons, it is often important to make the diagnostic distinctions among them. A specific diagnosis may become evident over time and can sometimes be aided by other clinical findings, symptoms, or family history.

Seborrheic Dermatitis

Seborrheic dermatitis (SD), referred to as *seborrheic eczema* in the United Kingdom, is a chronic inflammatory dermatitis. Its characteristic distribution involves areas that have the greatest concentration of sebaceous glands: scalp, face, presternal, interscapular area, umbilicus, and body folds (intertriginous areas). Lesions may involve the eyebrows, external ear canals, presternal area, and upper back. Dandruff is the mildest form of SD. The cause of SD is unknown; however, some evidence indicates that the yeast *Pityrosporum ovale* may have a role in its pathogenesis. It is probably unrelated to infantile SD (see previous comments). The usual onset occurs during late puberty and is seen more commonly in males. Seborrheic dermatitis fluctuates in severity and generally persists for years. It is commonly aggravated by changes in seasons or emotional stress. It may worsen in Parkinson disease and in acquired immunodeficiency syndrome (AIDS).

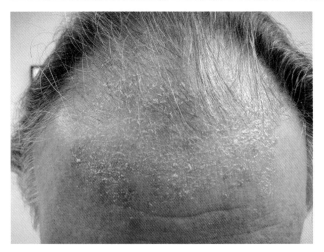

Figure 1-19 Seborrheic dermatitis.

DISTINGUISHING FEATURES
- Ranges from a mild scaling (dandruff) and/or erythema and diffuse scaling (Fig. 1-19) with minimally elevated plaques to thick, armorlike plaques that are indistinguishable from psoriasis ("sebopsoriasis")
- Pruritus is common

DIAGNOSIS
- Clinical

MANAGEMENT
- Mild scalp SD (dandruff) generally responds to the numerous commercially available antidandruff, antiseborrheic shampoos that contain one or more of the following ingredients: zinc pyrithione, coal tar, salicylic acid, selenium sulfide, ciclopirox, ketoconazole, and sulfur
- For itching and inflammation, a medium-strength (class 3 or 4) topical steroid in a gel, foam, or solution formulation may be used, only if necessary (see Appendix A)
- Topical antifungal creams, gels, lotions, or foams: **Loprox, Xolegel,** or **Extina,** and generic ketoconazole (see Appendix A)
- Severe scalp seborrheic dermatitis (sebopsoriasis) is often managed in the same manner as psoriasis of the scalp (see following discussion)

Psoriasis

Psoriasis is a common inflammatory disorder characterized by scaly red papules and plaques that may involve the scalp alone, or the scalp may be affected along with other areas of the body (addressed in Chapter 11, Axillae; Chapter 12, Arms, Elbows; Chapter 13, Hands and Fingers; Chapter 15, Trunk; Chapter 20, Inguinal Area; Chapter 21, Legs, Knees). When psoriasis involves only the scalp and retroauricular areas, it is sometimes referred to as *sebopsoriasis* or *seborrhiasis*. Psoriasis does not cause permanent alopecia.

DISTINGUISHING FEATURES
- Thick plaques, often anchored by hairs, with an overlying whitish, or classic "silvery" scale (Fig. 1-20)
- Scales are thicker and more clearly demarcated and more brightly erythematous than seen in SD (see previous discussion)
- May affect elbows and knees and other places on the body
- Itching varies

DIAGNOSIS
- Clinical

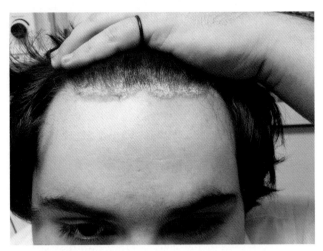

Figure 1-20 Psoriasis.

MANAGEMENT (see Appendices A and B)
Mild Cases
- For minimal scaling and thin plaques, similar to what is seen in SD (see previous discussion), managed with antipsoriasis, antidandruff shampoos and a low- (class 4 to 6) or mid-potency (class 3 or 4) topical steroid used as needed for itching

- Over-the-counter options include shampoos that contain tar (**Zetar, T/Gel**), selenium sulfide (**Selsun Blue, Head and Shoulders**), or salicylic acid (**T/Sal**)

Severe Cases
- Potent (class 2) and superpotent (class 1) topical steroids are frequently preceded by keratolytic agents to remove thick scale (see next point) to allow the medications to penetrate the scalp before the underlying inflammatory plaques can be effectively treated
- Thick scales and plaques are removed with keratolytics such as **Salex** cream or lotion, **Keralyt gel 6%,** or salicylic acid in petrolatum followed by a medium-to-high-potency (class 2, 3, or 4) topical steroid is under shower cap occlusion as needed overnight, or for 3 to 4 hours during the day. If necessary, a superpotent (class 1) topical steroid such as clobetasol propionate lotion, foam, or gel can be used with or without occlusion
- Calcipotriene (**Dovonex Scalp Solution**) 0.005%
- **Taclonex Scalp Suspension** contains calcipotriene hydrate and betamethasone dipropionate
- Intralesional corticosteroid injections

☑ **TIP: "Soak and Smear" (see Appendix B)**

Atopic Dermatitis

Atopic dermatitis (AD) of the scalp in adults, often misdiagnosed as SD, tends to be a very pruritic, recurrent problem and is exacerbated by frequent shampooing. Atopic dermatitis occurs in patients who have an atopic history, and it may also first appear in the elderly who have no apparent atopic history.

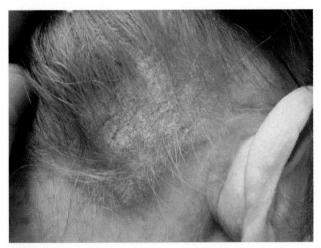

Figure 1-21 Atopic dermatitis.

DISTINGUISHING FEATURES
- Pruritus and scale, particularly in the occipital region (Fig. 1-21)
- Eczematous lesions may be present elsewhere on the body
- In chronic cases, lichenification of the occiput, retroauricular areas, and posterior neck
- The eruption is generally less well defined and has less scale than seen in SD and psoriasis

DIAGNOSIS
- History and physical examination
- Depends on excluding tinea capitis, SD, psoriasis, and pediculosis

MANAGEMENT
- Minimal shampooing
- **Class 1 to 4 topical steroids** depending on severity and clinical response (see Appendix A)

☑ **TIP: "Soak and Smear" (see Appendix B)**

👉 **ALSO CONSIDER**
- Tinea amiantacea
- Tinea capitis in children

RARELY
- Tinea capitis in adults

Seborrheic Keratosis vs Solar Keratosis vs Squamous Cell Carcinoma

Seborrheic Keratosis

A seborrheic keratosis (SK) is an extremely common benign skin growth that becomes apparent in people after age 40 (see Chapter 2, Forehead and Temples; Chapter 15, Trunk; Chapter 21, Legs). Seborrheic keratoses are the most common neoplasms in the elderly, and they have virtually no malignant potential. On the scalp, the temporoparietal area along the hairline is a common site. Patients often report a positive family history. Seborrheic keratoses have been whimsically described as "barnacles in the sea of life," and "maturity spots," metaphors intended to allay patients' anxieties. They are primarily a cosmetic concern, except when they become inflamed or irritated.

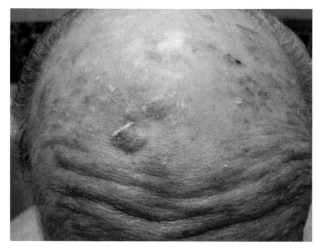

Figure 1-22 Seborrheic keratosis.

DISTINGUISHING FEATURES
- Warty, "stuck-on" appearance ranging from tan to dark brown to black with a "dry," crumbly, keratotic surface (Fig. 1-22)
- Characteristics of individual lesions tend to vary considerably, even on the same patient—they may be warty, tortoise shell-like, scaly, or flat
- Variable color even within a single lesion

DIAGNOSIS
- With experience, SKs are easily recognized clinically
- If necessary, a shave biopsy or curettage (see Appendix B) may be performed for histologic confirmation

MANAGEMENT (see Appendix B)
- Liquid nitrogen (LN$_2$) cryosurgery for thinner lesions
- Curettage with or without light electrocautery and curettage
- Excisional surgery, which results in scar formation, is unnecessary

Solar Keratosis

Solar keratosis, also known as *actinic keratosis*, is the most common sun-related skin growth (see Chapter 2, Forehead and Temples; Chapter 5, Nose and Perinasal Area; Chapter 12, Arms; Chapter 21, Legs). They occur in persons who are fair-skinned, burn easily, tan poorly, and result from cumulative sun exposure. Chiefly at risk are people who are bald and have outdoor occupations such as farmers, sailors, athletes, and gardeners, especially fair-skinned white males. Whether this lesion is benign (premalignant) or malignant (squamous cell carcinoma in situ) from its onset is controversial. What is accepted, however, is that solar keratoses have the potential to develop into invasive squamous cell carcinomas (SCCs). It is estimated that 1 in 20 lesions eventually becomes an SCC. It is also accepted that the invasive carcinomas that develop from actinic keratoses are of a very slow-growing, indolent, unaggressive type, and the prognosis usually is excellent.

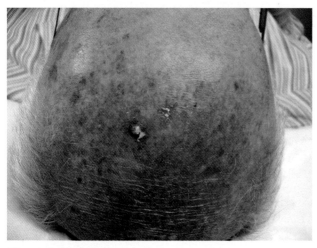

Figure 1-23 Solar keratosis.

DISTINGUISHING FEATURES
- Single or multiple discrete, flat, or elevated scaly lesions that arise on a background of sun-damaged skin (Fig. 1-23)
- Typically have an erythematous base covered by a white, yellowish, or brown scale (hyperkeratosis)
- Usually asymptomatic or may become slightly tender
- Often gradually enlarge, thicken, and become elevated and develop into a hypertrophic solar keratosis or a cutaneous horn (a hornlike projection of keratin)

- Sometimes tan or dark brown (pigmented solar keratosis) clinically indistinguishable from a solar lentigo ("liver spots") or a flat SK (see previous discussion)
- Advanced lesions are clinically difficult to distinguish from SCCs (see following discussion)

DIAGNOSIS
- Palpation reveals a gritty rough to the touch sandpaperlike texture
- A shave biopsy is performed when the diagnosis is in doubt or to rule out an SCC (see Appendix B)
- Cellular atypia is present, and the keratinocytes vary in size and shape. Mitotic figures are common

MANAGEMENT (see Appendices A and B)
- Limit sun exposure: use sunscreens, protective clothing, and headwear
- LN$_2$ cryosurgery
- Biopsy followed by electrocautery or electrocautery alone for thick hyperkeratotic lesions
- Chemical peels
- Dermabrasion
- Pharmaceutical agents: imiquimod (**Aldara**) cream, **Efudex** or **Carac** cream, diclofenac sodium (**Solarase**), topical tretinoin (**Retin-A**)
- Photodynamic therapy

Squamous Cell Carcinoma

Cutaneous SCC is a malignant tumor arising from keratinocytes of the epidermis. In adults, especially, the elderly, the sun-exposed scalp is a common site for these lesions (see also Chapter 2, Forehead and Temples; Chapter 5, Nose and Perinasal Area; Chapter 12, Arms; Chapter 21, Legs). After basal cell carcinoma, SCC is the second most common type of skin cancer; however, in contrast to basal cell carcinoma, it carries a risk of metastasis. It occurs in an older age group than does basal cell carcinoma; it is rare in dark-skinned people.

Most SCCs arise in solar keratoses (see previous discussion) with the identical epidemiologic profile. Such SCCs are slow-growing, minimally invasive, unaggressive, and the prognosis is usually excellent because distant metastases are rare. In situ SCC (**Bowen disease**) also has a low incidence of metastasis. Slow-growing, firm lesions with the ability to produce scale (keratinization) are less likely to metastasize.

⚠ **ALERT: Metastases are much more likely to arise from lesions that appear de novo without a preceding solar keratosis. Lesions that are softer, nonkeratinizing, or ulcerated also carry a greater risk. Poorly differentiated, deeper lesions, and especially for lesions that arise in the following locations and circumstances are more likely to spread:**
- Mucous membrane lesions (see Chapter 7, Lips and Perioral Area)
- Sites that received ionizing radiation
- The skin of organ transplant recipients
- Chronic inflammatory lesions (e.g., discoid lupus erythematosus)
- Long-standing scars or cutaneous ulcers (e.g., venous stasis ulcers) or other nonhealing wounds

⚠ **ALERT: An SCC is capable of locally infiltrative growth, spread to regional lymph nodes, and distant metastasis, most often to the lungs.**

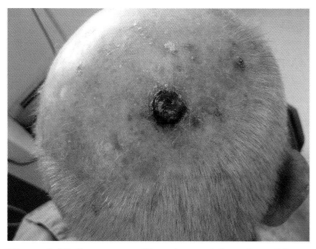

Figure 1-24 Squamous cell carcinoma (ulceration with thick crust).

DISTINGUISHING FEATURES
- Tend to arise on the bald areas of the scalp in elderly white men
- Scaly papules (often indistinguishable from solar keratoses), plaques, or nodules that grow slowly with a smooth or thick hyperkeratotic surface
- Ulceration and/or crusting may be the only finding (Fig. 1-24)
- As with solar keratoses (see previous discussion), an SCC may also produce a cutaneous horn on its surface
- Often indistinguishable from a hypertrophic solar keratosis or a basal cell carcinoma

DIAGNOSIS
- A shave or excisional biopsy (see Appendix B)
- Various degrees of cellular atypia are present, and the keratinocytes vary in size and shape

MANAGEMENT (see Appendices A and B)

- Limit sun exposure: use sunscreens, protective clothing, and headwear
- In most patients local treatment is usually curative
- Electrocautery and curettage for small lesions (generally <1 cm)
  - LN$_2$ cryosurgery
  - Total excision is the preferred method of therapy
- Micrographic (Mohs) surgery (see Appendix B) is useful for excessively large or invasive SCCs, for recurrent lesions, and for lesions with poorly delineated clinical borders. It is also a treatment of choice for lesions in an area of late radiation change
- **Aldara cream** may also have some utility in treating selected patient who have highly differentiated SCCs and in some renal transplant patients who tend to develop numerous SCCs
- Radiation therapy

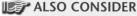

ALSO CONSIDER
- Basal cell carcinoma
- Lentigo maligna/malignant melanoma
- Melanocytic nevus, nevus sebaceous, epidermal nevus
- Warts/verrucous acanthoma

RARELY
- Scalp metastases

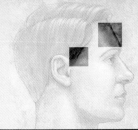

CHAPTER 2

Forehead and Temples

The forehead and temples are often home to lesions of molluscum contagiosum, most often noted in toddlers, and flat warts that tend to appear in young adults. Adolescent acne vulgaris and the acne-like lesions of rosacea in adults also occur here. Benign neoplasms such as various types of nevi, seborrheic keratoses, sebaceous hyperplasia, arise at different stages of life. In older individuals, the forehead and temples are particularly susceptible to sun-related dermatoses, solar keratoses, basal cell carcinomas, and squamous cell carcinomas.

There are few inflammatory skin disorders that are confined to the forehead and temples alone. For example, seborrheic dermatitis and psoriasis (see Chapter 1, Hair and Scalp) may extend beyond the hairline to involve the forehead and temples.

IN THIS CHAPTER

- Molluscum contagiosum *vs* flat warts versus milia
- Acne vulgaris *vs* rosacea
- Seborrheic dermatitis *vs* psoriasis
- Melanocytic nevus *vs* seborrheic keratosis *vs* solar lentigo
- Basal cell carcinoma *vs* sebaceous hyperplasia
- Solar keratosis *vs* squamous cell carcinoma

Molluscum Contagiosum

Molluscum contagiosum (MC) is a common superficial viral infection of the epidermis. Spread by skin-to-skin contact and caused by a large DNA-containing poxvirus, MC is seen most often in three clinical contexts: young, healthy children (infants and preschoolers), particularly in those who have atopic dermatitis; in the genital region (see Chapter 18, Genital Area) in sexually active young adults; and in patients with human immunodeficiency virus (HIV)/acquired immunodeficiency syndrome (AIDS).

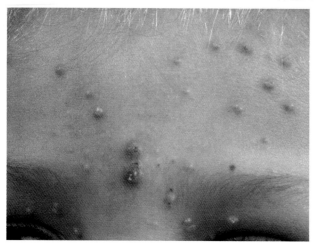

Figure 2-1 Molluscum contagiosum. (From Burkhart C, Morell D, Goldsmith LA, et al. *VisualDx: Essential Pediatric Dermatology.* Philadelphia, PA: Lippincott Williams & Wilkins; 2009.)

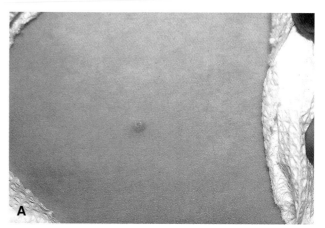

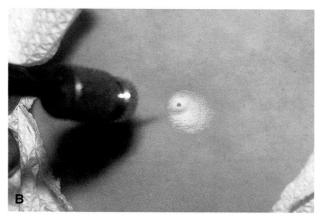

Figure 2-2 A, Molluscum contagiosum. **B,** Molluscum contagiosum; LN_2 accentuates the central core. (Both figures from Goodheart HP. *Goodheart's Photoguide to Common Skin Disorders: Diagnosis and Management.* 3rd ed. Philadelphia, PA: Lippincott Williams & Wilkins; 2009.)

DISTINGUISHING FEATURES
- Dome-shaped, waxy, or pearly papules with a central white core (umbilication); less frequently, lesions are pink to flesh-colored (Fig. 2-1)
- Generally 1 to 3 mm in diameter but may coalesce into double or triple lesions and become "giant" mollusca
- Often grouped via autoinoculation; often widely disseminated to trunk, extremities, and genital areas
- Often involves the face, forehead, eyelids, and conjunctiva (see Chapter 3, Eyelids and Periorbital Area)
- May appear in young children who have eczema that decreases skin barrier integrity
- The number of lesions varies from 1 to 20 up to hundreds.
- Generally asymptomatic; may itch and become inflamed and crusted
- In children, the course is most often self-limiting; lesions resolve within 6 to 8 months. Recurrences are rare in immunocompetent persons

DIAGNOSIS
- Clinical
- A handheld magnifier often reveals the central core
- A short application of cryotherapy with liquid nitrogen (LN_2) accentuates the central core (Fig. 2-2)
- Shave or curettage biopsy if diagnosis is in doubt ("molluscum bodies") (see Appendix B)

MANAGEMENT (see Appendices A and B)
- Wait for spontaneous resolution
- Cantharidin (**Cantharone**), a blister-producing agent (vesicant), is applied in an office setting. The preparation is applied to individual warts in a thin coat, using a cotton-tipped applicator or a toothpick. A waterproof bandage is used to cover the lesion(s). The procedure is painless. The occlusive dressing is left in place for 4 to 6 hours, and the skin is washed with soap and water. The cantharidin may cause the skin under the wart to blister, and the wart is thus lifted off the skin
- Cryotherapy with LN_2

- Electrocautery
- Curettage
- Patient- or parent-applied topical over-the-counter antiwart preparations
- Imiquimod 5% cream (**Aldara cream**) applied at bedtime

- Antiretroviral therapy and/or trichloroacetic acid peels for refractory lesions patients infected with HIV/AIDS
- Systemic griseofulvin and oral cimetidine have been anecdotally reported to be effective

Flat Warts

Flat warts (verrucae planae) are frequently noted on the face as well as on the arms, dorsa of hands, and legs (women). Most often seen in children and young adults.

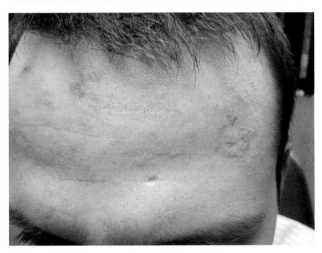

Figure 2-3 Verrucae planae (flat warts).

DISTINGUISHING FEATURES
- Small, flat-topped (planar), slightly elevated, skin-colored or tan papules, (1 to 3 mm) in diameter (Fig. 2-3)
- Lesions are subtle (side lighting may be necessary to see them)
- May present in a linear configuration caused by autoinoculation
- Tend to resolve spontaneously but may persist

DIAGNOSIS
- Clinical
- Shave biopsy, if necessary (see Appendix B)

MANAGEMENT (see Appendices A and B)
- Cautious, short applications of LN$_2$ therapy
- Light electrodesiccation
- Imiquimod (**Aldara cream**)
- Benzoyl peroxide or retinoids applied topically
- Over-the-counter lactic-salicylic acid (**Duofilm**) or **Occlusal-HP,** a salicylic acid preparation

Milium

Milium (plural, milia) is a very common tiny variant of an epidermoid cyst that contains keratin. Milia can occur in people of any age. They may arise in traumatic scars or in association with certain scarring-skin conditions, such as porphyria cutanea tarda (see Chapter 13, Hands, Dorsal Surface).

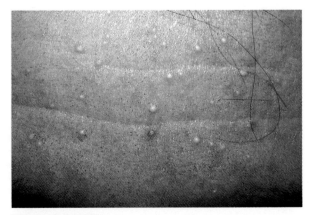

Figure 2-4 Milia.

DISTINGUISHING FEATURES
- 1.0 to 2.0 mm in diameter and are white to yellowish asymptomatic papules (Fig. 2-4)
- Most often noted on the face, especially around the eyes (see Chapter 3, Eyelids and Periorbital Area), cheeks, and forehead

DIAGNOSIS
- Clinical

MANAGEMENT
- In contrast to closed comedones, whiteheads (which they resemble), milia must first be incised (usually with a No. 11 blade or 20-gauge needle) before their contents can be expressed

ALSO CONSIDER
- Syringoma
- Xanthoma

RARELY
- Disseminated cryptococcosis and toxoplasmosis in patients infected with HIV/AIDS

Acne Vulgaris

Acne vulgaris (AV), typical teenage acne, is a condition that involves the pilosebaceous apparatus of the skin when androgenic hormones cause abnormal follicular keratinization that blocks the sebaceous duct. This blockage results in a *microcomedo* (the microscopic primary lesion of adolescent acne). The microcomedo enlarges to become the visible comedo, the noninflammatory blackhead or whitehead. Alternatively, the microcomedo may become an inflammatory lesion, such as a papule or pustule. Acne vulgaris most commonly erupts in areas of maximal sebaceous gland activity—the face, neck, chest, shoulders, back, and upper arms.

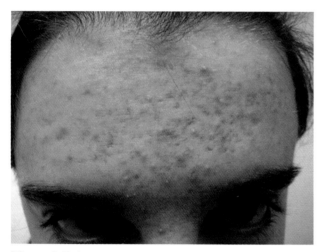

Figure 2-5 Acne.

DISTINGUISHING FEATURES (Fig. 2-5)
Inflammatory Lesions
- Papules, pustules, macules: "acne cysts" (nodules)
- Postinflammatory hyperpigmentation particularly in patients with darker skin

Noninflammatory (Comedonal) Lesions
- Open comedones (blackheads) closed comedones (whiteheads)

DIAGNOSIS
- Clinical

MANAGEMENT (also see Appendix C)
- A patient should be advised not to squeeze or pick lesions
- Gentle mild cleansing twice daily is usually adequate

- Patients who have moderate-to-severe acne that is unresponsive to topical treatment alone or acne that tends to scar are generally prescribed systemic as well as topical therapy

Mild
- Topical (see Appendix A): benzoyl peroxide, retinoids, topical antibiotics, combination of topical antibiotic and benzoyl peroxide (e.g., **Benzamycin, BenzaClin,** and **Duac** gels)
- Alternative topical prescription drugs: azelaic acid (**Azelex 20%**), as well as preparations that contain sulfur and sodium sulfacetamide such as **Sulfacet-R lotion, Novacet lotion,** and **Klaron lotion**

Moderate to Severe
- Oral antibiotics tetracycline derivatives such as generic tetracycline, minocycline, or doxycycline
- Oral retinoids. Isotretinoin (13-*cis*-retinoic acid) (**Accutane**) is an oral synthetic derivative of vitamin A that promotes long-term remissions in severe acne
- ⚠ **ALERT: Isotretinoin (Accutane) can cause severe birth defects if taken by a woman who is pregnant**
- In female patients, hormonal agents, such as oral contraceptives, and antiandrogenic drugs, such as spironolactone, may be prescribed in carefully selected situations
- Second-line oral antibiotics: erythromycin, amoxicillin (can be used during pregnancy), azithromycin (**Zithromax),** clindamycin, cephalosporins, oral sulfonamides
- Other therapeutic modalities
  - Comedo extraction (acne surgery)
  - Office-based chemical peels
  - Intralesional corticosteroid injections
  - Lasers, lights, and other newer technologies

Rosacea

Rosacea (see also Chapter 5, Nose and Perinasal Area; Chapter 6, Cheeks) arises later in life than AV, usually between 30 and 50 years of age. It occurs most commonly in fair-skinned people with an ethnic background of Great Britain, Ireland, Germany, Scandinavia, and certain areas of Eastern Europe. Women are more likely to be affected than men. Although the precise cause of rosacea remains a mystery, it is believed that certain environmental factors contribute to its development and progression. Precipitating factors that may exacerbate rosacea include sun exposure, excessive washing of the face, and irritating cosmetics.

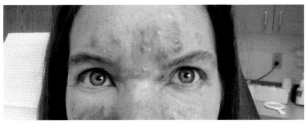

Figure 2-6 Rosacea.

DISTINGUISHING FEATURES
- Acnelike erythematous papules, pustules, and telang-iectasias, typically seen on the central third of the face—the forehead, nose, cheeks, and chin (the so-called "flush/blush" areas) (Fig. 2-6)
- Lacks the comedones ("blackheads" or "whiteheads") that are seen in acne
- No relationship to androgenic hormones
- Nonscarring
- May begin with (erythema) on the forehead and cheeks
- Cosmetic problem; however, burning and flushing can be quite uncomfortable
- Progression with papules and, sometimes, pustules
- May also have ocular involvement (see Chapter 3, Eyelids and Periorbital Area)

DIAGNOSIS
- Clinical
- Rarely, a biopsy may be necessary in atypical cases

MANAGEMENT
- See Chapter 6, Cheeks, and Appendix C

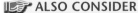 **ALSO CONSIDER**
- Systemic lupus erythematosus
- Seborrheic dermatitis
- Tinea faciei
- Polymorphous light eruption
- Acnelike disorders such as
  - Periorificial dermatitis
  - Drug-induced acne
  - Endocrinopathic acne
  - Physically induced and occupational acne
  - Demadex folliculitis
  - Bacterial folliculitis
  - Pityrosporum folliculitis

RARELY
- Chloracne
- Carcinoid syndrome
- Lupus vulgaris

Seborrheic Dermatitis

Seborrheic dermatitis (SD) often involves the face, whereas psoriasis tends to spare the face, except when involvement of the scalp extends beyond the hairline to the forehead. The pathogenesis of SD appears to be a combination of excessive sebum production, the activity of *Malassezia furfur*, as well as inflammatory, genetic, and immunologic factors (see Chapter 1, Hair and Scalp; Chapter 5, Nose and Perinasal Area).

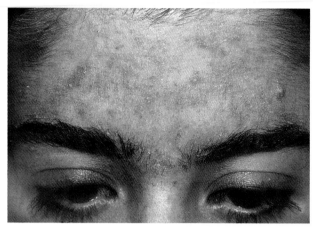

Figure 2-7 Seborrheic dermatitis.

DISTINGUISHING FEATURES
- Affects males more than females
- Mild scaling and/or erythema
- Often involves the scalp, eyebrows, nasal creases, and ears (Fig. 2-7)
- Pruritus is common

DIAGNOSIS
- Clinical

MANAGEMENT (see also Chapter 1, Hair and Scalp)
- Antiseborrheic shampoos
- Rapid response to low-potency topical steroids
- To minimize unwanted steroid reactions, topical steroids may be alternated with antifungals such as ketoconazole cream 2% **(Nizoral)** or ciclopirox 0.77% gel **(Loprox)** (see Appendix A)
- Tacrolimus **(Protopic ointment)** 0.1% and pimecrolimus **(Elidel cream)** 1% may also be effective
- **Promiseb Topical Cream (Sebclair** in Europe): a nonsteroidal cream that has both anti-inflammatory as well as antifungal effects. It is applied twice daily

Psoriasis

Psoriasis may extend to the forehead and temples from scalp involvement (see Fig. 1-20).

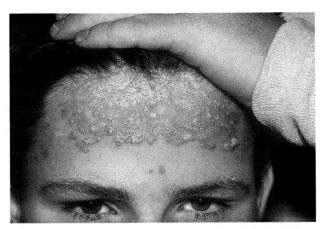

Figure 2-8 Psoriatic plaque of forehead and scalp.

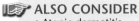 **ALSO CONSIDER**
- Atopic dermatitis
- Contact dermatitis
- Tinea faciei/capitis

Melanocytic Nevus

Melanocytic nevus (MN), a mole or "beauty mark" most often is a benign proliferation of nevus cells that are derived from melanocytes. *Congenital nevi* may be present at birth or in the neonatal period. During childhood and adolescence, acquired nevi appear. As adulthood approaches, the development of new lesions tapers off, and at middle age many existing lesions gradually lose their capacity to form melanin, become skin-colored, or disappear completely. Congenital and acquired nevi are much more often seen in patients with light or fair skin than in blacks or Asians. Large congenital nevi (see Chapter 12, Arms; Chapter 15, Trunk) are associated with a low, but real risk of malignant transformation and the development of melanoma.

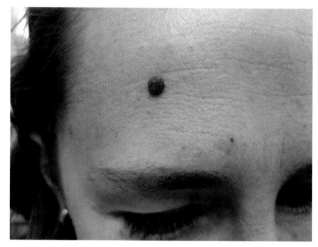

Figure 2-9 Melanocytic nevus.

DISTINGUISHING FEATURES
Compound Melanocytic Nevi
- Elevated, dome-shaped papules or papillomatous nodules that are uniformly brown to dark brown; may contain hairs (Fig. 2-9)
- Seen most often on the face, arms, legs, and trunk

Dermal Melanocytic Nevi
- May be elevated and dome-shaped, wartlike, or pedunculated

- Tan or brown, or dappled with pigmentation
- With age they often become skin-colored.
- Most seen mainly on the face and neck

Junctional Melanocytic Nevi
- Small, macular (flat), frecklelike; uniform in color
- Vary from brown to dark brown to black
- Acquired or congenital, junctional nevi are most prevalent on the face, arms, legs, trunk, genitalia, palms, and soles

DIAGNOSIS
- Based on clinical appearance or, if necessary, a histopathologic evaluation after removal

MANAGEMENT
- All MN should be carefully examined and considered for biopsy, particularly if there is any suggestion of clinical atypia
- Removal for cosmetic purposes or because of repeated irritation by clothing, such as a bra strap
- Shave removal/shave biopsy (see Appendix B). Elliptical excision is performed with the intent of removing lesions completely, including hairs.

Seborrheic Keratosis

A **seborrheic keratosis (SK)** is an extremely common benign skin growth seen in people after age 40. It is the most common neoplasm in the elderly and has no malignant potential. There is often a positive family history. Males are affected as often as females. SKs are whimsically described as "barnacles in the sea of life." Lesions are most often located on the back, chest (see Chapter 15, Trunk), arms (see Chapter 12, Arms, *Extensor Forearms*) legs (see Chapter 21, Legs), and face, particularly along the frontal hairline and scalp (see Chapter 1, Hair and Scalp). SKs are mainly a cosmetic concern, except when they are inflamed or irritated.

DISTINGUISHING FEATURES
- Typically a warty, "stuck-on" appearance (Fig. 2-10)
- Color ranges from tan to dark brown to black
- "Dry," crumbly, keratotic surface
- Appearance of individual lesions tends to vary considerably, even on the same patient: warty, tortoise shell-

like, scaly, flat or almost flat (a flat SK is often indistinguishable from solar keratoses or a solar lentigo) (see following discussion)
- Clinical variant: **dermatosis papulosa nigra**
  - Common manifestation that is diagnosed primarily in African Americans, African Caribbeans, and

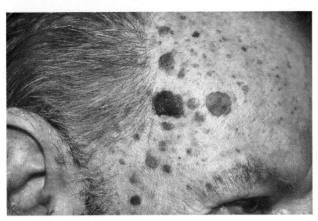

Figure 2-10 Seborrheic keratosis.

- It is histopathologically identical to SKs and are considered to be of autosomal dominant inheritance
- Lesions are darkly pigmented and, in contrast to typical SKs, they have minimal, if any, scale

DIAGNOSIS
- With experience, SKs are easily recognized
- A biopsy (generally a shave biopsy) is performed if necessary to confirm the diagnosis
- ⚠ **ALERT: To the untrained eye, however, these lesions may resemble melanomas. An excisional biopsy is necessary whenever malignant melanoma is suspected**

MANAGEMENT (see Appendix B)
- Cryosurgery performed with LN$_2$ spray or cotton swab
- Light electrocautery and curettage

sub-Saharan African blacks; however, it is also seen in other darker-skinned persons (e.g., Indians, Pakistanis)
- Generally seen on the face, especially the upper cheeks and lateral orbital areas (see Fig. 3-13)

Solar Lentigo

Solar lentigo (plural, lentigines), "liver spot," is a small, acquired tan macule that occurs on sun-exposed areas. They arise during middle and elderly years, primarily in whites (see Chapter 6, Cheeks; Chapter 13, Hands, Dorsal Surface). Lentigines are extremely common on the face, extensor forearms, dorsal hands, and anterior legs. The hyperpigmentation develops from an increase in melanocytes. Lentigo simplex (juvenile lentigines) lesions are permanent and have no relation to sun exposure.

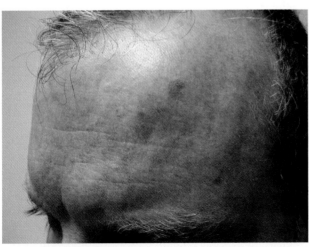

Figure 2-11 Solar lentigo.

DISTINGUISHING FEATURES
- Flat (not palpable)
- Uniformly pigmented oval to geometric macules (Fig. 2-11)
- Sharply circumscribed tan to dark brown

DIAGNOSIS
- Clinical

MANAGEMENT (see Appendix B)
- Sun protection, camouflage
- No treatment is necessary
- For cosmesis: light cryotherapy, trichloroacetic acid peels, topical hydroquinone, azelaic acid, retinoids, laser ablation

☞ ALSO CONSIDER
- Pigmented basal cell carcinoma
- Freckles (ephelides) vary with sun exposure
- Neurofibromas
- Skin tags (acrochordons)
- Angiofibroma (fibrous papules)
- Verruca vulgaris
- Pigmented solar keratosis
- ⚠ **ALERT: Lentigo maligna/melanoma (see Chapter 6, Cheeks)**

Basal Cell Carcinoma

Basal cell carcinoma (BCC) is the most common skin cancer. A BCC is slow-growing and very rarely metastasizes, but it can cause significant local invasion and considerable destruction if it is neglected or treated inadequately. Many of the same risk factors that predispose to solar keratoses and squamous cell carcinomas (SCCs) are responsible for the development of BCCs (see Chapter 1, Hair and Scalp, Chapter 4, Ears, and Chapter 5, Nose and Perinasal Area) and following discussion), although BCC tends to occur at a younger age.
Risk factors:
- Age older than 40 years
- Male sex
- Positive family history
- Light complexion with poor tanning ability (rare in blacks and Asians)
- Long-term sun exposure

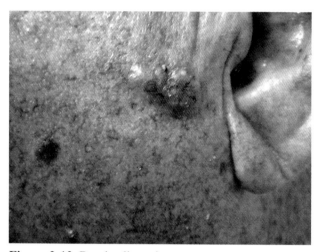

Figure 2-12 Basal cell carcinoma.

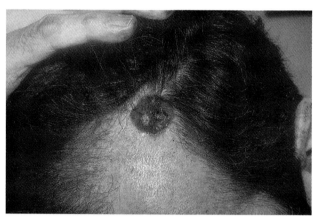

Figure 2-13 Basal cell carcinoma (pigmented).

DISTINGUISHING FEATURES
▲ Nodular BCC (most common type)
  - Occurs most commonly on the head, neck, and upper back
  - Pearly, shiny, semitranslucent papule or nodule with "rolled" (raised) border
  - Telangiectases over the surface account for a history of bleeding after very mild trauma (Fig. 2-12)
  - Occurs on sun-exposed areas (e.g., the face, especially on the nose, cheeks, forehead, periorbital area, lower face, and the back of the neck)
  - Erosion or ulceration ("rodent ulcer") because of its "gnawed" appearance
  - Asymptomatic but may ulcerate ("the sore that will not heal") and loose its characteristic appearance

- Variants
  ▲ Pigmented BCC
    - Brownish to blue-black pigmentation in more darkly pigmented persons (Fig. 2-13)
  - Morpheaform BCC (sclerosing BCC): least common and most aggressive form of BCC
    - Borders difficult to discern; resembles scar tissue
    - Lesions appear as whitish, scarred atrophic plaques with surrounding telangiectasia
    - Generally more difficult to treat than other BCCs

DIAGNOSIS
- Shave or excisional biopsy

MANAGEMENT
- Treatment options depend on histologic subtype and location (see Appendix B)
- Sun avoidance and use of sunscreens; wearing of protective clothing

Sebaceous Hyperplasia

Sebaceous hyperplasia, a common benign proliferation of enlarged sebaceous glands, is seen on the forehead and cheeks of the middle-aged and elderly. It is often confused with BCC.

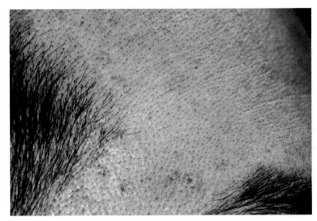

Figure 2-14 Sebaceous hyperplasia.

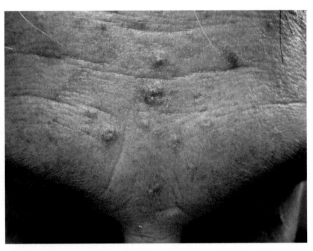

Figure 2-15 Sebaceous hyperplasia. Note yellowish papules with dells.

DISTINGUISHING FEATURES

- Yellow, yellow-orange, or cream-colored papules; often doughnut-shaped with a dell (umbilication) in the center (Figs. 2-14 and 2-15)
- 1 to 3 mm in size
- Telangiectasias are present on the raised borders
- Lesions occur on the forehead, temples, and cheeks

DIAGNOSIS

- Typical clinical appearance ("little bagels")
- Shave biopsy is indicated if BCC is suspected (see Appendix B)

MANAGEMENT

- Treatment is for cosmetic reasons includes electrodesiccation and curettage, CO_2 laser, photodynamic therapy, and trichloroacetic acid (see Appendix B)

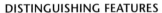

ALSO CONSIDER
- Squamous cell carcinoma
- Solar keratosis
- Angiofibroma
- Seborrheic keratosis, which may be indistinguishable from a pigmented basal cell carcinoma (see previous discussion)
- Melanocytic nevi

RARELY
- Merkel cell carcinoma
- Sebaceous carcinoma
- Sebaceous adenoma

Solar Keratoses

Solar keratoses and squamous cell carcinomas (SC) are extremely common on the forehead and temples of elderly, fair-complexioned men and are becoming increasingly more common in women. See further discussion in Chapter 1, Hair and Scalp.

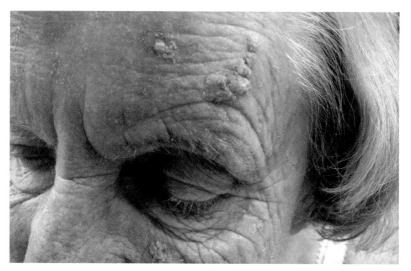

Figure 2-16 Solar keratosis and squamous cell carcinoma. This elderly woman has a squamous cell carcinoma and solar keratoses. Both types of lesions have hyperkeratotic surfaces, and they are often clinically indistinguishable. A shave biopsy is necessary to make the diagnosis.

DISTINGUISHING FEATURES
- Affects men more than women
- Elderly whites with fair skin
- Single or multiple discrete, flat, or elevated scaly papules
- Palpation reveals a gritty rough to the touch; sandpaperlike texture
- Typically erythematous base covered by a white, yellowish, or brown scale (hyperkeratosis)
- Usually asymptomatic or become slightly tender
- May evolve into hypertrophic solar keratosis or a cutaneous horn (see Chapter 4, Ears; Chapter 12, Arms); and Chapter 21, Legs
- A small percentage progress to SCC (see following discussion) (Fig. 2-16)

DIAGNOSIS
- Clinical
- A shave biopsy when diagnosis in doubt or to rule out an SCC

MANAGEMENT
- See Chapter 1, Hair and Scalp, and Appendix B

Squamous Cell Carcinoma

Most cutaneous **squamous cell carcinomas** (SCCs) arise in solar keratoses. The forehead and temples are common sites for these lesions to appear.

DISTINGUISHING FEATURES
- Increasing incidence in men
- Elderly whites with fair skin
- Scaly papule, plaque, or nodule with a smooth or thick hyperkeratotic surface
- Ulceration may be the only finding
- As with solar keratoses (see previous discussion), an SCC, as well as an SCC in situ (**Bowen disease** see Chapter 4, Ears; Chapter 12, Arms; and Chapter 21, Legs) may also produce a cutaneous horn on its surface
- Often indistinguishable from a hypertrophic solar keratosis or a BCC

DIAGNOSIS
- Shave or excisional biopsy

MANAGEMENT
- See Chapter 1, Hair and Scalp, and Appendix B

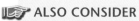 **ALSO CONSIDER**
- Basal cell carcinoma
- Wart
- Seborrheic keratosis
- Adnexal neoplasm
- Melanoma

RARELY
- Merkel cell carcinoma
- Atypical fibroxanthoma
- Granulomatous diseases such as tuberculosis, leishmaniasis, coccidioidomycosis

CHAPTER 3

Eyelids and Periorbital Area

Besides being subject to various inflammatory dermatoses such as atopic and contact dermatitis (AD and CD), seborrheic dermatitis, and rosacea, the skin of the eyelids and the surrounding periorbital area is repeatedly exposed to the environment. The sun, makeup, airborne substances (pollens, fragrance sprays), finger and toenail products, and contact lenses all have potential aggravating and allergenic potential in this area.

The eyelids readily swell and become edematous from internal complications such as urticaria (angioedema). The lids and periorbital region may also serve as clinical indicators of hyperlipidemia (xanthelasma) and dermatomyositis (heliotrope sign). In addition, this area is also subject to various benign and malignant neoplasms.

IN THIS CHAPTER

- Atopic dermatitis *vs* contact dermatitis
- Ocular rosacea *vs* seborrheic blepharitis
- Cutaneous sarcoidosis *vs* xanthelasma
- Syringoma *vs* molluscum contagiosum *vs* milium
- Skin tag *vs* seborrheic keratosis
- Stye (hordeolum) *vs* meibomian cyst (chalazion)
- Basal cell carcinoma *vs* hydrocystoma

Atopic Dermatitis

Atopic Dermatitis (AD) [atopic eczema] (see Chapter 1, Hair and Scalp; Chapter 12, Arms; Chapter 13, Hands and Fingers; Chapter 21, Legs) of the eyelids commonly appears in children. By definition, AD occurs in association with a personal or family history of hay fever, asthma, allergic rhinitis, sinusitis, or AD itself. The patient may present with itchy or irritated eyes, as well as AD elsewhere on the body. Most cases begin in childhood (often in infancy); however, AD may start at *any* age. Children with asthma as well as African Americans and Asians, particularly those living in an urban setting, tend to develop AD at an earlier age. In adults, particularly women, some cases of eyelid eczema may represent an allergic contact dermatitis. AD frequently remits spontaneously—reportedly in 40% to 50% of children—but it may return in adolescence or adulthood, and possibly persist for life.

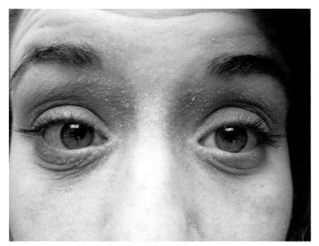

Figure 3-1 Atopic dermatitis: lichenification.

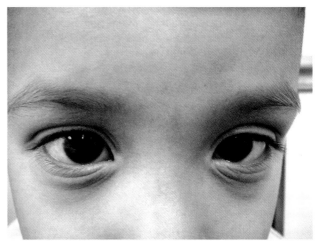

Figure 3-2 Atopic dermatitis: Dennie-Morgan lines.

DISTINGUISHING FEATURES
- Habitual rubbing results in lichenification (exaggerated skin lines)
- Dennie-Morgan lines are a characteristic double fold that extends from the inner to the outer canthus of the lower eyelid (Fig. 3-1)
- "Allergic shiners" refers to a darkened, violaceous, or tan coloring in the periorbital areas. Along with Dennie-Morgan lines, this dark coloring may be an instant clue to atopy (Fig. 3-2)

DIAGNOSIS
- There are usually features of AD at other sites (e.g., flexural creases)
- Personal and/or family history of atopy

MANAGEMENT (see Appendix A)
Topical Steroids

⚠ **ALERT: It should be noted that the thin eyelid skin that protects the underlying eyes warrants extra caution and requires the least potent topical preparations (particu-**
larly topical steroids) for the shortest period of time. Only nonfluorinated, mild topical steroids should be applied, ideally, only for very short periods, to avoid atrophy and absorption (e.g., over-the-counter hydrocortisone 1% or 0.5% cream or ointment).

Topical Immunomodulators (calcineurin inhibitors)
- "Topical steroid-sparing agents" are approved only for the treatment of eczema
- They are best used in areas of high risk where skin thinning (atrophy) tends to occur, such as the eyelids
  - Tacrolimus **(Protopic ointment)** 1% for adults; 0.03% in children
  - Pimecrolimus **(Elidel cream)** is available in a 1% formulation
  - Moisturizers such as petroleum jelly and/or barrier creams/lotions/emulsions
  - Ceramide-containing barrier creams such as **CeraVe, Atopiclair,** and **Epicerum** applied twice daily provide moisturization and enhance and restore the skin's protective barrier function

Contact Dermatitis

In **contact dermatitis (CD)** the thin skin of the eyelids contributes to its sensitivity and susceptibility to allergic and irritant reactions (e.g., poison ivy, cosmetics, nickel). Allergic contact dermatitis (ACD) is an itchy skin condition caused by an allergic reaction to material in contact with the skin. Not uncommonly, ACD of the eyelids may occur from use of artificial acrylic nails (Fig. 3-3). Allergic contact dermatitis is also distinct from irritant contact dermatitis (ICD), in which a similar skin condition is caused by excessive contact with a substance. Irritants include water, soaps, detergents, solvents, acids, alkalis, and friction. Irritant contact dermatitis may affect any individual, providing he or she has had enough exposure to the irritant, but those with AD (see previous discussion) are particularly sensitive.

Chemicals in the air may produce airborne CD (see Chapter 6, Cheeks). Airborne CD usually occurs maximally on the eyelids, but it may affect other exposed areas, particularly the head and the neck.

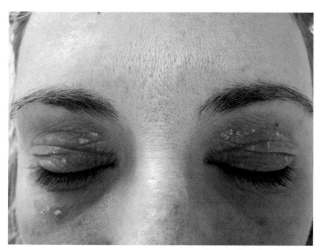

Figure 3-3 Contact dermatitis from acrylic nails.

DISTINGUISHING FEATURES
- Erythema, edema, and pruritus
- With or without scale
- If chronic, may lichenify
- Adult
- Predominantly female

DIAGNOSIS
- History of contact, which may be work- or occupation-related, or exposure to such irritants allergens as poison ivy and poison, oak

MANAGEMENT
- Avoidance of contactant
- Low-potency topical steroids (see Appendix A)

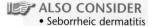

ALSO CONSIDER
- Seborrheic dermatitis
- Seborrheic blepharitis

EYELIDS AND PERIORBITAL AREA

Ocular Rosacea

Ocular rosacea frequently develops concurrently with cutaneous rosacea (see Chapter 6, Cheeks) but may precede the skin manifestations. Ocular symptoms result most often in blepharitis or conjunctivitis. Inflammation of meibomian glands, interpalpebral conjunctival hyperemia, and conjunctival telangiectasias may also occur. Episcleritis and keratoconjunctivitis sicca are rare complications.

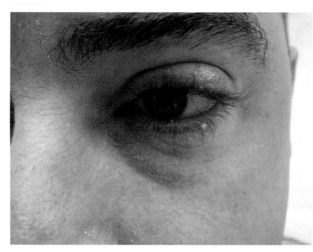

Figure 3-4 Rosacea.

DISTINGUISHING FEATURES
- Erythema (Fig. 3-4)
- Eye stinging or burning, dryness, photophobia, excessive tears, or a foreign body sensation

DIAGNOSIS
- Clinical; laboratory studies are not indicated.
- Often rosacea is elsewhere on face

MANAGEMENT (see Appendix A)
Topical Therapy
- Artificial tears
- Antibiotic ophthalmic ointment preparation such as erythromycin ointment
- Topical metronidazole 1% (**MetroGel**) is effective in treating skin lesions in rosacea (not approved for ophthalmic use, but may effective in treating eyelid involvement)
- Most cases can be treated and controlled with topical agents alone; however, if topical treatment is ineffective, an oral antibiotic is generally prescribed
- Referral to ophthalmology, if necessary

Oral Antibiotics
✔ **TIP: Short-term treatment with oral antibiotics typically delivers a rapid therapeutic response and often helps confirm the diagnosis of ocular rosacea.**
- Compared with topical therapy, systemic therapy has a more rapid onset of action
- Tetracycline in dosages ranging from 250 to 500 mg bid (twice daily), tapered when the inflammation has improved (usually after 2 to 3 weeks)
- If tetracycline is ineffective, minocycline (50 to 100 mg bid), doxycycline (50 to 100 mg bid), or erythromycin (250 mg bid to 250 mg 4 times a day) may be tried

Topical Immunomodulator
- Example: cyclosporine (**Restasis**)

Seborrheic Blepharitis

Seborrheic blepharitis (seborrheic dermatitis of the eyelid margins) may be a component of seborrheic dermatitis or it may also occur as a feature of atopic dermatitis, contact dermatitis, rosacea, or psoriasis. Seborrheic dermatitis is also commonly noted on the eyebrows and on the edges of the eyelids.

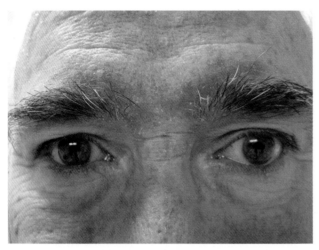

Figure 3-5 Seborrheic blepharitis.

DISTINGUISHING FEATURES
- Scale with or without erythema (Fig. 3-5)
- Evidence of seborrheic dermatitis elsewhere (e.g., scalp, eyebrows, nasal creases, behind ears) (see Chapter 1, Hair and Scalp; Chapter 4, Ears)

DIAGNOSIS
- Clinical

MANAGEMENT (see Appendix A)
- Hydrocortisone 1% ointment or cream (a very low-potency class 7 topical steroid is used, with caution; applied up to twice daily for 1 to 2 days or more, if necessary)
- Sulfacetamide and prednisolone ophthalmic (**Blephamide**) and tobramycin and dexamethasone ophthalmic ointment (**Tobradex**) is an antibiotic and steroid combination for topical ophthalmic use
- Ketoconazole or ciclopirox cream once daily for 2 to 4 weeks, repeated as necessary
- Topical immunomodulators such as tacrolimus (**Protopic ointment**) 1% for adults; 0.03% in children or pimecrolimus (**Elidel cream**) 1% may be effective

EYELIDS AND PERIORBITAL AREA

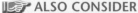 **ALSO CONSIDER**
- Atopic dermatitis
- Chalazion
- Dry eye syndrome
- Allergic conjunctivitis
- Bacterial conjunctivitis
- Viral conjunctivitis

RARELY
- Cicatricial pemphigoid
- Kawasaki syndrome in children

Cutaneous Sarcoidosis

Sarcoidosis is an inflammatory multisystem granulomatous disease of unknown etiology. Risk is increased threefold in African Americans compared with whites; Asians are rarely affected. Sarcoidosis is diagnosed when the classic clinical and radiologic findings are supported by histologic evidence of widespread noncaseating epithelioid granulomas that affect any organ system, most commonly the lungs. Besides thoracic involvement, ocular, neurologic, and extrapulmonary manifestations of sarcoidosis may cause complications such as blindness, meningitis, arthritis, renal disease, systemic morbidity, dermatitis, and death. Lymph nodes, liver, spleen, heart, central and peripheral nervous systems, musculoskeletal system, and salivary glands may be involved.

In ocular sarcoidosis, symptoms from uveitis include blurred vision, photophobia, floaters, redness, scotomata, and pain. Periocular lesions may produce dry eye symptoms, as well as periocular and adnexal lesions. Orbital involvement by a mass lesion may cause proptosis and diplopia. Other mucocutaneous locations include the lips and the mucous membranes of the mouth.

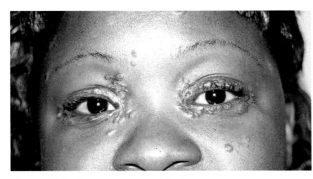

Figure 3-6 Cutaneous sarcoidosis.

DISTINGUISHING FEATURES
- Lesions usually begin on the nasal portion and, in more extensive cases, may encircle the eyes
- "Apple jelly" lesions
- Reddish, purple-brown infiltrative plaques (Fig. 3-6)
- May involve scars

DIAGNOSIS
- Skin biopsy (see Appendix B)

MANAGEMENT (see Appendix A)
- Topical steroids
- Intralesional corticosteroid injection
- Systemic steroids
- Plaquenil
- Steroid-sparing agents (e.g., methotrexate, azathioprine, cyclosporine, thalidomide)

Xanthelasma

Xanthelasma (xanthelasma palpebrarum) is the most common type of xanthoma. It is associated with hyperlipidemia in about 50% of cases, usually with hypercholesterolemia and increased low-density lipoprotein levels. The condition may be seen in light-skinned and dark-skinned individuals.

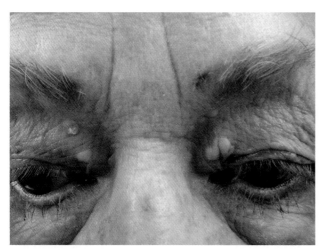

Figure 3-7 Xanthelasma.

DISTINGUISHING FEATURES

- Typically occurs in people older than 40 years of age; and women are affected nearly twice as often as men
- Arises symmetrically on upper and lower eyelids

- Yellowish-orange, flat papules or plaques (Fig. 3-7)
- Most commonly, lesions are noted near the inner canthus of the upper eyelid, although they may be seen on the lower lid as well
- Gradually grow larger over several months
- May or may not be associated with hyperlipidemia; however, younger individuals with xanthelasma have a proportionally greater likelihood of hyperlipidemia and hypercholesterolemia than do older individuals

DIAGNOSIS
- Clinical

MANAGEMENT (see Appendix B)
- Dietary and lifestyle modifications as well as the treatment of the underlying lipid disorder seem to have little impact on the xanthomas
- Surgery or locally destructive modalities may be necessary
  - Topical trichloroacetic acid
  - Electrodesiccation
  - Laser destruction
  - Excision

 ALSO CONSIDER
- Granuloma annulare
- Lichen planus
- Foreign body granuloma
- Systemic lupus erythematosus

RARELY
- Amyloidosis
- Juvenile xanthogranuloma
- Lymphoma
- Pseudolymphoma
- Granuloma faciale
- Leprosy
- Lupus vulgaris

EYELIDS AND PERIORBITAL AREA

Syringoma

Syringomas are small, benign, eccrine duct tumors that appear predominantly in women and are often hereditary. They generally first appear around puberty. More commonly seen on Asian skin, they are most often found in clusters on the eyelids but they may also arise elsewhere on the face. They are often a common incidental finding on the eyelids.

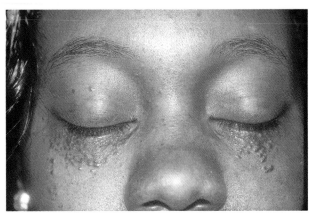

Figure 3-8 Syringoma.

DISTINGUISHING FEATURES
- Multiple asymptomatic skin, colored or yellowish firm, rounded papules 1 to 3 mm in diameter (Fig. 3-8)
- Most often appear on the lower lids

DIAGNOSIS
- Clinical
- Shave biopsy if diagnosis is in doubt (see Appendix B)

MANAGEMENT
- Cosmetic issue
- Often treated by electrosurgery or laser. This may or may not prove successful and may result in small scars
- Recurrences are common

Molluscum Contagiosum

Molluscum contagiosum (see Chapter 2, Forehead and Temples; Chapter 18, Genital Area) may appear on or around the eyelids or eyelid margins. This is most often seen in the pediatric age group and in patients who have human immunodeficiency virus (HIV)/acquired immunodeficiency syndrome (AIDS).

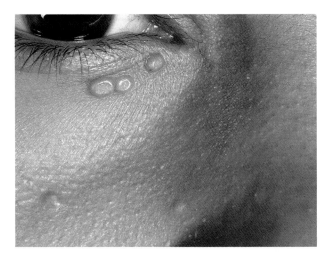

Figure 3-9 Molluscum contagiosum. (Used with permission from Burkhart C, Morell, D, Goldsmith LA, et al. *VisualDx: Essential Pediatric Dermatology.* Philadelphia, PA: Lippincott Williams & Wilkins; 2009.)

DISTINGUISHING FEATURES
- Dome-shaped, waxy or pearly papules with a central white core (umbilicated); less frequently, lesions are pink to flesh-colored (Fig. 3-9)

MANAGEMENT (see Appendices A and B)
- In this sensitive location, wait for spontaneous resolution in healthy, immunocompetent persons
- Electrocautery in adults
- Imiquimod 5% cream (**Aldara**) applied at bedtime
- Systemic griseofulvin and cimetidine have been anecdotally reported to be effective

Milium

Milium (plural, milia) (see Chapter 2, Forehead and Temples) is most often noted on the face, especially around the eyes, eyelids, cheeks, and forehead. Milia occur at almost any age. They are very common epidermal cysts that contain keratin.

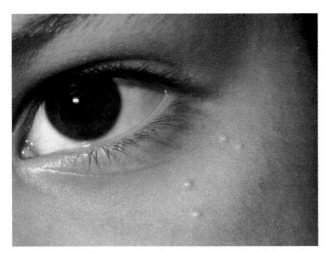

Figure 3-10 Milium. (Used with permission from Burkhart C, Morell, D, Goldsmith LA, et al. *VisualDx: Essential Pediatric Dermatology*. Philadelphia, PA: Lippincott Williams & Wilkins; 2009.)

DISTINGUISHING FEATURES
- 1.0 to 2.0 mm in diameter, white or yellow cysts (Fig. 3-10)

DIAGNOSIS
- Clinical

MANAGEMENT
- No treatment is medically necessary
- For cosmetic reasons, incision and extraction or electrocautery in adults

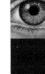

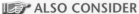 **ALSO CONSIDER**
- Closed comedones (whiteheads)
- Trichoepithelioma
- Flat warts (see Chapter 2, Forehead and Temples)

RARELY
- Disseminated cryptococcosis, toxoplasmosis in patients infected with HIV/AIDS

Skin Tag

A **skin tag** (acrochordon) is an extremely common benign, quite harmless lesion often seen in the body folds. When large, they are referred to as fibroepithelial polyps "soft fibromas" or "pedunculated lipofibromas" Besides eyelids, they are often seen in any skin fold including the neck and axillae (see also Chapter 10, Neck; Chapter 11, Axillae), groin (see Chapter 20, Inguinal area), and inframammary areas. An association with type 2 diabetes mellitus and obesity has been observed.

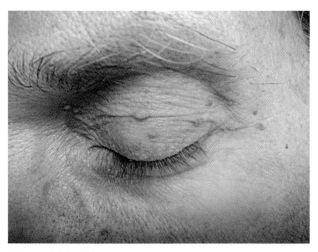

Figure 3-11 Skin tags.

DISTINGUISHING FEATURES
- Small, soft, often pedunculated or sessile papules (Fig. 3-11)
- Skin-colored or darker than the patient's skin
- Most vary in size from 2 to 5 mm in diameter, although larger ones up to 5 cm in diameter (fibroepithelial polyp) are sometimes evident
- A family history often exists
- Primarily of cosmetic concern
- Usually asymptomatic unless inflamed or irritated by friction, jewelry, or clothing
- During pregnancy, lesions tend to grow larger and are more numerous

DIAGNOSIS
- Clinical
- Easy to recognize; a skin biopsy is rarely necessary

MANAGEMENT
- May be disregarded; occasionally they spontaneously self-destruct (become necrotic and autoamputate)
- Snip excision (see Appendix B). Very small skin tags are easily removed by snipping them off at their base using an iris scissors, with or without prior local anesthesia. The crushing action of the scissors results in little bleeding or pain

✔ **TIP: A rapid and painless treatment for small skin tags is to dip a needle holder or nontoothed forceps into LN_2 for 15 seconds and then gently grasp each skin tag for about 10 seconds. There is little or no collateral damage, just a narrow rim of erythema ensues. Multiple lesions can be treated by this method. The frozen skin tag will be shed in approximately 10 days. This is a good approach for skin tags on the eyelids.**

Seborrheic Keratosis

Seborrheic keratoses (see Chapter 1, Hair and Scalp; Chapter 2, Forehead and Temples; Chapter 15, Trunk; Chapter 16, Breasts and Inframammary Area; Chapter 21, Legs) are sometimes noted in the periorbital area, where they tend to be small and are often in the company of pigmented skin tags, which they closely resemble. They are benign, harmless lesions.

DISTINGUISHING FEATURES
- Most vary in size from 2 to 5 mm in diameter (Fig. 3-12)
- Flat or pedunculated (indistinguishable from skin tags; see previous discussion)
- Often multiple light brown or black
- Clinical variant: **dermatosis papulosa nigra** (see also Chapter 2, Forehead and Temples; Chapter 6, Cheeks)
  - Located on the lateral orbital areas (Fig. 3-13)
  - May be filiform (wartlike)

DIAGNOSIS
- Clinical
- Snip or shave biopsy if the diagnosis is in doubt (see Appendix B)

MANAGEMENT
- Mainly a cosmetic concern
- Snip excision (see Appendix B)
- Electrocautery

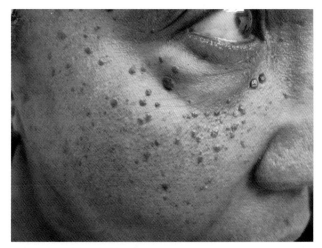

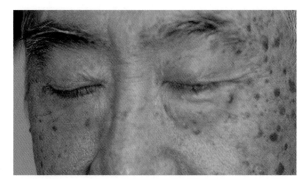

Figure 3-12 Seborrheic keratosis.

Figure 3-13 Dermatosis papulosa nigra.

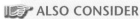 **ALSO CONSIDER**
- Wart
- Neurofibroma
- Melanocytic nevus

Stye (Hordeolum)

A **hordeolum** (stye) is a common disorder of the eyelid. It is an acute focal infection (usually *Staphylococcus aureus*) involving either the glands of Zeis (external hordeola, or styes) or, less frequently, the meibomian glands (internal hordeola). Essentially, a hordeolum represents an acute focal infectious process, and a chalazion represents a chronic, noninfectious granulomatous reaction (see following discussion). The patient may have a history of risk factors for hordeola, such as meibomian gland dysfunction, chronic blepharitis, or rosacea.

DISTINGUISHING FEATURES
- Painful, warm, swollen, red papule on the eyelid margin (Fig. 3-14)
- May cause blurring of vision

DIAGNOSIS
- Clinical examination
- Differentiating hordeola from acute chalazia may be difficult because they both are similar in appearance; however, hordeola are very tender and painful

MANAGEMENT
- Usually self-limited; spontaneously resolves in 1 to 2 weeks
- Warm compresses and massages of the lesions
- Topical antibiotic ointment if the lesion is draining or if there is an accompanying blepharoconjunctivitis
- Systemic antibiotics if necessary (e.g., a tetracycline derivative)
- Internal hordeola may occasionally evolve into chalazia, which may require topical steroids, oral antibiotics, intralesional steroids, or surgical incision and curettage

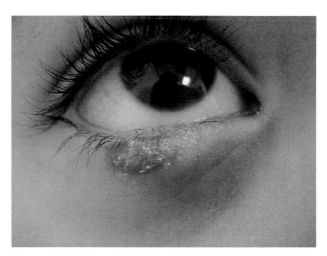

Figure 3-14 Stye (hordeolum).

Meibomian Cyst (Chalazion)

A **chalazion,** or meibomian cyst, is a common granulomatous inflammatory response of either a meibomian gland or a Zeis gland. It may develop because of a blockage of a gland orifice. The resulting mass of granulation tissue and chronic inflammation (with lymphocytes and lipid-laden macrophages) distinguishes a chalazion from an internal or external hordeolum (see previous discussion), which is primarily an acute pyogenic lesion. Chalazia form when underlying meibomitis results in stasis of gland secretions and the contents of the glands (sebum) are released into the tarsus and adjacent tissues to incite a noninfectious inflammatory reaction. Chalazia are sometimes associated with seborrhea, chronic blepharitis, and rosacea.

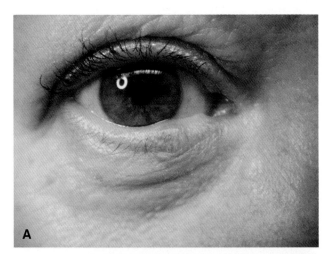

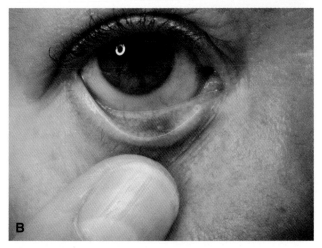

Figure 3-15 A, Meibomian cyst (chalazion).
B, Meibomian cyst. Eversion of the lid may reveal the dilated meibomian gland.

DISTINGUISHING FEATURES
- Nontender, firm papule located deep within the lid or the tarsal plate (Fig. 3-15A)
- Lid discomfort, redness, tenderness, swelling
- Eversion of the lid may reveal the dilated meibomian gland (Fig. 3-15B)
- More common on the upper lid

DIAGNOSIS
- Clinical

MANAGEMENT
- Small, asymptomatic chalazia may be ignored
- Conservative treatment with lid massage, moist heat, and topical mild steroids can be helpful in minimizing inflammation and in reducing edema
- Topical antibiotics are not effective
- An oral tetracycline (e.g., doxycycline 100 mg or minocycline 50 mg daily for 10 days)
- Secondarily infected chalazion (i.e., internal hordeolum) includes heat and topical and/or systemic antibiotics
- Ophthalmologic surgery by incision and curettage is performed only if medical therapy fails

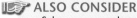 **ALSO CONSIDER**
- Sebaceous neoplasm
- Mucocele
- Hydrocystoma (see following discussion)

RARELY
- Orbital cellulitis

Basal Cell Carcinoma

In **basal cell carcinoma (BCC),** the lower eyelid is more exposed than the upper lid to sun, which accounts for the development of BCCs in this location. Squamous cell carcinomas and other malignant neoplasms are unusual in this site.

DISTINGUISHING FEATURES
- Pearly papule, often very small (Fig. 3-16)
- Middle-aged or elderly individuals are usually affected
- Telangiectasias may be difficult to visualize
- With or without crusting or ulceration

DIAGNOSIS
- Shave biopsy
- Excisional biopsy by an ophthalmologist

MANAGEMENT
- Lesions on or near the eyelids may require Mohs micrographic surgery (see Appendix B), often followed by an oculoplastic reconstruction
- ⚠ **ALERT: A hydrocystoma (see following discussion) and a BCC of the eyelid are clinically very similar (see Figs. 3-16 and 3-17). A biopsy may be necessary to distinguish them from one another.**

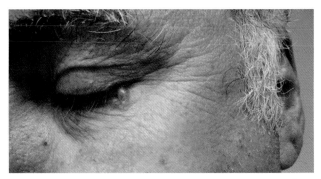

Figure 3-16 Basal cell carcinoma. (Image courtesy of Benjamin Barankin, MD.)

Hydrocystoma

Hydrocystoma (apocrine hidrocystoma) is a benign cystic proliferation of the apocrine secretory glands. These cysts most commonly appear as solitary, soft, dome-shaped, translucent papules or nodules and most frequently are located on the eyelids, especially the inner canthus.

DISTINGUISHING FEATURES
- Clear, translucent, shiny, jelly-like cyst (Fig. 3-17)
- Color varies from flesh-colored to blue or black
- Small; less than 5 mm in diameter
- Grow slowly and usually persist indefinitely

DIAGNOSIS
- Clinical
- Biopsy, if diagnosis is in doubt

MANAGEMENT
- Do not usually need treatment, but cysts can be readily removed by a minor surgical procedure
- Larger cysts may be removed if they are unsightly or because they have become inflamed

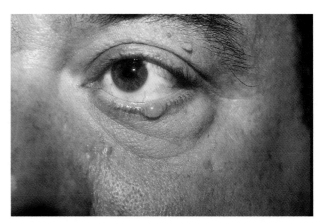

Figure 3-17 Hydrocystoma.

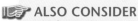 **ALSO CONSIDER**
- Melanocytic nevus
- Blue nevus
- Malignant melanoma
- Milia
- Syringoma
- Eccrine cystadenoma
- Follicular cyst

CHAPTER 4

Ears

The ears have a close relationship to the skin disorders of the scalp. In both sexes, the external ears (pinnae), auditory canals, and retroauricular areas are typical places for the appearance of inflammatory disorders such as seborrheic dermatitis, atopic dermatitis, and psoriasis. The ear lobes are subject to contact dermatitis, hypertrophic scars, and keloids from earrings. Discoid lupus erythematosus also occurs on the external ears, generally on the conchae. The diagnosis of these conditions is usually uncomplicated and made on clinical grounds, often aided by evidence of these dermatoses elsewhere on the body. Another inflammatory process, often mistaken for a solar keratosis, is chondrodermatitis nodularis helicis, a tender, inflammatory condition of the skin and underlying cartilage of the ears.

Ears that are not protected from the sun are also common sites for the development of solar keratoses, basal cell carcinomas, and squamous cell carcinomas. Such lesions are noted predominantly in fair-complexioned, elderly men whose hairstyles or lack of hair generally has not afforded protection of the ears from ultraviolet radiation (see Chapter 1, Hair and Scalp). In contrast, women historically tend to have fewer neoplasms on the external ears by virtue of longer hairstyles. No doubt the current fashion of shorter hair styles that leave unprotected, sun-exposed ears will, in time, lead to more of these lesions in women.

IN THIS CHAPTER

Helix and Antihelix
- Chondrodermatitis nodularis helicis *vs* solar keratosis/cutaneous horn
- Keratoacanthoma *vs* squamous cell carcinoma *vs* basal cell carcinoma

Auditory Canals, Conchae, and Retroauricular Areas (Folds)
- Seborrheic dermatitis *vs* psoriasis *vs* eczema (atopic dermatitis)

Chondrodermatitis Nodularis Helicis
vs Solar Keratosis/Cutaneous Horn

Chondrodermatitis Nodularis Helicis

Chondrodermatitis nodularis helicis (CNH) is a common, benign, tender, painful condition of the helix or antihelix of the ear. Chondrodermatitis nodularis helicis can be difficult to distinguish from a solar keratosis and an early squamous cell carcinoma (SCC). It occurs most commonly in fair-skinned persons, usually affecting middle-aged or older men. About 10% to 35% of cases involve women.

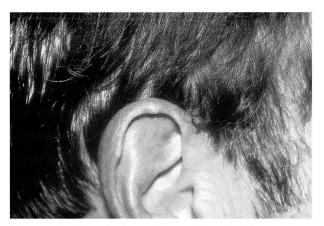

Figure 4-1 Chondrodermatitis nodularis helicis.

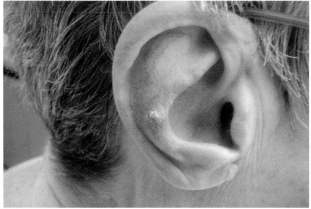

Figure 4-2 Chondrodermatitis nodularis helicis on the antihelix.

DISTINGUISHING FEATURES
- Spontaneously appearing tender or painful firm papule with or without a central crust or umbilication
- Most often located on the apex of the helix (Fig. 4-1), less commonly on the antihelix of ear (Fig. 4-2)
- The papule is usually reaches a maximum size of 4 to 6 mm and remains stable
- The affected ear is tender when compressed, such as when the patient sleeps on the affected side or talks on the telephone
- ☑ **TIP: Lesions are generally located on the lateral edge of the helix (where there is less direct sun exposure)**

DIAGNOSIS
- Clinical: however, a shave biopsy (see Appendix B) is indicated if the diagnosis is in doubt

MANAGEMENT
- Suggest sleeping on other side using a soft pillow or a foam "donut" cut from a block of foam or a **CNH Ear Protector,** which can be ordered from www.delasco.com
- Some resolve after one or more intralesional corticosteroid injections
- Shave excision that includes some of the underlying cartilage (this may be curative)
- Wedge excision if these options fail

Solar Keratosis

Solar keratoses (actinic keratoses) and **cutaneous horns** are common findings on the sun-exposed ears of elderly fair-skinned men. Both also arise on the scalp (see also Chapter 1, Hair and Scalp; Chapter 2, Forehead and Temples; Chapter 5, Nose and Perinasal Area; Chapter 12, Arms; Chapter 21, Legs), on other sun-exposed areas, particularly the face, nose, forearms, and dorsal hands. Malignant lesions at the base of the cutaneous horn usually are SCCs.

Solar keratoses on the ear may gradually enlarge, thicken, become more elevated, and develop into a hypertrophic solar keratosis or a cutaneous horn (a fingernail platelike keratinization produced by either a solar keratosis or an SCC). This frequently occurs in patients aged 70 or older.

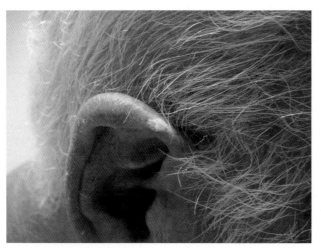

Figure 4-3 Solar keratosis.

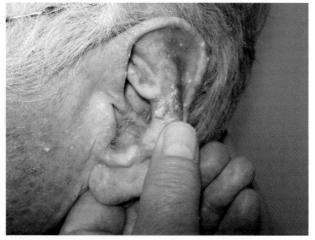

Figure 4-4 Cutaneous horn on the antihelix.

DISTINGUISHING FEATURES
- Elderly male predominance
- Scaly (hyperkeratotic) papule (Fig. 4-3)
- Palpation reveals a gritty, sandpaperlike texture
- Most often located on helix or antihelix of ear (Fig. 4-4)
- Actinic (sun) damage elsewhere is usually noted
- ✔ **TIP: Lesions are generally located on the superior edge of the helix (where there is direct sun exposure)**

DIAGNOSIS
- Shave biopsy when the diagnosis is in doubt or to rule out an SCC
- Advanced lesions may be clinically difficult to distinguish from SCC (see following discussion)
- **Cutaneous horn**
  - A shave biopsy that includes the base is generally performed
  - A solar keratosis or a malignancy such as SCC or an SCC in situ (**Bowen disease**) is often noted at the base of the horn
  - Less often, a wart or a basal cell carcinoma (BCC) is found

MANAGEMENT (see Appendix B)
- **Prevention** begins with educating the patient to limit sun exposure by using sunscreens and wearing protective head wear that shades the ears (e.g., wearing a broad-brimmed hat)
- **Treatment** includes methods such as the following:
  - Liquid nitrogen (LN$_2$) applied to individual lesions for 3 to 5 seconds
  - Biopsy, followed by electrocautery of individual lesions, or electrocautery alone
- Cutaneous horn
  - Shave biopsy
  - Cryotherapy or curettage with or without electrodesiccation

👉 **ALSO CONSIDER**
- Seborrheic keratosis
- Wart
- Keratoacanthoma
- Gouty tophus

RARELY
- Rheumatoid nodule
- Endochondral pseudocyst

EARS

Keratoacanthoma *vs* Squamous Cell Carcinoma *vs* Basal Cell Carcinoma

Keratoacanthoma

A **keratoacanthoma (KA)** is a unique lesion with a characteristic clinical appearance (see also Chapter 5, Nose and Perinasal Area; Chapter 12, Arms). This condition occurs in individuals who are generally over 65. If ignored, the lesion reportedly regresses spontaneously. There is controversy about the benign versus malignant nature of this lesion. A KA resembles an SCC histologically and is considered by some dermatologists and dermatopathologists to be a low-grade variant of an SCC.

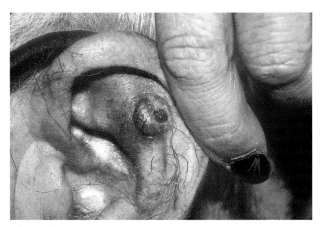

Figure 4-5 Keratoacanthoma.

DISTINGUISHING FEATURES
- Affects males more than females
- Rapidly growing; usually taking 3 to 4 weeks to appear
- Occurs as a single dome-shaped erythematous or skin-colored nodule plus a central keratin core with an overlying crust (central crater) (Fig. 4-5)

- May attain a diameter of 1.0 to 2.5 cm
- Lesions appear on the sun-exposed face, ears, neck, dorsa of hands, and forearms
- Spontaneous regression may result in scarring
- May be indistinguishable from an SCC

DIAGNOSIS
- An excisional or incisional biopsy is often recommended so that the complete architecture of the lesion can be evaluated histologically. (An insufficient biopsy, such as a shave biopsy, may result in a histology that is indistinguishable from an SCC.)
- However, because these lesions often appear in areas where it is difficult to perform an excisional biopsy (i.e., on the external ears and nose), a deep shave biopsy may be adequate to obtain sufficient tissue

MANAGEMENT (see Appendix B)
- Deep shave biopsy
- Electrodesiccation and curettage
- Excision
- Intralesional 5-fluorouracil
- Micrographic (Mohs) surgery for recurrences

Squamous Cell Carcinoma

Often clinically similar to solar keratosis (see previous discussion), a **squamous cell carcinoma (SCC)** on the external ear can represent a more difficult problem. Softer, nonkeratinizing, or ulcerated lesions are generally less well differentiated and are more likely to spread. Slow-growing, firm papules with the ability to produce scale (keratinization) tend to be more clearly differentiated and less likely to metastasize (e.g., an SCC underlying a cutaneous horn). Frequently, an SCC is often indistinguishable from a hypertrophic solar keratosis, a KA, or a BCC.

⚠ **ALERT: When metastases from SCC do occur, they are more likely to result from lesions that appear on the ears or on the vermillion border of the lips or from tumors more than 2 cm in diameter (see Chapter 1, Hair and Scalp; Chapter 2, Forehead and Temples; Chapter 5, Nose and Perinasal Area; Chapter 7, Lips and Perioral Area; Chapter 12, Arms; Chapter 21, Legs).**

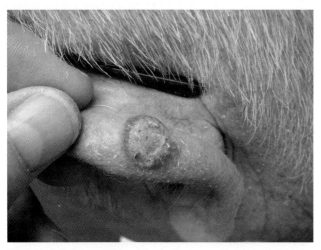

Figure 4-6 Squamous cell carcinoma.

DISTINGUISHING FEATURES
- As on other locations, an early SCC (Fig. 4-6) is clinically similar to a precursor solar keratosis
- As it evolves, an SCC may ulcerate

DIAGNOSIS
- A shave or excisional biopsy
- Histologically, various degrees of cellular atypia are present, and the keratinocytes differ in size and shape

MANAGEMENT (see Appendix B)
- Limit sun exposure: use sunscreens and protective clothing
- Electrocautery and curettage for small lesions (generally <1 cm) and SCC in situ (Bowen disease)
- Total excision, which is the preferred method of therapy for SCC, permitting histologic diagnosis of the tumor margins
- Cryosurgery with LN_2 in selected lesions
- Micrographic (Mohs) surgery is useful for excessively large or invasive carcinomas, for recurrent lesions, for those with poorly delineated clinical borders (e.g., ear canals)
- Radiation therapy is used for those patients who are physically debilitated or are unable to, or refuse to, undergo, excisional surgery

Basal Cell Carcinoma

Basal cell carcinomas (BCCs) also occur on the sun-exposed parts of the ears. At times, the lesion is ulcerated and may be difficult to distinguish from an SCC (see Chapter 2, Forehead and Temples; Chapter 6, Nose).

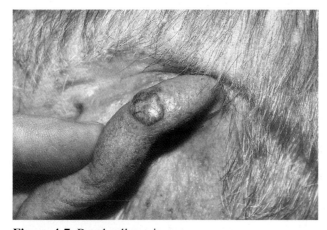

Figure 4-7 Basal cell carcinoma.

DISTINGUISHING FEATURES
- Classically, a pearly papule with telangiectasias and a central crust ("rodent ulcer") (Fig. 4-7)
- Most often located on helix of ear
- Middle-aged or elderly men
- Lesion may be hyperkeratotic or ulcerated
- A shave biopsy is necessary to clarify the diagnosis

MANAGEMENT (see Appendix B)
- Electrocautery and curettage or cryosurgery with LN_2
- Total excision
- Micrographic (Mohs) surgery for morpheaform, recurrent, or large lesions or those in the ear canal
- Radiation therapy for elderly debilitated patients or for those who are physically unable to undergo excisional surgery

DIAGNOSIS
- Shave biopsy

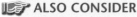 **ALSO CONSIDER**
- Verruca vulgaris
- Solar keratosis
- Seborrheic keratosis

Seborrheic Dermatitis vs Psoriasis vs Eczema (Atopic Dermatitis)

Seborrheic Dermatitis

Seborrheic dermatitis (SD) is the most common inflammatory skin condition that affects the ears. The usual onset occurs during puberty and is seen more commonly in males. Seborrheic dermatitis often bears a very close resemblance to both atopic dermatitis and psoriasis (see Chapter 1, Hair and Scalp; and Chapter 2, Forehead and Temples).

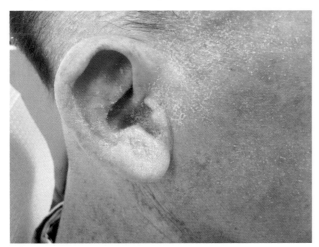

Figure 4-8 Seborrheic dermatitis (scalp, ears, and ear canals).

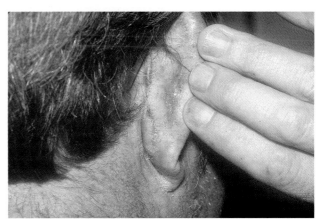

Figure 4-9 Seborrheic dermatitis behind ears.

DISTINGUISHING FEATURES
- May also have dandruff of scalp and/or face
- Erythema with or without overlying whitish or yellowish scaling (Fig. 4-8)
- With or without fissuring of retroauricular folds (Fig. 4-9)
- Lesions occur particularly around the external acoustic meatus, retroauricular areas, and may involve the entire pinna
- Pruritus is common, but usually not as severe as in atopic dermatitis

DIAGNOSIS
- Clinical

MANAGEMENT (see Appendix A)
- Intermittent application of low- to mid-potency topical steroids depending on severity and clinical response
- Topical antifungal gels, lotions, or foams such as ciclopirox cream **(Loprox), Xolegel, Extina,** and generic 2% ketoconazole cream
- **Promiseb,** a nonsteroidal cream, has both an anti-inflammatory as well as antifungal effects

Psoriasis

It is not uncommon for **psoriasis** to be present in the auditory canals and external ears. When psoriasis involves only the scalp and retroauricular areas, it is sometimes referred to as "sebopsoriasis" or "seborrhiasis" (see Chapter 1, Hair and Scalp; and Chapter 2, Forehead and Temples).

DISTINGUISHING FEATURES
- Thicker plaques, often silvery, or with a whitish scale and more brightly erythematous than seen in SD and eczema (atopic dermatitis) and is generally more difficult to treat (Fig. 4-10)
- Similar to SD, it often involves the external auditory canal
- May not cause any symptoms at all or may be somewhat itchy

DIAGNOSIS
- Clinical

MANAGEMENT (see Appendix A)
Mild Cases
- For minimal scaling and thin plaques similar to that is seen in SD (see previous discussion), psoriasis can often be managed with antipsoriasis-antidandruff shampoos and a low-potency (class 4 to 6) or mid-potency (class 3 or 4) topical steroid used as needed for itching
- Over-the-counter options include shampoos that contain tar **(Zetar, T/Gel),** selenium sulfide **(Selsun Blue, Head and Shoulders),** or salicylic acid **(T/Sa)**
- Calcipotriol cream **(Dovonex)** or ointment or **Vectical** (calcitriol) ointment, a vitamin D analog

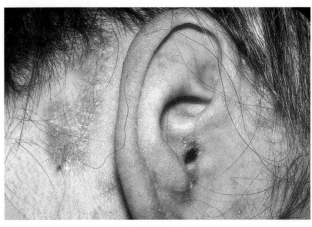

Figure 4-10 Psoriasis.

Severe Cases

- Potent (class 2) and superpotent (class 1) topical steroids are frequently preceded by keratolytic agents to remove thick scale, to allow the medications to penetrate the scalp before the underlying inflammatory plaques can be effectively treated
- Keratolytics: **Salex** cream or lotion, **Keralyt gel 6%,** or salicylic acid in petrolatum to remove scale (see Appendix B) followed by a medium- to high-potency (class 2, 3, or 4) topical steroid **Dovonex lotion** or **Vectical** (calcitriol) ointment
- **Taclonex ointment (**combines betamethasone and calcipotriene)

Eczema (Atopic Dermatitis)

Eczema or **atopic dermatitis** is a common manifestation on the external ears in both children and adults who have an atopic diathesis (see Chapter 1, Hair and Scalp; Chapter 3, Eyelids and Periorbital Area; Chapter 12, Arms; Chapter 21, Legs).

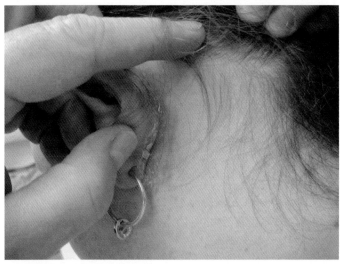

Figure 4-11 Atopic dermatitis. It is markedly pruritic. Note the scale, erythema of the retroauricular area, and similarity to seborrheic dermatitis (Fig 4-9).

DISTINGUISHING FEATURES

- Scale, erythema
- May involve the ear canal, conchae, or retroauricular areas (Fig. 4-11)
- Pruritus is significant
- With or without fissuring of retroauricular areas and lobular crease
- Eczematous lesions may be present elsewhere on the body and help distinguish it from seborrheic dermatitis and psoriasis

DIAGNOSIS

- History and physical examination

MANAGEMENT (see Appendix A)

- Class 1 to 4 topical steroids depending on severity and clinical response
- Tacrolimus **(Protopic ointment)** 1% for adults; 0.03% in children; or pimecrolimus **(Elidel cream)** is available in a 1% formulation

ALSO CONSIDER
- Contact dermatitis
- Tinea capitis/tinea faciale
- Intertrigo

EARS

CHAPTER 5

Nose and Perinasal Area

The nose has two outstanding features—its prominence and its abundance of sebaceous glands—both of which make it and its surrounding area a site prone to develop the most common inflammatory conditions: acne vulgaris, rosacea, seborrheic dermatitis, and periorificial dermatitis, as well as sun-related dermatoses. Also, the central location of the nose makes it and the cheeks cosmetic features of prime importance.

Many benign neoplasms occur on the nose. They can be easily recognized, particularly in younger patients. Melanocytic nevi, or moles, are extremely common benign facial papules that appear in childhood. Fibrous papules of the nose are acquired benign lesions that first appear in adulthood.

The prominence of the nose also presents it as a prime target for photosensitive disorders (e.g., systemic lupus erythematosus) and the development of ultraviolet-induced premalignant and malignant neoplasms such as solar keratoses, squamous cell carcinomas, and basal cell carcinomas. Pigmentary lesions such as solar lentigines, and much less commonly, an early in situ melanoma known as lentigo maligna, may be seen on the nose in the elderly.

> ## IN THIS CHAPTER
> ### Nasal Bridge and Ala Nasi
> - Rosacea/rhinophyma *vs* adult-onset acne
> - Melanocytic nevus *vs* fibrous papule *vs* basal cell carcinoma
> - Solar keratosis *vs* squamous cell carcinoma *vs* keratoacanthoma
>
> ### Nasal Creases and Perinasal Area
> - Perioral (periorificial) dermatitis *vs* seborrheic dermatitis

Rosacea/Rhinophyma *vs* Adult-Onset Acne

Rosacea/Rhinophyma

Rosacea (see also Chapter 3, Eyelids and Periorbital Area; Chapter 6, Cheeks) is frequently mistaken for acne. When acnelike lesions appear on the nose, it is sometimes difficult to distinguish between the two conditions; however, if there is evidence of acne or rosacea elsewhere on the face, it can be of diagnostic significance. **Rhinophyma** is an unsightly manifestation of rosacea. This condition usually occurs in men over 40. It is quite uncommon and is rarely seen in women. There is no evidence that alcohol ingestion causes it.

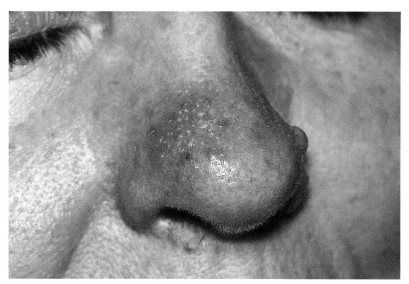

Figure 5-1 Rosacea.

DISTINGUISHING FEATURES
- Appears later in life than acne (30 to 50 years of age)
- Persistent acnelike erythematous papules, pustules, and telangiectasias against a background of erythema (Fig. 5-1)
- No association with menstrual cycle
- Evidence of rosacea may be seen elsewhere on the face or eyelids
- Lacks the comedones ("blackheads" or "whiteheads") that are seen in acne

DIAGNOSIS
- Clinical
- Rarely, a biopsy may be necessary in atypical cases

MANAGEMENT
- See Chapter 6, Cheeks, and Appendix C
- Sunscreens/sun avoidance

Rhinophyma

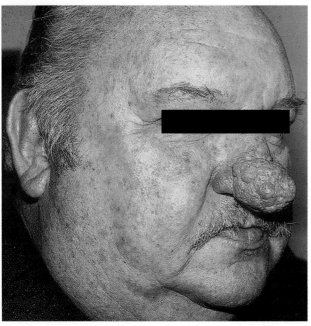

Figure 5-2 Rhinophyma.

DISTINGUISHING FEATURES
- Men over 40
- Consists of knobby nasal papules that tend to become larger and swollen over time (Fig. 5-2)

DIAGNOSIS
- Clinical

MANAGEMENT
- The usual treatments that are described to treat rosacea are not effective for rhinophyma
- Recontouring procedures with a scalpel or a carbon dioxide laser have been used to remove the excess nose tissue of rhinophyma by "sculpting" it down to a more normal shape and appearance. This may also be accomplished by electrocautery and dermabrasion

Adult-Onset Acne

Adult-onset acne (postadolescent acne) is overwhelmingly a condition of females (see also Chapter 6, Cheeks; Chapter 9, Chin and Mandibular Area). When acnelike lesions appear on the nose of adults who have never had acne, the diagnosis is most likely rosacea.

MANAGEMENT
- Discussed in Chapter 6, Cheeks (see also Chapter 2, Forehead and Temples, and Appendix C)

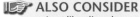 **ALSO CONSIDER**
- Acnelike disorders
  - Endocrinopathic acne
- Physically induced and occupational acne
- Demadex folliculitis
- Bacterial folliculitis
- Pityrosporum folliculitis

RARELY
- Chloracne

Melanocytic Nevus

Melanocytic nevus (common mole) may be evident on the nose. Most of these nevi are either the compound or dermal types (see Chapter 2, Forehead and Temples). Such lesions may appear to be clinically similar to a basal cell carcinoma (BCC); however, the history of a lesion is often an important differentiating feature because melanocytic nevi on the nose typically have been apparent since adolescence.

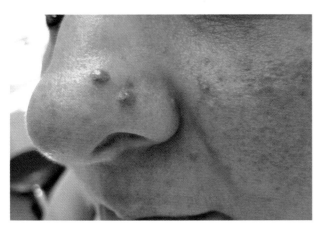

Figure 5-3 Melanocytic nevus.

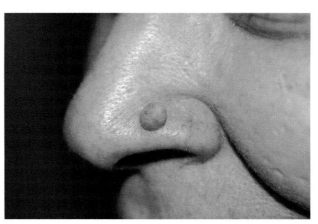

Figure 5-4 Melanocytic nevus.

DISTINGUISHING FEATURES
- Dome-shaped papule; sometimes with hairs (Fig. 5-3)
- Size remains stable
- Flesh-colored (less translucent than BCC) or vary from dark brown to black; pigmentation can be uniform or speckled
- May have telangiectasias but not as apparent as BCC (see following discussion)
- Lesions tend to loose their capacity to form melanin and become flesh-colored during adulthood (Fig. 5-4)

DIAGNOSIS
- Clinical
- Shave biopsy if diagnosis is in doubt (see Appendix B)

MANAGEMENT
- No treatment required
- Shave removal for cosmetic reasons

Fibrous Papule

Fibrous papule, of the nose (angiokeratoma), is an acquired benign lesion that arises in adults. They are very common. Located on, or sometimes near, the nose, as solitary or multiple lesions. Most often the diagnostic confusion is between a melanocytic nevus and a basal cell carcinoma (BCC)

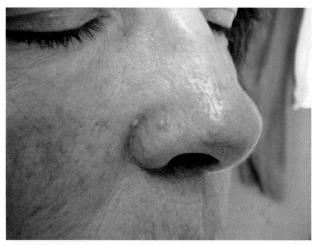

Figure 5-5 Fibrous papule (angiofibroma).

DISTINGUISHING FEATURES
- Firm, dome-shaped, flesh-colored, or slightly erythematous papule 2 to 4 mm in size (Fig. 5-5)
- Hairless
- Most often occurs on the nose; less commonly, elsewhere on the face
- Develop during late adolescence or early adult life
- Similar in appearance to a skin-colored dermal nevus (see previous discussion)
- Harmless, but persists unchanged lifelong

DIAGNOSIS
- Clinical
- Shave biopsy if diagnosis is in doubt (see Appendix B)

MANAGEMENT
- No treatment required
- ⚠ **ALERT: It is important to distinguish fibrous papules from BCC (see following discussion), which may also present as a firm shiny papule**

Basal Cell Carcinoma

Basal cell carcinoma (BCC), the most common malignancy of the skin, is commonly seen on the nose. Basal cell carcinoma is locally invasive and slow-growing, and it very rarely metastasizes. It has many of the same risk factors that predispose to solar keratoses and squamous cell carcinomas (see Chapter 2, Forehead and Temples).

Risk factors:
- Age over 40
- Male sex
- Positive family history
- Light complexion with poor tanning ability (rare in blacks and Asians)
- Cumulative sun exposure (primary risk factor)

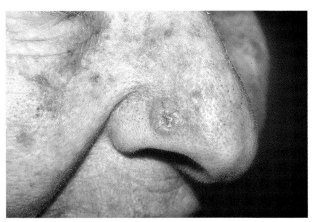

Figure 5-6 Basal cell carcinoma.

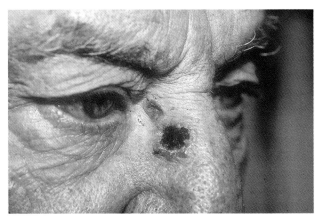

Figure 5-7 Basal cell carcinoma (pigmented).

DISTINGUISHING FEATURES

- Nodular BCC is the most common type
  - Pearly, papule, or nodule with rolled raised border (Fig. 5-6)
- Appear most often on the ala nasi, nasal creases, nasal tip, and bridge of nose
- Telangiectases
- No visible hairs (follicles usually destroyed)
- Size progressively increases
- Erosion or ulceration ("rodent ulcer")

- Variant: pigmented BCC contains melanin; brownish to blue-black pigmentation seen in more darkly pigmented persons (Fig. 5-7)

DIAGNOSIS

- Shave biopsy; excisional biopsy is rarely necessary

MANAGEMENT (see Appendix B)

- Treatment options depend on histologic subtype and specific location on the nose (see Appendix B)
- Micrographic (Mohs) surgery is the best treatment for large or recurrent lesions, especially those that arise on the nasal alae or tip of the nose
- Sun avoidance and use of sunscreens; wearing protective clothing

---

ALSO CONSIDER
- Squamous cell carcinoma
- Solar keratosis
- Warts
- Sebaceous hyperplasia
- Neurofibroma
- Seborrheic keratosis, which may be indistinguishable from a pigmented basal cell carcinoma

RARELY
- Merkel cell tumor

Solar Keratosis *vs* Squamous Cell Carcinoma *vs* Keratoacanthoma

Solar Keratosis

Solar keratoses, as well as squamous cell carcinomas (SCCs) and BCCs, occur in persons who are fair-skinned, burn easily, and tan poorly (see also Chapter 1, Hair and Scalp; Chapter 2, Forehead and Temples; Chapter 5, Nose and Perinasal Area; Chapter 12, Arms; Chapter 21, Legs). They are the result of cumulative sun exposure. Those who have worked at outdoor occupations, such as farmers, sailors, athletes, and gardeners, especially fair-skinned white males who are bald, are chiefly at risk. A solar keratosis, if left untreated, may progress into a squamous cell carcinoma in 2% to 5% of cases.

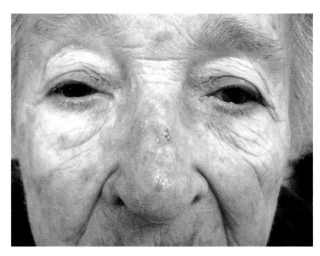

Figure 5-8 Solar keratosis.

DISTINGUISHING FEATURES

- Scaly, rough-textured papule or papules with or without an erythematous base covered by a white, yellowish, or brown scale (hyperkeratosis). Lesions may be subtle and not visible but palpable (Fig. 5-8)
- Usually 3 to 8 mm in size; can gradually enlarge, thicken, and become more elevated and develop into a hypertrophic solar keratosis or a **cutaneous horn** (a hornlike projection of keratin) (Fig. 5-9)
- Advanced lesions may be clinically difficult to distinguish from SCC
- On occasion, a solar keratosis is tan or dark brown (**pigmented solar keratosis**) and is clinically indistinguishable from a solar lentigo ("liver spot") (Fig. 5-10)

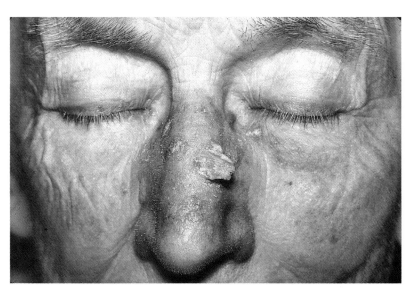

Figure 5-9 Solar keratosis and a squamous cell carcinoma underlying a cutaneous horn.

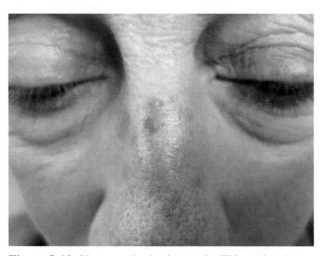

Figure 5-10 Pigmented solar keratosis. This patient has a solar keratosis (slightly palpable) and solar lentigines.

DIAGNOSIS
- Palpation reveals a gritty, spiky, sandpaper-like texture
- A shave biopsy is performed when the diagnosis is in doubt or to rule out an SCC (see Appendix B)

MANAGEMENT (see Appendices A and B)
- Limit sun exposure; use sunscreens
- Liquid nitrogen (LN$_2$) cryosurgery
- Biopsy followed by electrocautery or electrocautery alone for thick hyperkeratotic lesions
- Topical imiquimod **(Aldara),** 5-fluorouracil **(Efudex and Carac),** or diclofenac sodium **(Solarase)** for multiple lesions
- Photodynamic therapy

Squamous Cell Carcinoma

Squamous cell carcinoma (SCC) is a malignant epithelial tumor arising from keratinocytes of the epidermis (see also Chapter 1, Hair and Scalp; Chapter 2, Forehead and Temples; Chapter 5, Nose and Perinasal Area; Chapter 12, Arms; and Chapter 21, Legs). Second to BCC, the sun-exposed nose is a common site for an SCC to appear. An SCC occurs in an older age group than does BCC and it very rare in dark-skinned persons. Most SCCs on the nose arise in solar keratoses. Such SCCs are slow-growing, and metastases are rare.

DISTINGUISHING FEATURES
- May present as an ulcer, a papule, a plaque, or a nodule
- Slow-growing and may be scaly or ulcerated
- Often indistinguishable from a precursor solar keratosis and may underlie a cutaneous horn (see Fig. 5-9)
- May at times be indistinguishable from BCC

DIAGNOSIS
- Shave biopsy; excisional biopsy is rarely necessary

MANAGEMENT (see also Chapter 1, Hair and Scalp)
- Limit sun exposure; use sunscreens
- Treatment options depend on histologic subtype and specific location on the nose (see Appendix B)
- Electrocautery and curettage for small lesions (generally smaller than 1 cm)
  - LN$_2$ cryosurgery
  - Total excision is the preferred method of therapy
- Micrographic (Mohs) surgery is useful for excessively large or invasive SCCs, for recurrent lesions, and for lesions with poorly delineated clinical borders. It is also a treatment of choice for lesions in an area of late radiation change
- Imiquimod **(Aldara)** 5% cream may also have some utility in treating selected patients who have highly differentiated SCCs and in some renal transplant patients who tend to develop numerous SCCs. Imiquimod is approved for the treatment of solar keratoses, superficial BCCs, and is now being used "off-label" for SCC in situ **(Bowen disease)**
- Radiation therapy

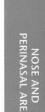

Keratoacanthoma

A **keratoacanthoma (KA)** (see also Chapter 4, Ears and Chapter 12, Arms) is a lesion about which there is controversy: is it benign or malignant? A KA resembles an SCC histologically and is considered by some dermatologists and dermatopathologists to be a low-grade variant of an SCC. Keratoacanthomas occur in the elderly, generally individuals over 65.

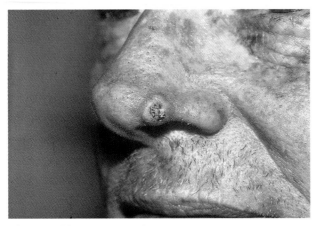

Figure 5-11 Keratoacanthoma.

DISTINGUISHING FEATURES

- Affects males more than females
- Rapidly growing; usually taking 3 to 4 weeks to appear
- Usually has a typical central crater (Fig. 5-11)
- Occurs as a single dome-shaped erythematous or skin-colored nodule plus a central keratin core with an overlying crust
- May attain a diameter of 1.0 to 2.5 cm
- Spontaneous regression may result in scarring
- May be indistinguishable from SCC

DIAGNOSIS

- A KA on the nose is located in a difficult area to perform an excisional biopsy; consequently, a deep shave biopsy is often adequate to obtain sufficient tissue

MANAGEMENT (see Appendix B)

- Deep shave biopsy
- Electrodesiccation and curettage
- Excision
- Intralesional 5-fluorouracil
- Mohs procedure for recurrences

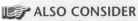

ALSO CONSIDER
- Basal cell carcinoma
- Wart
- Seborrheic keratosis

Perioral (Periorificial) Dermatitis
vs Seborrheic Dermatitis
(Nasal Creases and Perinasal Area)

Perioral (Periorificial) Dermatitis

Perioral (periorificial) dermatitis is a rosacea-like eruption seen primarily in young women and uncommonly in young boys and girls. It rarely occurs in men, unless due to the application of long-term topical steroids. It is usually found around the mouth, but it may be noted around the eyes as well as the nose, which explains the more inclusive term *periorificial*. Often idiopathic, however, it is exacerbated and sometimes caused by the application of potent of topical steroids or long-term use of less potent topical steroids (see also Chapter 7, Lips and Perioral Area).

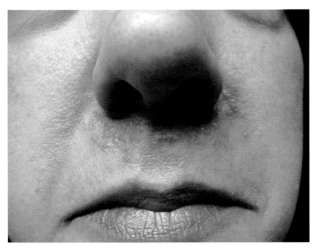

Figure 5-12 Perioral (periorificial) dermatitis.

DISTINGUISHING FEATURES
- Features that distinguish perioral dermatitis from rosacea:
  - Appears mostly in women between 15 and 40 years of age
  - Small (acnelike) erythematous papules or pustules without telangiectasias (Fig. 5-12)
  - Occasionally has superimposed seborrheic dermatitislike scaling
  - Infrequently recurs after effective treatment

DIAGNOSIS
- Clinical
- Excellent response to therapeutic trial with oral tetracycline

MANAGEMENT (see Appendix A)
- Gentle cleansing
- Discontinue applying all face creams including cosmetics and sunscreens
- Avoid topical steroids on face (discontinue or wean)
- Responds readily to oral tetracycline or one of its derivatives
- Topical antibiotics such as erythromycin, clindamycin, or metronidazole are less effective
- Azelaic acid (**Finacea**) or topical calcineurin inhibitors such as tacrolimus (**Protopic**) 1% ointment or pimecrolimus (**Elidel**) 1% cream may also be useful
- ✔ TIP: When caused by the application of potent of a topical steroid, its discontinuance may result in a worsening of the condition before it starts to improve ("one step forward, two steps backward").

Seborrheic Dermatitis

Seborrheic dermatitis (SD), also referred to as *seborrheic eczema* in the United Kingdom, is a condition that involves the area surrounding the nose and medial cheeks ("dandruff of the face"). Seborrheic dermatitis is an extremely common chronic inflammatory dermatitis (see Chapter 1, Hair and Scalp; Chapter 2, Forehead and Temples; Chapter 4, Ears; Chapter 6, Cheeks). It may appear at any age after puberty, fluctuating in severity and persisting indefinitely. It is generally considered to be idiopathic; however, some evidence indicates that *Pityrosporon ovale*, a small yeast, may play a part in its pathogenesis because SD occasionally responds to antifungal medications (see following discussion). Seborrheic dermatitis is not related to diet, but it may be aggravated by illness, psychological stress, and change of season. Persons with immunodeficiency (especially infection with human immunodeficiency virus [HIV]/acquired immunodeficiency syndrome [AIDS]), neurologic disorders such as Parkinson disease, and stroke are particularly prone to develop SD. This condition is often confused with rosacea (see Chapter 6, Cheeks), with which it may coexist in the same patient.

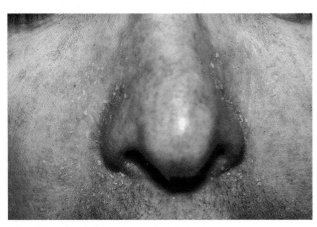

Figure 5-13 Seborrheic dermatitis.

DISTINGUISHING FEATURES
- Begins in young adulthood
- Affects males more than females
- Affects the nasolabial creases and paranasal area (Fig. 5-13)
- Similar lesions may be present elsewhere: scalp, eyebrows, ears, eyelid margins (see Fig. 3-5)

DIAGNOSIS
- Clinical

MANAGEMENT (see Appendix A)
- Low-potency topical steroids
- Topical steroids may be alternated with antifungals such as ketoconazole cream 2% (**Nizoral**) or ciclopirox 0.77% gel (**Loprox**)
- Tacrolimus (**Protopic ointment**) 0.1% and pimecrolimus (**Elidel cream**) 1% may also be effective
- **Promiseb Topical Cream**, a nonsteroidal cream, has both an anti-inflammatory as well as antifungal effects. It is applied twice daily

☞ ALSO CONSIDER
- Erythrotelangiectatic rosacea
- Acne
- "Butterfly rash" of systemic lupus erythematosus
- Tinea faciale
- Eczematous dermatitis, such as atopic dermatitis
- Contact dermatitis to cosmetics or airborne allergens photosensitivity

RARELY
- Adenoma sebaceum
- Leprosy

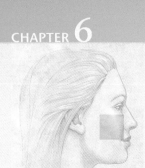

CHAPTER 6

Cheeks

The cheeks, visible from the front and the sides, constitute the largest area of the face and may be affected by a number of conditions that are often signs of underlying systemic diseases (e.g., systemic lupus erythematosus, carcinoid syndrome, fifth disease). Also, various benign, premalignant, and malignant lesions are found on this sun-exposed location.

In infants, atopic dermatitis occurs commonly on the cheeks and often appears at less than 1 year of age. In teens and adults, acne vulgaris, rosacea and various acne imitators such as keratosis pilaris, as well as pigmentary disorders such as vitiligo, pityriasis alba, and melasma are often noted on the cheeks. Infections such as impetigo and tinea also appear on the cheeks and paranasal regions. In adults, seborrheic dermatitis is the most common inflammatory dermatosis of the face.

IN THIS CHAPTER

- Impetigo *vs* tinea faciale
- Keratosis pilaris *vs* acne vulgaris
- Adult-onset acne *vs* rosacea
- Seborrheic dermatitis *vs* systemic lupus erythematosus
- Atopic dermatitis/eczema *vs* contact dermatitis
- Vitiligo vulgaris *vs* pityriasis alba *vs* postinflammatory hypopigmentation
- Melasma *vs* postinflammatory hyperpigmentation
- Solar lentigo *vs* flat seborrheic keratosis *vs* lentigo maligna/lentigo maligna melanoma
- Solar keratosis *vs* squamous cell carcinoma *vs* basal cell carcinoma

Impetigo *vs* Tinea Faciale

Impetigo

Impetigo is a highly contagious superficial bacterial infection of the superficial layers of the epidermis, caused most often by *Staphylococcus aureus* and less often by group A beta-hemolytic streptococci. In fact, both organisms can be present at the same time. Impetigo mainly affects infants and children; however, it may occur at any age. Participation in sports that involve skin-to-skin contact, such as football or wrestling, is a potential cause. Impetigo rarely progresses to systemic infection, although poststreptococcal glomerulonephritis is a very rare complication.

Impetigo traditionally has been divided into bullous and nonbullous varieties, but because they are clinically more or less indistinguishable, it is probably less confusing to use the term *impetigo* to describe both. Secondary impetiginization can, and often does, emerge as a secondary infection of preexisting skin disease or traumatized skin. An example is impetiginized eczema.

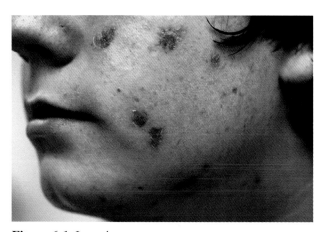

Figure 6-1 Impetigo.

DISTINGUISHING FEATURES

- Begins as a crust or thin-roofed, fragile vesicle or bulla that ruptures and often leaves a peripheral collarette of scale or the flaccid remains of bullae with a hemorrhagic crusted border (Fig. 6-1)
- Intact bullae are not usually present because they are very fragile
- Oozing serum dries and gives rise to the classic golden-yellow "honey-crusted" lesion
- In time, a varnishlike, "stuck on" crust develops
- The infection is generally self-limiting even without treatment

DIAGNOSIS

- Usually made on clinical grounds

- Bacterial culture and sensitivity testing are recommended if standard topical or oral treatment does not result in improvement

MANAGEMENT (see Appendix A)

- Antibacterial soaps such as povidone-iodine (**Betadine**) or chlorhexidine (**Hibiclens**)
- Mupirocin 2% (**Bactroban, Centany**) ointment or cream, or retapamulin ointment (**Altabax**), applied 3 times daily, may be used alone to treat very limited cases of impetigo. It is used until all lesions are cleared
- For widespread involvement, an oral antistaphylococcal penicillinase-resistant antibiotic, such as cephalosporin, dicloxacillin, or erythromycin, may be used alone or in conjunction with topical antibiotics
- **ALERT: An emerging problem is methicillin-resistant *S. aureus* (MRSA), which may appear in both immunocompromised and immunocompetent patients. If infectious skin lesions do not improve during treatment intended for presumptive *S. aureus*, the diagnosis of MRSA should be considered and definitive antibacterial therapy should be determined on the basis of in vitro antibiotic sensitivity. Tetracyclines, trimethoprim-sulfamethoxazole (Bactrim), clindamycin, and linezolid are effective oral antibiotics for MRSA**
- In patients who are determined to be chronic nasal carriers and have recurrent impetigo, mupirocin 2% cream or ointment can be applied inside the nostrils 3 times daily for 5 days each month to reduce bacterial colonization in the nose
- Chronic nasal carriers also can be treated with rifampin
- Family members should be evaluated as potential nasal carriers of *S. aureus* and treated, if necessary
- A young child can usually return to school or a child care setting as soon as he or she is not contagious—often within 24 hours of starting antibiotic therapy

Tinea Faciale

Tinea faciale (same as tinea faciei) is most often acquired by contact with an infected animal, usually kittens and occasionally dogs. *Microsporum canis*, *Trichosporum rubrum*, and *Trichosporum mentagrophytes* are the usual pathogens. It may also spread from other infected humans, or it may be autoinoculated from other areas of the body that are infected by tinea such as tinea pedis or tinea capitis. As with impetigo (see previous discussion), transmission of tinea may be seen in wrestlers (tinea gladiatorum).

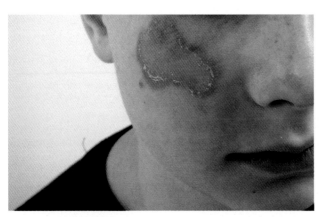

Figure 6-2 Tinea faciale.

DISTINGUISHING FEATURES

- Lesions often annular ("ringworm") with peripheral enlargement and central clearing (Figure 6-2)
- Single or multiple lesions; if multiple, the distribution is typically asymmetric
- May be pruritic or asymptomatic

DIAGNOSIS

- A history of a newly adopted kitten or of another infected contact is helpful
- Diagnosis is confirmed by a positive potassium hydroxide examination or fungal culture best taken from the border (it is especially easy to find hyphae in those patients who have been previously treated with topical steroids) (see Appendix B)

MANAGEMENT

- Topical antifungal agents are useful (see Appendix A)
- Systemic antifungal agents such as griseofulvin, terbinafine **(Lamisil),** or itraconazole **(Sporanox)** are sometimes necessary when multiple lesions are present or in areas that are repeatedly shaved, such as men's beards (tinea barbae) or, especially, women's legs (see Chapter 21, Legs), in which granulomatous lesions (Majocchi granuloma) may appear
- If pets appear to be the source of infection, they may also need antifungal treatment after evaluation by a veterinarian

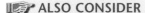

ALSO CONSIDER
- Atopic dermatitis
- Granuloma annulare
- Contact dermatitis
- Seborrheic dermatitis
- Herpes virus infection
- Varicella
- Urticaria
- Acute lyme disease (erythema migrans)
- Psoriasis
- Rosacea
- Subacute lupus erythematosus and systemic lupus erythematosus
- Thermal or chemical burn
- Cutaneous candidiasis
- Ecthyma, which is a more serious form of impetigo in which the infection penetrates deeper into the dermis

Keratosis Pilaris *vs* Acne Vulgaris

Keratosis Pilaris

Keratosis pilaris (KP) is an extremely common finding that looks and feels like "goose bumps." Keratosis pilaris appears most often in adolescence during the teen years and is frequently mistaken for acne, particularly when it involves the malar area of the face. It is more commonly seen on the deltoid and posterolateral upper arms (see Chapter 12, Arms), the shoulders, upper back, buttocks, and thighs. KP is also known as "allergic bumps" because is it often seen in individuals who have allergies and/or ichthyosis vulgaris. It often improves, especially during the summer months and with the passage of time. KP runs in families, especially families that tend to have hay fever, asthma, sinusitis, some allergies, or atopic dermatitis.

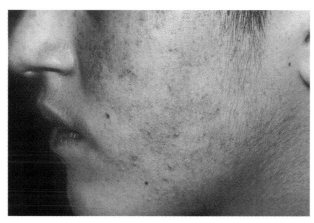

Figure 6-3 Keratosis pilaris.

DISTINGUISHING FEATURES
- In children, the lateral sides of the cheeks are frequently involved
- Tiny, whitish, red, or tan, spiny papules
- Distributed in a gridlike pattern (Fig. 6-3)
- "Goose flesh," "sandpaperlike" appearance and texture
- When erythematous and inflamed, KP resembles acne
- Usually worse during the winter months

DIAGNOSIS
- Clinical

MANAGEMENT (see Appendix A)
- There is no cure or very effective treatment; however, the roughness can be lessened temporarily by applying certain moisturizers, exfoliating or barrier creams, or lotions such as:
  - Ammonium lactate **(Lac-Hydrin),** available in a cream or lotion, reduces roughness and softens the keratin plugs. It does not, however, lessen the redness caused by the condition
  - Urea-containing products such as **Carmol** and **Keralac** moisturize and soften dry, rough skin. It also helps loosen and remove the dead skin cells
  - Topical retinoids may be an effective temporary treatment, but they can cause bothersome skin irritations, such as severe dryness, redness, and exfoliation. Tretinoin **(Retin-A Micro, Avita)** and tazarotene **(Tazorac)** are examples of topical retinoids

Acne Vulgaris

Teenage **acne vulgaris** may resemble and often coexist with keratosis pilaris.
✔ **TIP: However, the primary lesions are quite different (see Chapter 2, Forehead and Temples).**

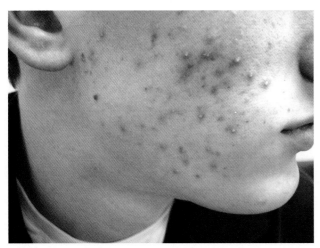

Figure 6-4 Acne vulgaris.

DISTINGUISHING FEATURES
- **Inflammatory lesions:** papules, pustules, macules (Fig. 6-4)

DIAGNOSIS
- Clinical

MANAGEMENT (see Appendix C)

MANAGEMENT (see Appendix C)

ALSO CONSIDER
- Erythromelanosis faciei

RARELY
- Keratosis pilaris atrophicans (ulerythema ophryogenes)
- Vitamin A deficiency
- Darier disease

Adult-Onset Acne

Adult-onset acne (postadolescent acne) is overwhelmingly a condition of females (see Chapter 9, Chin and Mandibular Area). In fact, women often break out with acne in their 20's and early 30's, sometimes for the first time, and some women continue to have acne into their 40's and 50's. The prevalence of female adult acne has increased significantly in the past several generations. Proposed hypotheses to explain this apparent increase include:
- The entry of women into the workforce and its attendant stresses
- The use of low estrogen-containing oral contraceptives
- The proliferation of food additives and the injection of hormones and antibiotics into livestock
- The increased use of makeup
- Several investigators have suggested that milk and other dairy products may be exacerbating factors.

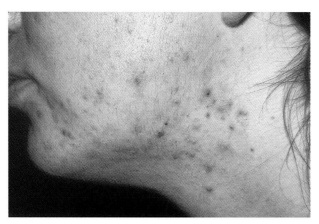

Figure 6-5 Adult-onset acne (note lesions mostly on lower face and neck).

DISTINGUISHING FEATURES
- Affects women much more often than men
- Evanescent, inflammatory red papules and/or pustules
- Lesions are more prevalent on the lower face, neck, and cheeks (Fig. 6-5)
- Relatively or totally comedo-free
- In general, lesions tend to be few in number
- Premenstrual or (less commonly) midcycle flares
- Lesions last for several days; sometimes they persist for a month or longer; sometimes occur without any pattern
- May occur on the perioral area, along the jaw line, or on the chin; also the hairline, neck, and upper trunk

DIAGNOSIS
- Clinical; however, in those not responding to treatment or who have other signs of hormonal excess such as male characteristics (e.g., facial hair) or irregular menstrual periods, hormonal tests are indicated

MANAGEMENT (see Appendix C)
- Skin care should be kept simple and gentle with the use of mild soaps

Topical
- Benzoyl peroxide, retinoids, topical antibiotics, combination of topical antibiotic and benzoyl peroxide (e.g., **Benzamycin, BenzaClin**, and **Duac** gels)
- Alternative topical prescription drugs
  - Azelaic acid (**Azelex 20%**), as well as preparations that contain sulfur and sodium sulfacetamide such as **Sulfacet-R lotion, Novacet lotion**, and **Klaron lotion**
  - Intralesional corticosteroid injection (see Appendix B)

Systemic
- Oral antibiotics (see Appendix A)
- Oral contraceptives
- Oral antiandrogens
- Spironolactone (**Aldactone**)

✔ **TIP: Every female acne patient should be questioned about her menstrual history.**

⚠ **ALERT: A hormonal and gynecologic evaluation is appropriate for a small number of acne patients, particularly women in their mid-20s or older who have treatment-resistant acne, a sudden onset of severe acne, virilizing signs or symptoms, irregular menstrual periods, or hirsutism**

Rosacea

Rosacea occurs most commonly in fair-skinned people with an ethnic background from Northern Europe (see Chapter 2, Forehead and Temples; Chapter 5, Nose and Perinasal Area). Frequently mistaken for acne; in fact, as recently as 20 years ago, rosacea was referred to as *acne rosacea*. Both conditions look alike, often respond to the same treatments, and may coexist in the same patient. Rosacea is rare in all dark-skinned people, including Hispanic, African, and African American populations. Patients may also have ocular involvement (see Chapter 3, Eyelids and Periorbital Area). Although sun exposure, irritating soaps, and facial products are known to exacerbate rosacea, there is no convincing evidence that alcohol ingestion, spicy foods, or caffeine are triggers.

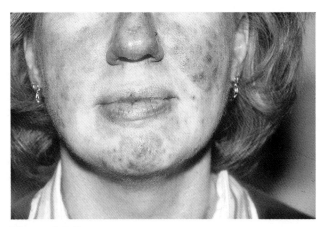

Figure 6-6 Rosacea.

DISTINGUISHING FEATURES

- Appears later in life than acne (30 to 50 years of age)
- May coexist with acne that began in teens or adulthood
- Women affected more than men
- Acnelike erythematous, beefy red papules, pustules, and telangiectasias, typically seen on the central third of the face—the forehead, nose, cheeks, and chin against a background of erythema (Fig. 6-6)
- Lacks the comedones ("blackheads" or "whiteheads") that are seen in acne
- Often flushing and blushing
- No relationship to androgenic hormones

- Nonscarring
- Primarily a cosmetic problem; however, burning and flushing can occur

DIAGNOSIS

- Clinical
- Rarely, a biopsy may be necessary in atypical cases

MANAGEMENT (see Appendix C)

- Skin care should be kept simple and gentle with the use of mild soaps
- Sunscreens/sun avoidance

Topical

- **Noritate** (metronidazole) 1% cream, and **MetroGel** 1% gel, applied once daily
- **Azelex** cream and **Finacea** gel 15% both contain azelaic acid.
- **Rosula** and **Klaron** (contain sulfacetamide and 5% sulfur)

Systemic

- If topical treatment is ineffective, an oral antibiotic is generally prescribed
  - Tetracycline and tetracycline derivatives, such as minocycline and doxycycline, are the first-line oral drugs; azithromycin, clarithromycin, or amoxicillin are used as second-line alternatives when a tetracycline fails or is not tolerated
  - Pulse dye lasers and intense pulsed light as well as electrocautery with a small needle is used to destroy small telangiectasias (see Appendix B)

☞ ALSO CONSIDER

- Normal flushing reactions, "rosy cheeks," "vasomotor instability," and "hot flash" menopausal symptoms
  - ✓ **TIP: Physiologic flushing and blushing reactions and facial telangiectasias tend to be seen in fair-skinned people. These conditions should be distinguished from rosacea; in fact, they are often misdiagnosed by health care providers as rosacea. Sometimes these patients may simply have "rosy cheeks"; furthermore, in many instances, rosacea can be difficult to distinguish from weathered, sun-damaged skin that is seen in many fair-skinned farmers, gardeners, sailors, or in many people who have worked or spent long periods of their lives outdoors and have developed multiple facial telangiectasias.**
- Acnelike disorders
  - Perioral/periorificial dermatitis
  - Neonatal acne
  - Topical steroid-induced rosacea; drug-induced acne

- Endocrinopathic acne
- Bacterial folliculitis
- Pityrosporum folliculitis
- Systemic lupus erythematosus
- Seborrheic dermatitis
- Tinea faciei
- Polymorphous light eruption
- Physically induced and occupational acne
- Demadex folliculitis

RARELY

- Chloracne
- Lupus vulgaris
- Conditions that may have flushing symptoms such as renal cell tumor, carcinoid syndrome, pheochromocytoma, mastocytosis, polycythemia vera

Seborrheic Dermatitis *vs* Systemic Lupus Erythematosus

Seborrheic Dermatitis

Seborrheic dermatitis (SD) often involves the medial cheeks and perinasal area (see Chapter 1, Hair and Scalp; Chapter 5, Nose and Perinasal Area) as well as the scalp, forehead, eyebrows, and eyelashes. Seborrheic dermatitis is often confused with rosacea, with which it may coexist in the same patient. Also, it may suggest systemic lupus erythematosus (see following discussion). Its characteristic distribution involves areas that have the greatest concentration of sebaceous glands: scalp, face, presternal region, interscapular area, umbilicus, and body folds (intertriginous areas).

There appears to be a hereditary predisposition to the development of SD. When it presents in patients who are infected with the human immunodeficiency virus, severe SD may serve as an early marker of the acquired immunodeficiency syndrome.

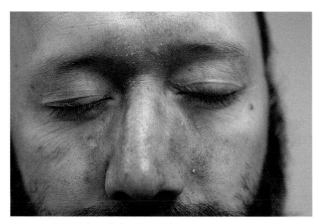

Figure 6-7 Seborrheic dermatitis.

DISTINGUISHING FEATURES
- Affects males more than females
- Begins in young adulthood after puberty
- On the face, lesions are erythematous, (Fig. 6-7) with or without an overlying whitish scale; sometimes SD presents with orange-yellow greasy patches
- Affects the medial cheeks as well as the nasolabial creases, perinasal area, and eyelid margins (**seborrheic blepharitis**) (see Chapter 3, Eyelids and Periorbital Area)
- Tends to be bilaterally symmetric in its distribution
- Scaly, rather than papulopustular, as seen in rosacea

- May itch or burn
- Typical SD may be present elsewhere (e.g., scalp [dandruff], ears, eyebrows, axillae, groin, upper chest)
- Facial SD usually flares in the winter and improves in the summer; however, many patients report provocation of the condition after sun exposure

DIAGNOSIS
- Clinical

MANAGEMENT (see Appendix A)
- Rapid response to low- and very low-potency topical steroids (class 6 and 7)
- To minimize unwanted topical steroid reactions, the topical steroids may be alternated with topical antifungals such as ketoconazole cream 2% (**Nizoral**), or ciclopirox 0.77% gel (**Loprox**)
- Limited use of tacrolimus (**Protopic ointment**) 0.1% and pimecrolimus (**Elidel cream**) 1% may also be effective
- **Promiseb,** a nonsteroidal cream, is a recent addition to therapy for SD. It has both an anti-inflammatory as well as antifungal effects
- ⚠ **ALERT: Topical steroids should be used only for brief periods on the face**
- ✔ **TIP: Topical steroids reduce the inflammation of SD, but do not confer antifungal effects. Consequently, using an antifungal agent as adjunctive therapy with a topical steroid is a sensible long-term treatment approach**

Systemic Lupus Erythematosus

Systemic lupus erythematosus (SLE) is a chronic, idiopathic, multisystemic, autoimmune disease associated with polyclonal B-cell activation. Fibrinoid degeneration of connective tissue and the walls of blood vessels associated with an inflammatory infiltrate involving various organs may result in arthralgia or arthritis, kidney disease, liver disease, central nervous system disease, gastrointestinal disease, pericarditis, pneumonitis, myopathy, and splenomegaly, as well as skin disease. The cutaneous manifestations of SLE result from the production of multiple autoantibodies that deposit immune complexes at the dermal–epidermal junction. The classic malar "butterfly" rash is one of the 4 of the 11 American Rheumatologic Association (ARA) criteria for lupus (see Chapter 10, Neck, for ARA criteria).

DISTINGUISHING FEATURES

- Classic malar or "butterfly" rash, which includes the bridge of the nose fanning out over the cheeks; a *persistent* erythema over the cheeks that tends to spare the nasolabial creases (Fig. 6-8)
- Photosensitivity may be the initial symptom of SLE
- Fatigue, fever, and malaise may be the presenting non-specific symptoms
- Has a 9:1 female-to-male ratio; more common in blacks and Hispanics
- Flare of lupus is common during pregnancy

DIAGNOSIS

- Laboratory evaluation
  - Antinuclear antibody titers are positive in 95% of patients (most often in a peripheral rim pattern)
  - Antibody to native double-stranded DNA (anti-dsDNA) is present in 60% to 80% of patients and is more specific for SLE
  - Anti-Sm antibody has a strong specificity for SLE. This is particularly relevant in patients in whom anti-dsDNA results are negative and may help exclude underlying systemic involvement
  - Antiphospholipid antibodies are present in 25% of patients
  - The erythrocyte sedimentation rate is usually elevated
  - Hypocomplementemia occurs in 70% of patients and is noted especially when there is renal involvement in active SLE

MANAGEMENT (see Appendix A)

- Sun exposure should be avoided
- Prednisone is the mainstay of therapy

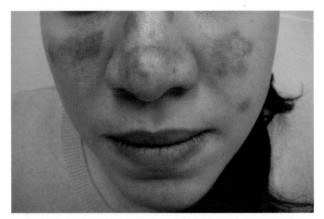

Figure 6-8 Systemic lupus erythematosus ("butterfly" rash).

- Oral antimalarials such as hydroxychloroquine (**Plaquenil**) and chloroquine (**Aralen**) are sometimes used as first-line therapy
- Other therapeutic agents:
  - Dapsone, gold, oral retinoids such as isotretinoin, and immunosuppressive drugs such as azathioprine (**Imuran**) and cyclophosphamide (**Cytoxan**) and methotrexate may be helpful. Such agents are used as adjuvant therapy because of their steroid-sparing effects
  - Mycophenolate (**CellCept**) as well as interferon alfa-2a and alfa-2b (**Roferon** and **Intron A**) may also be used
  - Thalidomide and intravenous gamma globulin are recalcitrant cases

---

ALSO CONSIDER
- Cutaneous sarcoidosis
- Rosacea and erythrotelangiectatic rosacea
- Tinea faciale
- Eczematous dermatitis, such as atopic dermatitis
- Polymorphous light eruption

RARELY
- Lupus miliaria disseminata faciei
- Lupus vulgaris (cutaneous tuberculosis)

Atopic Dermatitis/Eczema

Atopic dermatitis (atopic eczema) often starts in early infancy (from 2 months to 2 years) and may present as a widespread facial, scalp, and truncal eczema. The eruption may become generalized. In many cases, atopic dermatitis first manifests with severe "cradle cap" or severe recalcitrant intertriginous (groin, neck, axillae) rashes. It is characterized by pruritus, dry skin, and an association with other atopic diseases (asthma, allergic rhinitis). By 1 year of age, lesions begin to occur in the flexural creases, diaper area (see Chapter 10, Neck; Chapter 18, Genital Area). Later in life, distal extremities are affected; however, the cheeks and periorbital regions may also be involved in adults.

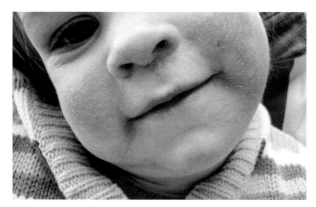

Figure 6-9 Atopic dermatitis.

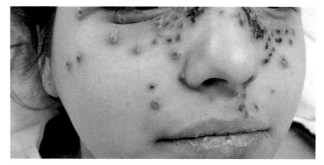

Figure 6-10 Kaposi varicelliform eruption.

INFANCY

DISTINGUISHING FEATURES
- Classic red, glazed, scaly cheeks (Fig. 6-9)
- Itchiness, disturbed sleep
- Bilaterally symmetric

DIAGNOSIS
- Clinical
- Atopic diathesis in family (first- or second-degree relative)
- Eczematous lesions are often present elsewhere on the body

MANAGEMENT (see Appendix A)
- Low-potency topical steroids
- **Protopic ointment** 0.03% and pimecrolimus cream **(Elidel)** 1% is designated for treatment in children
- Emollients, barrier creams/lotions such as **CeraVe** and **EpiCeram**

CHILDREN AND ADULTS

DISTINGUISHING FEATURES
- Itchy, scaly, erythematous cheeks; occasionally, oozing, impetiginized, plaques
- In children, Dennie-Morgan lines and "allergic shiners" may be present (see Chapter 3, Eyelids and Periorbital Area)

- Lesions may also occur on the, lips, scalp, and behind the ears
- Secondary infection with *S. aureus* may trigger relapses of atopic dermatitis; also herpes simplex virus may result in eczema herpeticum (Kaposi varicelliform eruption), which is more commonly seen in childhood (Fig. 6-10)

DIAGNOSIS
- Clinical
- Atopic diathesis in family
- A history of eczema and/or eczematous lesions are often present elsewhere on the body
- The diagnosis also depends on excluding conditions such as fungal infections, SD, psoriasis, scabies, contact dermatitis, ichthyosis, and, less often, cutaneous T-cell lymphoma

MANAGEMENT (see Appendix A)
- Low-potency topical steroids
- Emollients, barrier creams/lotions such as **CeraVe** and **EpiCeram**
- Tacrolimus ointment **(Protopic)** 0.1% in adults. A lower 0.03% concentration is designated for treatment in children
- Pimecrolimus cream **(Elidel)** in a 1% formulation

Contact Dermatitis

There are two types of **contact dermatitis (CD):** irritant contact dermatitis **(ICD),** caused by excessive contact with such materials as water, soaps, and makeup, and **allergic contact dermatitis (ACD),** which is a true allergic reaction to material in contact with the skin. The industrial workplace and other "hands-on" jobs commonly afford environments that tend to result in ICD or ACD. Chemicals in the air may produce an airborne ICD or ACD (e.g., insecticide sprays or from the burning residue of rhus dermatitis [poison ivy or poison oak]). Irritant contact dermatitis in infants tends to occur in the diaper area (diaper rash, napkin dermatitis).

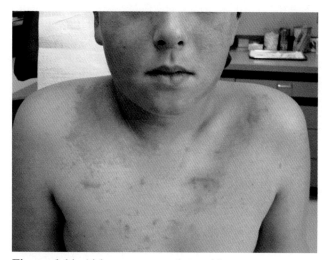

Figure 6-11 Airborne contact dermatitis.

INFANT/CHILD

DISTINGUISHING FEATURES
- Red, glazed, scaly cheeks (similar to atopic dermatitis (see previous discussion)
- Mostly seen in neck folds and diaper area (see Chapter 18, Genital Area)
- Males and females equally affected
- May have atopic diathesis in family
- Generally non–immune-mediated (ICD)

DIAGNOSIS
- History

MANAGEMENT (see Appendix A, Formulary)
- Avoidance of contactant
- Low-potency topical steroids
- Petrolatum, combination of 13% zinc oxide, aloe, and vitamin E **(Desitin Rapid Relief Cream),** barrier creams/lotions such as **CeraVe** and **EpiCram**

ADULT

DISTINGUISHING FEATURES
- Affects predominantly females
- Immune-mediated (ACD) or non–immune-mediated (ICD)
- Erythematous, pruritic, eczematous eruption in areas of contact (Fig. 6-11)

DIAGNOSIS
- History of contactant (e.g., makeup, hair dye, airborne allergen)
- Patch testing (see Appendix B), if necessary

MANAGEMENT (see Appendix A)
- Avoidance of contactant
- Low- to mid (short-term)-potency topical steroids
- Barrier creams/lotions such as **CeraVe** and **EpiCeram**

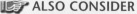**ALSO CONSIDER**
- Infant/child
  - Seborrheic dermatitis
  - Impetigo
  - Fungal infections

RARELY
- Histiocytosis X (Langerhans cell histiocytosis)
- Adult
  - Seborrheic dermatitis, psoriasis
- Systemic lupus erythematosus

Vitiligo Vulgaris *vs* Pityriasis Alba *vs* Postinflammatory Hypopigmentation

Vitiligo Vulgaris

Vitiligo vulgaris is an acquired disorder of skin depigmentation that affects 1% to 2% of the world's population. It is characterized by depigmentation of the epidermis due to a partial or complete loss of melanocytes. Thirty percent of patients have a positive family history. The cause is unknown, but is thought to result from an autoimmune process resulting in the loss of melanocytes. Vitiligo may develop in patients with other diseases that are believed to have an autoimmune basis (e.g., thyroid dysfunction, Addison disease, alopecia areata, diabetes mellitus, pernicious anemia).

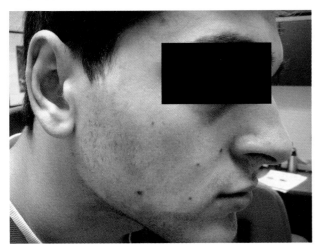

Figure 6-12 A, Vitiligo.

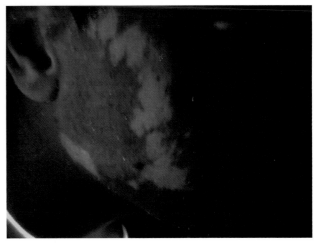

Figure 6-12 B, Vitiligo (Wood's lamp).

DISTINGUISHING FEATURES
- Hypopigmented or depigmented, chalk-white macules (Figure 6-12A)
- Occasionally have various shades of color (trichrome vitiligo)
- In dark-skinned people, pigmentary loss may be observed at any time of year, whereas in light-skinned people, the lesions may be most obvious in the summer because the tanning effects of the summer sun can accentuate the contrast between the light and dark skin
- Lesions tend to have a bilateral, symmetric distribution
- Occur on the hands and feet, body folds, bony prominences, and external genitals
- Lesions characteristically appear around orifices (e.g., the mouth, eyes, nose, and anus), but they may also involve the eyebrows, eyelashes, and scalp hair, resulting in white hairs (leukotrichia)

DIAGNOSIS
- Clinical
- Aided by Wood's lamp examination; this should reveal a "milk-white" fluorescence (Fig. 6-12B)

MANAGEMENT (see Appendices A and B)
- Some patients spontaneously experience partial repigmentation
- Response to repigmentation treatments is often disappointing
- Facial vitiligo responds better than do lesions on the back of hands and feet, which are very resistant to therapy

- For children who have light skin tones, sunscreens and observation may be the best course
- With limited disease, potent (class 2) and superpotent (class 1) topical corticosteroids are occasionally helpful in promoting repigmentation. Such treatment should be considered for a trial period of no more than 2 months
- A calcineurin inhibitor such as **Protopic** 0.1% ointment is especially useful on the face and neck, where strong steroid creams may cause skin thinning
- Sunscreens are suggested to avoid exacerbating the contrast between normal skin and lesions and to protect the lesions, which are sensitive to the sun
- Cosmetics that are formulated to match the patient's normal skin color (e.g., **Dermablend** or **Covermark**). Self-tanning compounds that contain dihydroxyacetone may effectively hide the white patches

Photochemotherapy
- Using psoralens and natural sunlight or psoralens and ultraviolet A (PUVA) light
- Narrow-band ultraviolet B and excimer laser therapy are expensive and not readily available.

Surgical Options
- Transplants in stable vitiligo include punch grafts and minigrafting
- Patients with extensive vitiligo (more than 50% loss of pigment) may elect to have the remaining skin "bleached" with 20% monobenzyl ether of hydroquinone (**Benoquin**). The results are permanent

Pityriasis Alba

Pityriasis alba is a common skin condition affecting children and occasionally young adults. The hypopigmented spots are commonly seen on the face and other areas of the skin in children who have atopic dermatitis. A history of preceding inflammation is generally absent. Pityriasis alba patches are more apparent in summer, especially in dark-skinned children, because they do not tan as well as the surrounding skin. Infrequently, the slightly scaly patches that precede the hypopigmentation may be seen.

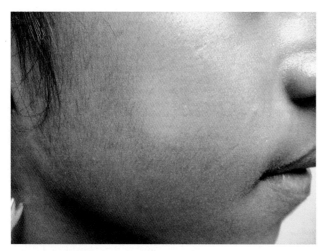

Figure 6-13 Pityriasis alba.

DISTINGUISHING FEATURES
- One or more round or oval pink patches appear, leaving pale marks after the presumptive inflammation has subsided (Fig. 6-13)
- Scale is often absent
- Lateral cheeks and lateral upper arms
- More obvious in summer months and in darker skin types
- Atopic diathesis in patient or family
- Atopic dermatitis may be noted elsewhere

DIAGNOSIS
- Clinical

MANAGEMENT
- Generally the color will return to normal after a few months, or in some cases persist 2 or 3 years
- No treatment is necessary, but a moisturizing cream may improve the dry appearance. If the patches are red or itchy, a mild topical steroid cream (hydrocortisone 1%) can be applied for a few days

Postinflammatory Hypopigmentation

Lightening of the skin may follow nearly any inflammatory cutaneous eruption (e.g., eczema, psoriasis, pityriasis alba [see previous discussion]). The reduction in melanin production or a loss of melanocytes results in pale patches (hypopigmentation or hypomelanosis) **Postinflammatory hypopigmentation** may also develop after an injury to the skin, such as a burn or surgical scar.

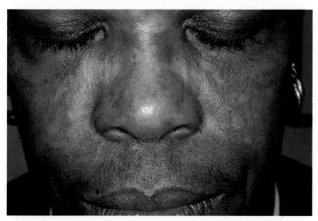

Figure 6-14 Postinflammatory hypopigmentation (secondary to seborrheic dermatitis).

DISTINGUISHING FEATURES
- Areas of hypopigmentation that roughly correspond to the location and shape of the antecedent eruption (Fig. 6-14)

DIAGNOSIS
- Clinical

MANAGEMENT
- Areas often repigment after the passage of time

ALSO CONSIDER
- tinea versicolor (more common on trunk)
- Inherited pigmentary disorders (e.g., nevoid hypomelanosis)

RARELY
- Tuberous sclerosis
- Leprosy
- Albinism

Melasma *vs* Postinflammatory Hyperpigmentation

Melasma

Melasma, formerly known as chloasma, appears as a blotchy, brownish pigmentation on the face that develops slowly. The pigmentation is due to overproduction of melanin. It is seen most frequently in young women during their reproductive years, particularly in those who have darker complexions and live in sunny climates such as Asia, the Middle East, South America, Africa, and the Indian subcontinent. In North America, melasma is most prevalent among Hispanics, African Americans, and immigrants from countries in which it is common.

Melasma may result from pregnancy, oral contraceptive use, menopause, or it may arise de novo for no apparent reason. It is exacerbated by exposure to sunlight. Melasma is rare before puberty. When men are affected (mainly in Pakistani and Indian men), the clinical and histologic picture is identical; however, the explanation is unknown.

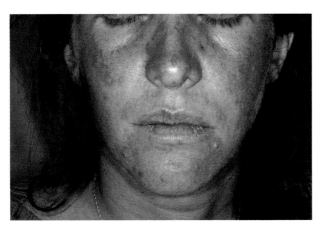

Figure 6-15 Melasma.

DISTINGUISHING FEATURES

- Females affected much more than males
- Hyperpigmented macules are found mainly on the cheeks (malar prominences), angles of the jaw, forehead, nose, chin, and above the upper lip (Fig. 6-15)
- Lesions are tan to brown, often symmetric, well-demarcated patches
- During pregnancy, the darkening of the skin often occurs in the second and third trimesters and spontaneously fades after termination of pregnancy
- Tends to fade on discontinuance of oral contraceptives or avoidance of sunlight; however, it may persist indefinitely

DIAGNOSIS (see Appendix B)

- Clinical
- Wood's lamp examination accentuates epidermal pigmentation

MANAGEMENT (see Appendix A)

☑ **TIP: Without year-round, daily sun protection the strict avoidance of sunlight, potentially successful treatments are doomed to failure**

- Discontinuing hormonal contraception, if appropriate
- Treatment involves a combination approach using one or more bleaching agents and cosmetic camouflage
- Over-the-counter preparations such as **Ambi** and **Esoterica** contain 2% hydroquinone
- Preparations of 3% hydroquinone (**Melanex**) and 4% hydroquinone (**Eldoquin-forte**) are available by prescription only. **Lustra,** a 4% hydroquinone agent, other lightening agents include the tyrosinase inhibitor, azelaic acid (**Azelex 20% cream**), which may be used in addition to hydroquinone (azelaic acid is safe even in pregnancy); also kojic acid, another tyrosinase inhibitor may be effective
- Topical tretinoin (do not use this during pregnancy) can also be used in combination with both hydroquinone and a topical steroid (**Tri-Luma cream**)
- Topical alpha hydroxy acids including glycolic acid and lactic acid, as creams or as repeated superficial chemical peels

⚠ **ALERT: Dermabrasion and microdermabrasion may increase pigment production and darken the melasma**

- Laser resurfacing and intense pulsed light

Postinflammatory Hyperpigmentation

Postinflammatory hyperpigmentation, a darkening of the skin, may occur after almost any inflammatory eruption, including eczema, lichen planus, or acne. It also may develop after an injury such as a burn or a therapeutic intervention. The hyperpigmentation stems from the melanocytes' exaggerated response to cutaneous insult, which results in an increased or abnormal distribution of the pigment melanin. As with melasma, postinflammatory hyperpigmentation tends to develop more often in people with dark complexions.

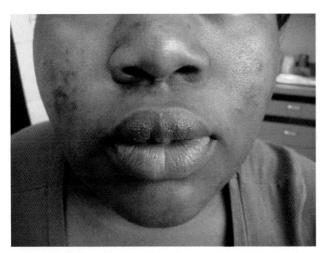

Figure 6-16 Postinflammatory hyperpigmentation (secondary to acne).

DISTINGUISHING FEATURES
- Irregular, light brown-to-black macules and/or patches (Fig. 6-16)
- Hyperpigmented lesions tend to conform in location and shape to the preceding eruption or injury; on occasion, they may mimic the exact shape of the inciting insult

DIAGNOSIS
- Clinical

MANAGEMENT
- Often, the passage of time, coupled with sun protection, affords a gradual lightening of darkened areas
- Patients should be advised to use a good broad-spectrum sunscreen daily to reduce further darkening
- Avoidance of the inciting event may prevent future lesions
- When lesions persist, many of the measures used to treat melasma (see previous discussion) may be tried; however, persistent postinflammatory hyperpigmentation tends to be much more recalcitrant than is melasma to therapeutic measures, and cosmetic coverups may be used

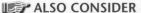

ALSO CONSIDER
- Inherited pigmentary disorders (e.g., nevoid hypermelanosis)
- Solar lentigo
- Drug-induced hyperpigmentation

RARELY
- Ochronosis
- Lichen planus actinicus
- Cutaneous mercury deposits

Solar Lentigo *vs* Flat Seborrheic Keratosis *vs* Lentigo Maligna/Lentigo Maligna Melanoma

Solar Lentigo

Solar lentigo (plural, lentigines) or "liver spot," "sun spot" is a small, extremely common, acquired tan macule(s) associated with sun exposure in fair-skinned people. Lentigines arise during the middle and elderly years. In contrast to freckles (ephelides), they persist even in the absence of sunlight. Most often, they appear on the face, and dorsal hands (see Chapter 13, Hands and Fingers) Lentigines are sometimes associated with photochemotherapy (PUVA) and local high-dose radiation therapy.

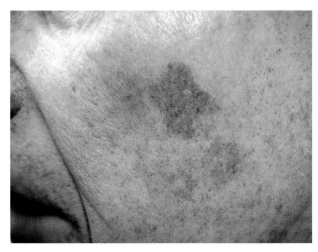

Figure 6-17 Solar lentigo.

DISTINGUISHING FEATURES
- Round or oval, uniformly colored tan-brown to black macules (Fig. 6-17)
- Sometimes coalesce to form larger patches
- PUVA lentigines are frecklelike in appearance and are persistent
- Radiation lentigines resemble sun-induced lentigines

DIAGNOSIS
- Clinical
- ⚠ **ALERT: When a lentigo begins to show a variegation in coloration, it may be impossible to distinguish from a lentigo maligna/lentigo maligna melanoma (see following discussion), and a shave or incisional biopsy should be performed**

MANAGEMENT (see Appendices A and B)
- Primarily a cosmetic concern
- A broad-spectrum sunscreen may help to prevent new lesions and lessen the darkening of older lesions
- Several creams may lighten lentigines if applied for a number of months, such as alpha-hydroxy acids, vitamin C, topical retinoids, azelaic acid, and mequinol and tretinoin (**Solagé**)
- Solar lentigines can be removed through the use of chemical peels, cryotherapy, or laser treatments

Flat Seborrheic Keratosis

Seborrheic keratosis (SK) on the face as well as on the legs (see Chapter 21, Legs) may be virtually flat, unlike the thicker more keratotic lesions noted on the trunk. On close inspection however, the surface is slightly rough or scaly. A solar lentigo (see previous discussion) has no surface scale. It may be impossible to distinguish the two clinically; however, this is of no great importance in light of the benign nature of both of these lesions.

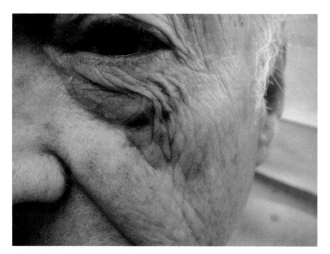

Figure 6-18 Flat seborrheic keratosis.

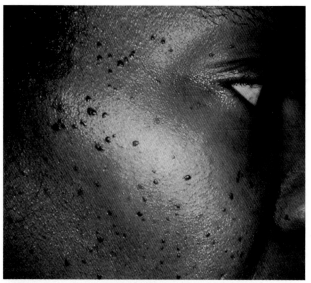

Figure 6-19 Dermatosis papulosa nigrans. (From Hall BJ, Hall JC, eds. *Sauer's Manual of Skin Diseases*. 10th ed. Philadelphia, PA: Lippincott Williams Wilkins; 2010.)

DISTINGUISHING FEATURES
- Round or oval, uniformly colored tan-brown to black macules that may be slightly scaly (Fig. 6-18)
- Located on sun-exposed and non–sun-exposed sites

DIAGNOSIS
- Clinical
- Biopsy only if a malignant neoplasm is suspected

MANAGEMENT (see Appendix B)
- Mainly a cosmetic concern
- Gentle cryosurgery is performed with liquid nitrogen spray or cotton swab
- Light electrocautery and curettage

VARIANT

▲ **Dermatosis papulosa nigrans (DPN)** is a common manifestation diagnosed primarily in African American, African Caribbean, and sub-Saharan African individuals; however, it may also be seen in darker-skinned persons of other races and nationalities. Lesions start appearing in adolescence and increase in number as persons age. DPNs are histopathologically identical to SKs and are considered to be of autosomal dominant inheritance.

DISTINGUISHING FEATURES
- Dermatosis papulosa nigrans, often multiple, are seen on the face, especially the upper cheeks and lateral orbital areas
- Lesions are flat, papular, or filiform (Fig. 6-19)
- Dermatosis papulosa nigrans are darkly pigmented and, in contrast to typical nonflat SKs, they have minimal, if any, scale

DIAGNOSIS
- Clinical
- Biopsy, if diagnosis is in doubt

MANAGEMENT
- Mainly a cosmetic concern
- Because some patients have numerous lesions, it is often difficult to remove all of them

⚠ **ALERT: Cryosurgery with liquid nitrogen can result in hypopigmentation**

Lentigo Maligna (LM)/Lentigo Maligna Melanoma

Lentigo maligna (LM)/lentigo maligna melanoma (LMM) is a type of lentigo that is found on the face of elderly patients with chronically sun-damaged skin. They comprise 5% to 10% of melanomas. Lentigo maligna and LMM have a predilection for the cheeks, nose, ears, and extensor forearms. Lentigo maligna is considered to be a potential precursor to melanoma. When an LM invades the dermis, it is then referred to as an LMM. The disease shows an increased worldwide incidence in fair-complexioned individuals living in sunny climates and nearer the equator, suggesting a causative role for ultraviolet radiation. The incidence of LM subtypes (in situ and invasive) appears to be rising in the United States.

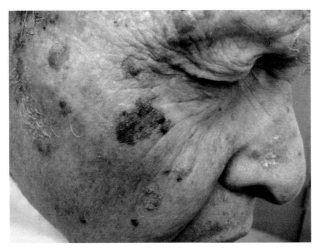

Figure 6-20 Lentigo maligna melanoma (note also seborrheic keratoses).

DISTINGUISHING FEATURES
- Elderly; older than 65 years of age
- More prevalent on the chronically sun-damaged skin of the head, neck, and arms
- The in situ precursor macular lesion is usually large (>1 to 3 cm in diameter), present for a minimum of 10 to 15 years, and demonstrates pigmentation ranging from dark brown to black (Fig. 6-20)
- As the lesion grows with a long radial growth phase, the border becomes irregular
- Both LM and LMM remain superficial and slowly evolve for many years before they progress to a vertical growth phase

- Dermal invasion (progression to LMM) is characterized by the development of raised blue-black nodules within the in situ lesion
- Generally, an LMM has a better prognosis than other melanomas

DIAGNOSIS
- A broad, paper-thin shave biopsy or multiple smaller biopsies may be the best technique

MANAGEMENT (see Appendices A and B)
- Surgical excision with 0.5-cm margin
- Mohs surgery may prove useful in completely removing subclinical tumor extension in certain subtypes of melanoma in situ, such as lentigo maligna
- **Aldara** 10% cream is sometimes effective for large, inoperable lesions

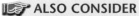

ALSO CONSIDER
- Melanocytic nevus
- Lentigo simplex
- Pigmented solar keratosis
- Melasma
- Drug-induced hyperpigmentation

RARELY
- Addison disease

Solar Keratosis *vs* Squamous Cell Carcinoma *vs* Basal Cell Carcinoma

Solar Keratosis

Solar keratosis (described in more detail in Chapter 2, Forehead and Temples, and Chapter 5, Nose and Perinasal Area) are extremely common on the cheeks as well as other sun-exposed areas.

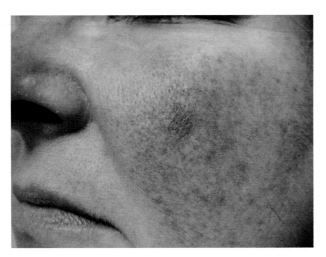

Figure 6-21 Lentigo maligna: This subtle lesion proved to be an early potentially invasive lentigo maligna melanoma.

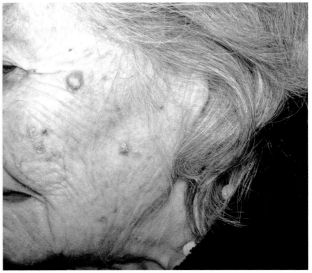

Figure 6-22 Squamous cell carcinoma and solar keratosis (larger lesion).

DISTINGUISHING FEATURES
- Males affected more than females
- Single or multiple discrete, flat, or elevated scaly lesions arise on a background of sun-damaged skin
- Typically have an erythematous base covered by a white, yellowish, or brown scale (hyperkeratosis)
- May enlarge and become hypertrophic solar keratosis or a cutaneous horn
- Often difficult to distinguish from squamous cell carcinoma (see following discussion) (Fig. 6-21)

DIAGNOSIS
- Palpation reveals a gritty rough to the touch sandpaperlike texture
- A shave biopsy is performed when the diagnosis is in doubt or to rule out a squamous cell carcinoma

MANAGEMENT
- The treatment of solar keratosis on the cheeks does not differ from treatment in other areas of the face and scalp (see Chapter 1, Hair and Scalp)

Squamous Cell Carcinomas

Most cutaneous **squamous cell carcinomas** arise in solar keratoses. Consequently, they arise in the same locations as solar keratoses.

DISTINGUISHING FEATURES
- Males affected more than females
- Elderly whites most often affected
- Scaly papule, plaque, or nodule with a smooth or thick hyperkeratotic surface
- Ulceration may be the only finding
- As with solar keratoses (see previous discussion), a squamous cell carcinoma, as well as a squamous cell carcinoma in situ (Bowen disease), may also produce a cutaneous horn on its surface
- Often indistinguishable from a hypertrophic solar keratosis (Fig. 6-21) or a BCC

DIAGNOSIS
- A shave or excisional biopsy (see Appendix B)

MANAGEMENT
- The treatment of squamous cell carcinoma does not differ from treatment in other areas of the face and scalp (see Chapter 1, Hair and Scalp)

Basal Cell Carcinomas

Basal cell carcinomas (BCCs) (described in more detail in Chapter 2, Forehead and Temples, and Chapter 5, Nose and Perinasal Area) are extremely common on the cheeks as well as other sun-exposed areas.

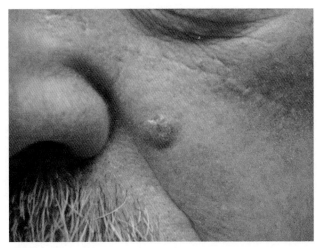

Figure 6-23 Basal cell carcinoma.

DISTINGUISHING FEATURES
- Age older than 40 years
- Males affected more than females
- Nodular BCC is the most common type on the cheeks
- Pearly, shiny, telangiectatic, semitranslucent papule or nodule with rolled (raised) border (Fig. 6-22)
- May be pigmented
- Erosion or ulceration ("rodent ulcer") due to its "gnawed" appearance
- When keratotic, a BCC may be impossible to distinguish from a squamous cell carcinoma (see previous discussion)

DIAGNOSIS
- Shave or excisional biopsy

MANAGEMENT (see Chapter 2, Forehead and Temples; Appendix B)
- Treatment options depend on histologic subtype and location
- Sun avoidance and use of sunscreens; wearing of protective clothing

ALSO CONSIDER
- Angiofibroma
- Seborrheic keratosis, which may be indistinguishable from a pigmented BCC
- Intradermal nevus

RARELY
- Merkel cell carcinoma

CHAPTER 7

Lips and Perioral Area

The term *cheilitis* refers to inflammatory lesions involving the mucous membranes of the lips. Many disorders of mucous membranes (see also Chapter 8, Oral Cavity and Tongue), both inflammatory, as well as neoplastic, are difficult to distinguish from one another when confined to the mucosa because they tend to look alike clinically. Some of these disorders (e.g., lichen planus and atopic dermatitis) are usually associated with more easily diagnosed characteristic coexisting lesions elsewhere on nonmucous membrane skin. Because the lower lip is in a more exposed position, sun-induced cheilitis (actinic cheilitis) and neoplasms such as solar keratoses and squamous cell carcinomas are more often seen here. The upper lip and its vermillion border are a common venue for herpes simplex virus infections. Benign lesions such as venous lake, labial melanotic macule, and pyogenic granuloma are also seen on the lips. Many of the conditions seen in the perioral region represent an extension of disorders noted elsewhere on the face such as acne, folliculitis, contact dermatitis, and various benign and malignant neoplasms.

IN THIS CHAPTER

- Atopic cheilitis *vs* irritant/allergic contact dermatitis
- Perioral (periorificial dermatitis) *vs* adult-onset acne
- Angular cheilitis (perlèche) *vs* candidiasis
- Primary herpes simplex virus *vs* recurrent herpes simplex virus
- Pyogenic granuloma *vs* venous lake *vs* labial melanotic macule
- Solar keratosis/solar cheilitis *vs* squamous cell carcinoma *vs* verruca vulgaris

Atopic Cheilitis

Atopic cheilitis is a variant of atopic dermatitis (see Chapter 1, Hair and Scalp; Chapter 3, Eyelids and Periorbital Area; Chapter 12, Arms; Chapter 21, Legs) As in atopic dermatitis elsewhere on the body, atopic cheilitis occurs in association with a personal or family history of atopy. It is exacerbated by frequent wet/dry cycles, lip licking, lip biting, and so on.

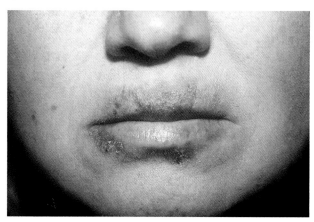

Figure 7-1 Atopic cheilitis.

DISTINGUISHING FEATURES
- Inflammation of the lips is characterized by redness, fissuring, and scaling
- The scaling and erythema of eczema may spread beyond the vermillion border, which becomes less distinct and blurred (Fig. 7-1)
- Worsened by lip licking, mouth breathing
- Frequently occurs in patients with eczema elsewhere on the body
- History of easy chapping in wintertime
- May be exacerbated by contact to irritant or sensitizing chemical agents, ultraviolet irradiation, and cold and windy weather

DIAGNOSIS
- Clinical

MANAGEMENT (see Appendix A)
- Low potency (class 6) ointment-based topical steroids
- Avoidance of identified irritants
- If indicated, psychological consultation for obsessive/compulsive lip licking

Irritant/Allergic Contact Dermatitis

Irritant contact dermatitis (ICD) and **allergic contact dermatitis (ACD)** may be caused by irritants or allergens (see Chapter 3, Eyelids and Periorbital Area; Chapter 6, Cheeks). Agents such as lipsticks, lip balms, sunscreen in lip cosmetics, toothpaste ingredients, dental prostheses, colophony in dental floss, nail varnish, cosmetics, and nickel in the mouthpiece of a musical instrument (e.g., flute) have been implicated in causing both ICD and ACD. Other allergens include fragrance, balsam of Peru, lanolin, and flavorings (strawberry and vanilla).

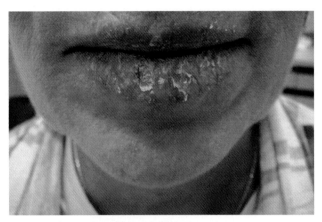

Figure 7-2 Irritant/allergic cheilitis.

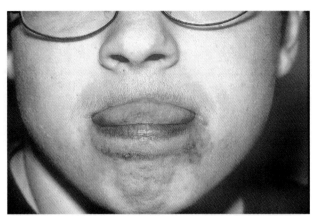

Figure 7-3 Irritant contact dermatitis due to lip licking.

DISTINGUISHING FEATURES
- Similar to atopic cheilitis, inflammation of the lips with redness, fissuring, and scaling (Fig. 7-2)
- History of easy chapping
- May also have coexistent atopic cheilitis and eczema elsewhere on the body

DIAGNOSIS
- Diagnostic clues have to be obtained from a careful history, which includes a review of oral rinses, toothpastes, cleansers, and so on
- Lip licking (ask family members if they observe patient licking lips); many patients are unaware or unable to self-report this habit (Fig. 7-3)

- Patch testing to a standard screening series in perioral allergic contact dermatitis is most useful to diagnose allergic contact dermatitis to medicaments (see Appendix B)

MANAGEMENT
- Avoidance of identified irritants/contactants
- Low-potency (class 6) ointment-based topical steroids
- Moisturize with petroleum jelly at bedtime

ALSO CONSIDER
- Chronic chapped lips

RARELY
- Cheilitis granulomatosa (Melkersson-Rosenthal syndrome)

Perioral Dermatitis

Perioral dermatitis, also known as *periorificial dermatitis* (see also Chapter 5, Nose and Perinasal Area), is a rosacealike eruption seen primarily in young women and uncommonly in young children. As with rosacea, the etiology of perioral dermatitis is unknown; tooth whiteners, and fluoridated toothpaste have occasionally been implicated, but without any consistent evidence. It is accepted, however, that frequent application of high-potency, and less commonly, low-potency topical corticosteroids have been reported to cause a **topical steroid-induced rosacea/perioral dermatitislike eruption** in some individuals.

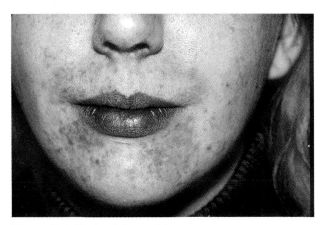

Figure 7-4 Perioral dermatitis.

DISTINGUISHING FEATURES
- Appears in women between the ages of 15 and 40
- Manifests in tiny 1- to 3-mm erythematous papules or pustules without comedones and telangiectasias
- Characteristically circles the mouth and spares the area beyond the vermilion border of the lips (Fig. 7-4)
- Occasionally there is superimposed scaling

- Usually this condition does not recur after successful treatment

DIAGNOSIS
- Clinical
- Inquire about topical steroid applications
- Diagnosis is confirmed by response to treatment with systemic antibiotic (usually a tetracycline derivative)

MANAGEMENT (see Appendix A)
- Discontinue applying all face creams, including cosmetics and sunscreens
- Avoid topical steroids on face (discontinue, or wean)
- Responds readily to low-dose oral tetracycline or one of its derivatives. It is tapered when the inflammation has improved (usually after 2 to 3 weeks)
- Azithromycin, clarithromycin, or amoxicillin are used as second-line alternatives when a tetracycline fails or is not tolerated
- Topical antibiotics such as erythromycin, clindamycin, or metronidazole are less effective
- ✔ **TIP: Topical steroid–induced rosacea/perioral dermatitislike eruption: When the steroid cream is discontinued, the eruption often flares before it starts to improve. This often prompts the patient to continue its application.**

Adult-Onset Acne

Adult-onset acne (postadolescent acne) is overwhelmingly a condition of women (see also Chapter 2, Forehead and Temples; Chapter 6, Cheeks; Chapter 9, Chin and Mandibular Area).

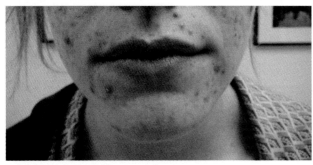

Figure 7-5 Adult-onset acne.

DISTINGUISHING FEATURES
- Affects women much more than men
- Evanescent, inflammatory red papules and/or pustules (Fig. 7-5)
- ✔ **TIP: Lesions characteristically occur on the perioral area, along the jaw line, or on the chin; also the hairline, neck, and upper trunk**
- Premenstrual or, less commonly, midcycle flares
- Relatively or totally comedo-free

DIAGNOSIS
- Clinical
- However, in those not responding to treatment or who have other signs of hormonal excess such as male characteristics (e.g., facial hair) or irregular menstrual periods, hormonal tests are indicated

MANAGEMENT (see Appendix C)
- ✔ **TIP: Every female acne patient should be questioned about her menstrual history**
- ✔ **TIP: A hormonal and gynecologic evaluation is appropriate for a small number of acne patients, particularly women in their mid-20s or older who have treatment-resistant acne, a sudden onset of severe acne, virilizing signs or symptoms, irregular menstrual periods, or hirsutism**

☞ **ALSO CONSIDER**
- Acnelike disorders
  - Endocrinopathic acne
  - Physically induced and occupational acne
- Rosacea
- Impetigo
- Overuse/misuse of topical steroids
- Demadex folliculitis
- Bacterial folliculitis

RARELY
- Sycosis barbae
- Gram-negative folliculitis
- Vesicular dermatophytosis
- Pityrosporum folliculitis
- Chloracne

Angular Cheilitis (Perlèche)

Angular cheilitis (angular stomatitis) is also known as *perlèche*. The word "perlèche," derived from the French "to lick," is an inflammation that occurs at the corners of the mouth. It is sometimes seen in young patients who have atopic dermatitis, specifically atopic cheilitis (see previous discussion). It also appears in the elderly, wherein aging and atrophy of the perioral muscles of facial expression results in "pocketing" at the corners of the mouth, an overhang of the upper lip over the lower lip, causing a moist deep furrow. In many instances, perlèche is often simply a form of **intertrigo,** a common inflammatory condition of skin folds that occurs when opposing moist skin surfaces are in constant contact with each other (see Chapter 11, Axillae; Chapter 20, Inguinal Area). Both yeasts (candidal) (see following discussion) and bacteria (especially *Staphylococcus aureus*) may be primarily or, more often, secondarily involved.

Other factors such as poor-fitting dentures, malocclusion, edentia, and bone resorption may lead to drooling or vertical shortening of the face, thus accentuating the melolabial crease. Lip licking in children, mouth breathing, and orthodontic devices are also risk factors. Vitamin deficiency is often blamed but rarely proved as a cause of angular cheilitis.

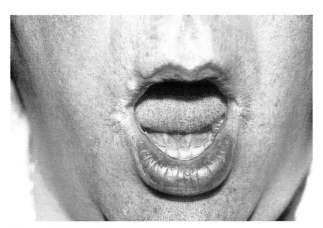

Figure 7-6 Angular cheilitis.

DISTINGUISHING FEATURES
- Redness, maceration, scaling, fissuring, and crusting occur at the corners (angles) of the mouth (Fig. 7-6)

DIAGNOSIS
- Clinical
- Fungal examination, bacterial cultures as needed

MANAGEMENT (see Appendix A)
- A mild topical steroid such as desonide (**DesOwen**) 0.05% or **Elocon** (mometasone furoate) ointment **0.1%,** or over-the-counter hydrocortisone 1% cream or ointment often helps resolve the inflammation
- Petrolatum or other ointments are used to protect and moisturize the area
- Topical anticandidal (ketoconazole, clotrimazole, nystatin) and antibacterial agents (mupirocin), alone or in combination with a class 6 topical hydrocortisone ointment, are often effective when candida is suspected or found on potassium hydroxide preparation or culture
- Topical immunomodulators such as topical calcineurin inhibitors such as tacrolimus (**Protopic**) 1% ointment or pimecrolimus (**Elidel**) 1% cream may also be tried
- If necessary, a dental referral is suggested to correct potential causative factors mentioned earlier

Candidiasis

The macerated "pockets" previously described as perlèche, a form of intertrigo, may serve as a nidus for the secondary overgrowth of *Candida albicans*. The condition is noted especially in diabetics and in male tobacco smokers over 60. Iron deficiency anemia and other vitamin deficiencies have been cited as other predisposing factors.

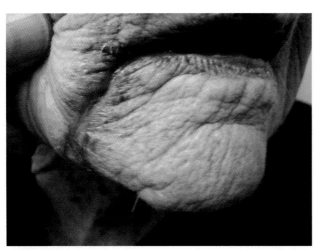

Figure 7-7 Candidal intertrigo.

DISTINGUISHING FEATURES
- Redness, maceration, scaling, fissuring, and crusting occur at the corners of the mouth (Fig. 7-7)

DIAGNOSIS
- Clinical
- Positive fungal examination

MANAGEMENT (see Appendix A)
- Topical anticandidal (ketoconazole 2%, clotrimazole 1%, nystatin) alone as well as antibacterial agents such as mupirocin, often in combination with a class 6 topical hydrocortisone ointment, are often effective when *Candida* is suspected or found on potassium hydroxide or culture
- Reduction of smoking
- Correction of vitamin deficiency, if indicated

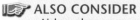

ALSO CONSIDER
- Lichen planus
- Leukoplakia

RARELY
- Human immunodeficiency virus infection (exfoliative cheilitis)
- Chronic multifocal oral candidosis
- Anemia or vitamin deficiency (vitamin B_{12})

Primary Herpes Simplex Virus

Primary labial herpes simplex virus (herpes simplex labialis) infections are caused most often by herpes simplex virus-1 (HSV-1) (see also Chapter 8, Oral Cavity and Tongue). Herpes simplex virus-1 is mainly associated with oral-facial infections ("cold sores" or "fever blisters"); however, HSV type 2 may also be the cause. Herpes simplex virus is highly contagious and is spread by direct contact with the skin or mucous membranes. Primary infections are acquired in infancy and early childhood and most are subclinical. The virus invades and replicates in neurons as well as in epidermal and dermal cells. Virions travel from the initial site of infection on the skin or mucosa to the sensory dorsal root ganglion, where latency is established.

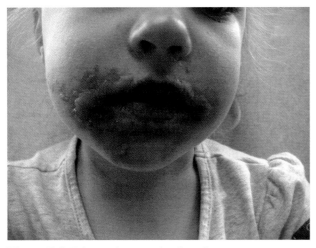

Figure 7-8 Primary herpes simplex virus.

DISTINGUISHING FEATURES

- Classic: a vesicle or a group of vesicles overlying an erythematous base (Fig. 7-8)
- Lesions become pustules crusts or erosions and generally heal without scarring
- Incubation period of 4 to 5 days; begins with fever, restlessness, and excessive drooling
- Oral cavity (lips, gums, buccal mucosa, fauces, face, tongue, and hard palate) are the areas generally affected
- Local lymph glands may be enlarged and tender (submandibular or cervical lymphadenopathy)
- Fever subsides after 3 to 5 days, and recovery is usually complete within 2 weeks
- Encephalitis and aseptic meningitis are very rare complications

DIAGNOSIS

- Usually based on clinical appearance and history
- When necessary, the following tests may be administered on fresh lesions:
  - The Tzanck preparation (see Appendix B), if positive, suggests HSV or varicella-zoster virus (VZV) infection. This test is used to rapidly determine the presence of HSV or VZV; it does not distinguish between these two viruses
  - Culture from intact vesicles
  - HSV tissue culture using monoclonal antibodies requires only 24 hours. The test is 90% sensitive, but it is expensive
  - Polymerase chain reaction for HSV DNA detection can be conducted; it also is expensive
  - Serologic tests for HSV are generally not very useful

MANAGEMENT

- Supportive
- If necessary, oral antiviral therapy (acyclovir, valacyclovir, or famciclovir) is given within 72 hours to reduce pain, viral shedding, and time to healing. These drugs inhibit the HSV multiplying once it reaches the skin or mucous membranes, but they cannot eradicate the virus from its resting stage within the nerve cells. They can therefore shorten and prevent attacks, but a single course cannot prevent future attacks
- Valacyclovir **(Valtrex)** (1 g twice daily for 7 to 10 days)
- Famciclovir **(Famvir)** (250 mg 3 times daily for 7 to 10 days)
- Acyclovir (200 mg 5 times daily or 400 mg 3 times daily for 10 days)
- ⚠ **ALERT: Immunocompromised hosts, patients with Kaposi varicelliform eruption, or those with HSV encephalitis may require intravenous antiviral therapy**

Recurrent Herpes Simplex Virus

After the primary infection resolves, the virus retreats to a dorsal root ganglion, where it becomes incorporated into the genetic material of the cell. It remains latent until it is reactivated by various triggers such as sunlight exposure, menses, immunosuppression, fever, common colds, dental surgery, and possibly stress. In many cases, no reason for the eruption is evident.

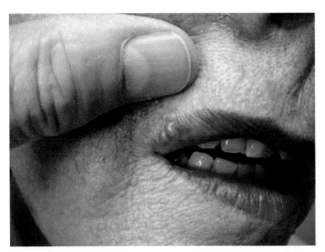

Figure 7-9 Recurrent herpes simplex virus.

DISTINGUISHING FEATURES

- Recurrent infections differ from primary infections; vesicles are smaller in size
- Lesions tend to recur at or near the same location within the distribution of a sensory nerve
- Seen on or near the vermilion border of the lip (herpes labialis) (Fig. 7-9)
- Generally milder and the number of lesions fewer than those associated with primary HSV
- Patients commonly experience a prodrome of itching, pain, or numbness
- Recurrent vesicular lesions eventually become pustular, ulcerate, or form a crust
- Over time, recurrences decrease in frequency and often stop altogether
- Persistent ulcerative or verrucous vegetative lesions may be seen in immunocompromised patients

- Most cases of recurrent erythema multiforme minor accompany, and appear to be caused by, recurrent clinical and subclinical HSV episodes (see following discussion)
- ☑ TIP: Viral shedding, leading to possible transmission, may occur during the period of primary infection, during subsequent recurrences, as well as periods of asymptomatic viral shedding.
- ⚠ ALERT: Lesions are contagious until they are completely crusted over. Patients must avoid contact with other children and pregnant women until all lesions are crusted.

DIAGNOSIS

- Usually based on clinical appearance and history of recurrences

MANAGEMENT (see Appendix A)

- Treatment should be initiated at the first sign of prodrome, which can often abort the lesions. Following are treatment options:
  - Valacyclovir (**Valtrex**) (2 g twice daily for 1 day taken about 12 hours apart)
  - Famciclovir (**Famvir**) 1500 mg as a single dose
- Suppressive therapy may be used for persistent or frequent recurrences (more than six recurrences per year) or recurrent erythema multiforme minor (see following discussion). After 1 year of treatment with these agents, the medication should be discontinued, to determine the recurrence rate, and the dosage can be adjusted as needed
  - Valacyclovir (1 g daily for 6 to 12 months; afterward, the clinician should attempt to taper the dose to 500 mg or to discontinue the agent)
  - Famciclovir (250 mg twice daily for 12 months)
  - Acyclovir (400 mg twice daily for 12 months)

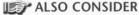 **ALSO CONSIDER**
- Impetigo
- Aphthous stomatitis
- Erythema multiforme
- Bullous pemphigoid (in the elderly)

RARELY
- Pemphigus vulgaris
- Behçet disease

Pyogenic Granuloma

Pyogenic granuloma (PG) is a relatively common benign skin growth that presents as a shiny red papule or nodule (see also Chapter 13, Hands, Distal Fingers, and Periungual Area). Pyogenic granuloma is a vascular hyperplasia that occurs most often in children and young adults. It is benign but can bleed profusely. The cause is unknown. The following factors have been identified as having a possible role to play in its development:

- Trauma: some cases develop at the site of a recent minor injury, such as a pinprick
- Hormonal influences: they occur in up to 5% of pregnancies
- Drug-induced: multiple lesions sometimes develop in patients on systemic retinoids (acitretin or isotretinoin) or protease inhibitors

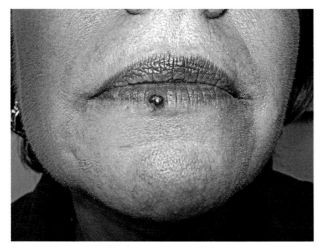

Figure 7-10 Pyogenic granuloma.

DISTINGUISHING FEATURES
- Generally solitary and first appear as a small pinhead-sized red, brownish-red, purple, or blue-black papule that grows rapidly to become 2 mm to 2 cm in diameter. It resembles a hemangioma or granulation tissue ("proud flesh")
- Lesions tend to occur on the lips, gums (Fig. 7-10), buccal mucosa, and fingers
- On nonmucous membrane skin, the base of the lesion is often surrounded by a collarette of skin (see Chapter 13, Hands and Fingers)

- Asymptomatic but tend to bleed readily even after minor trauma and may ulcerate and form crusts
- Women are affected more often than men because of the relationship with pregnancy; however, PG appears in equal frequency in boys and girls
- May arise during pregnancy (granuloma gravidarum): lesions tend to occur on the lips, gums, and buccal mucosa
- May occur in neonates (umbilical granuloma) (see Chapter 17, Umbilicus)

DIAGNOSIS
- Clinical appearance
- Shave biopsy, if there is any doubt about the diagnosis (see Appendix B)

MANAGEMENT
- A PG in pregnant women may go away on its own after delivery; therefore, waiting is the best strategy in many cases
- If due to a drug, they usually disappear when the drug is stopped
- The lesion is generally destroyed by curettage and electrocautery and the feeding blood vessel cauterized to reduce the chances of regrowth
- Laser therapy, cryosurgery, or excisional surgery are sometimes used
- Recurrences are not uncommon if the lesion is not completely removed

Venous Lake

Venous lake (venous varix) is a common benign angioma that usually occurs in patients older than 60 years. This neoplasm is characterized by a blood-filled vascular channel. It may also appear on the ears and eyelids.

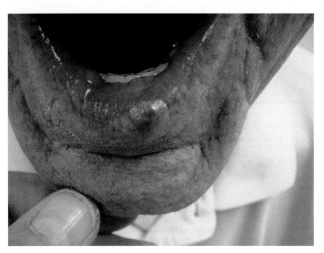

Figure 7-11 Venous lake.

DISTINGUISHING FEATURES

- Age greater than 60 years
- Typically seen on the lower lip
- Lesion is compressible
- Dome-shaped papule or macule generally dark blue to purple (Fig. 7-11)

DIAGNOSIS

- Clinical

MANAGEMENT

- Most often no treatment is necessary
- Electrodesiccation or laser ablation for cosmetic reasons

Labial Melanotic Macule

A **labial melanotic macule** is a benign, pigmented macule on the lower lip. It is noted most often on white adults. It is thought to be caused by sun exposure. This lesion is sometimes suspected to be a potential melanoma and can cause concern in both the patient and the health care provider. Fortunately, melanoma is very rare on the lip (but it can occur).

Similar freckles may also occur in areas that are not exposed to the sun:

- Inside the mouth (oral melanotic macule)
- On the vulva in women (vulval labial melanotic macule)
- On the penis in men (penile melanotic macule)

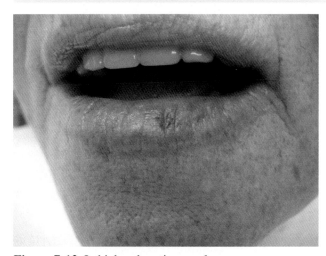

Figure 7-12 Labial melanotic macule.

DISTINGUISHING FEATURES

- Pigmented macule, most often on the lower lip
- Well-defined, oval, brown to black patch (Fig. 7-12)
- Usually solitary; most commonly seen in adult women
- Occasionally can be seen on the upper lip
- Size ranges from 1 to 8 mm. Once developed, the lesions usually remain unchanged in size and color

DIAGNOSIS

- Clinical; has a characteristic pattern when examined with the magnifying glass or dermatoscope
- Shave biopsy, if lesion shows progressive change or melanoma is suspected

MANAGEMENT (see Appendix B)

- No therapy is necessary
- Typical lesions can be observed
- If treatment is requested, the macules can be frozen (cryotherapy) or removed using a laser or intense pulsed light. Excision can also be performed but will leave a scar

☞ **ALSO CONSIDER**

- Hemangioma
  - Freckles (ephelides)
  - Lentigo simplex
  - Solar lentigo
  - Dental amalgam tattoo
  - Junctional melanocytic nevus (flat mole)
- Nonmelanoma skin cancer (e.g., basal cell carcinoma, squamous cell carcinoma)

RARELY

- Lentigo maligna
  - Superficial spreading melanoma
- Nodular (amelanotic) melanoma
- Kaposi sarcoma
- Multiple lentiginoses (various syndromes) such as:
  - Peutz-Jeghers syndrome
  - Addison disease

Solar Keratoses

Solar keratoses on the lip and its vermilion border are common lesions that arise in persons who are fair-skinned, burn easily, and tan poorly; these lesions are the result of cumulative sun exposure. They appear in adults and the elderly and are rare in dark-skinned persons. The lower lip is also a frequent target of sun exposure, and the appearance of **solar cheilitis** (actinic cheilitis) is most often noted here.

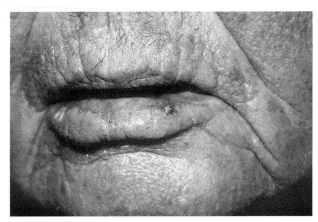

Figure 7-13 Solar keratosis.

DISTINGUISHING FEATURES
- Vermillion border of upper lip or mucous membrane of lower lip (Fig. 7-13)
- Early lesions may feel rough to palpation and be slightly white or yellowish in color
- Adult to elderly
- Affects males more than females

DIAGNOSIS
- Clinical or shave biopsy, if the diagnosis is in doubt

MANAGEMENT (see Appendix B)
- Limit sun exposure
- Liquid nitrogen (LN$_2$) cryosurgery
- Electrocautery and curettage

Solar Cheilitis

Solar Cheilitis describes wide spread solar keratoses on the lower lip due to chronic sun exposure.

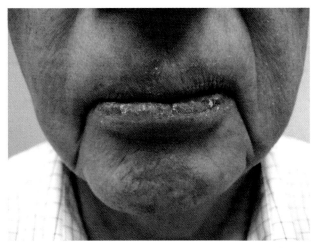

Figure 7-14 Solar cheilitis. (Image courtesy of Benjamin Barankin, MD.)

DISTINGUISHING FEATURES
- Lower lip; may involve entire length of lip; however, intraoral portion is spared
- Affects elderly men more than women
- A whitish discoloration, sometimes with erosions, crusts, and/or atrophy (Fig. 7-14)

DIAGNOSIS
- A shave biopsy of thickened or persistent localized areas

MANAGEMENT (see Appendix B)
- Cryosurgery with LN$_2$
- Topical imiquimod (**Aldara cream**), or 5- fluorouracil cream (**Carac, Efudex**) may also have some utility in treating selected patients (see Appendix A)
- Photodynamic therapy
- Laser ablation
- Surgical excision with mucosal advancement flap
- ⚠ ALERT: Solar keratosis and solar cheilitis may be precursors to squamous cell carcinoma (see following discussion)

Squamous Cell Carcinoma

Most **squamous cell carcinomas (SCCs)** arise in patients with the same epidemiologic profile as do solar keratoses (see previous discussion). Those that appear on the mucous membrane of the lips may arise in a preexisting solar keratosis or solar cheilitis; however, an SCC may appear de novo without any preceding solar dyskeratosis. Such lesions are much more likely to metastasize.

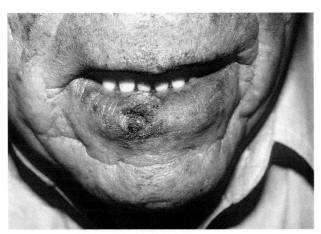

Figure 7-15 Squamous cell carcinoma.

DISTINGUISHING FEATURES

- Lower lip often with a history of solar keratosis
- Begins with a small, slightly raised, warty (verrucous), yellowish-brownish hyperkeratosis and enlarges in time (an exaggeration of solar keratosis or cheilitis)

- Alternatively, the presenting sign may be a small erosion, crust, or ulcer that fails to heal and bleeds recurrently
- It can progress rapidly when extensive ulcerative necrosis occurs into a nodule or tumor (Fig. 7-15)

DIAGNOSIS

- History
- Biopsy
- If indicated, sonographic examination of regional lymph nodes
- Chest x-ray

MANAGEMENT (see Appendix B)

- Must be referred to an oral/head and neck surgeon for management
- ⚠ **ALERT: Squamous cell carcinoma of the lip has the potential for metastasis. Any nonhealing lip erosion or ulcer should be biopsied**
- Excision with control of margins (e.g., Mohs micrographic surgery)
- Radiation therapy if inoperable or difficult to completely excise
- Neck dissection for lymph node involvement
- Chemotherapy for systemic involvement

Verruca Vulgaris

Verruca vulgaris is apt to occur anywhere on the body including mucous membranes. Warts on the lips tend to occur most often in children and in immunocompromised persons.

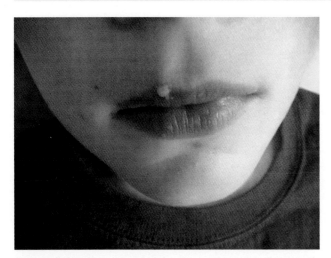

Figure 7-16 Verruca vulgaris. (From Burkhart C, Morell, D, Goldsmith LA, et al. *VisualDx: Essential Pediatric Dermatology.* Philadelphia, PA: Lippincott Williams & Wilkins; 2009.)

DISTINGUISHING FEATURES

- Hyperkeratotic papule(s) (Fig. 7-16)
- Flat or filiform
- Often flesh-colored

DIAGNOSIS

- Clinical
- Biopsy if diagnosis is in doubt

MANAGEMENT

- Benign neglect is sometimes the best option in young children
- Local destruction (electrocautery and cryodestruction with LN_2 are the usual approaches) (see Appendix B)

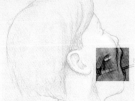

CHAPTER 8

Oral Cavity and Tongue

Oral mucous membrane lesions are often clues to the presence of systemic illnesses such as acquired immunodeficiency syndrome (AIDS), syphilis, and systemic lupus erythematosus. They may also be helpful in diagnosing dermatologic conditions, including lichen planus and pemphigus.

Lesions such as aphthous ulcers ("canker sores") are often seen as isolated phenomena but may also be an accompaniment or a precursor to a symptom complex, such as seen in Behçet syndrome or ulcerative colitis. Oral viral infections include herpes simplex (HSV) infections, oral hairy leukoplakia, and cytomegalovirus. It is often difficult to make a clinical diagnosis in the oral cavity. Lesions may resemble normal variants, or they may appear clinically identical to one another (also see Chapter 7, Lips and Perioral Area).

IN THIS CHAPTER

Buccal and Gingival Mucosa
- Oral mucous cyst *vs* oral fibroma *vs* verruca vulgaris
- Aphthous ulcers *vs* primary herpes gingivostomatitis *vs* erythema multiforme
- Oral candidiasis *vs* oral lichen planus
- Leukoplakia *vs* squamous cell carcinoma

Tongue
- Geographic tongue *vs* mucous patches of secondary syphilis
- Oral hairy leukoplakia *vs* lichen planus *vs* candidiasis

Oral Mucous Cyst (Mucocele)

An **oral mucous cyst (mucocele)** is a common, mucus-filled blisterlike lesion of the minor salivary glands. Such lesions are not true cysts; rather, they are "pseudocysts" due to the absence of a true epithelial lining. They are considered to be the result of trauma to the openings of salivary glands. An injury or rupture of these microscopic excretory ducts leads to an accumulation of mucus inside of the connective tissue of the lip. The trauma of lip biting or the sucking action of drawing the mucous membranes of the lower lip between the teeth are thought to be common causes. Patients are most often not aware of having had an injury. Oral mucous cysts are most commonly in infants, young children, and young adults.

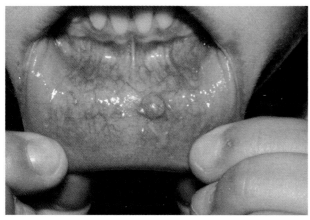

Figure 8-1 Oral mucous cyst.

DISTINGUISHING FEATURES
- Most commonly occur on the inner surface of the lower lip but may also appear on the floor of the mouth, gingiva, buccal mucosa, and tongue (Fig. 8-1)
- Painless, sometimes bothersome, bluish or clear, translucent, glistening, dome-shaped papule that contains mucoid material
- Bluish color is due the thin layer of epithelium that covers the capillaries. Deeper lesions are usually the same color as the rest of the lip because they are covered with a thicker layer of tissue

- Bleeding into the lesion may occasionally resemble a hemangioma
- Easily ruptured and may spontaneously disappear, particularly in infants
- May recur repeatedly

DIAGNOSIS
- Clinical
- Incision and drainage reveals mucoid material
- A biopsy may be performed to rule out other suspected mucosal neoplasms

MANAGEMENT
- Reassurance, because superficial mucoceles often resolve spontaneously
- Incision and drainage
- For frequent recurrences or if problematic to the patient, treatment options include cryosurgery with liquid nitrogen (LN_2) spray, intralesional injections of triamcinolone acetonide, and electrodesiccation (see Appendix B)
- Oral surgery is the treatment of choice for deeper, recalcitrant lesions. Excision should include the immediate adjacent glandular tissue
- Laser ablation and micromarsupialization are other options

Oral Fibroma

Oral fibroma is most often observed in adults. It is the most common oral neoplasm and it probably represents reactive fibrous hyperplasia resulting from trauma or local irritation.

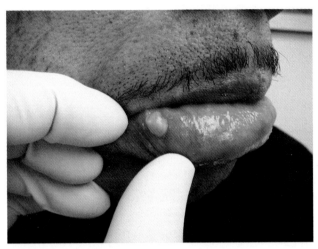

Figure 8-2 Oral fibroma.

DISTINGUISHING FEATURES
- Seen most often on the buccal mucosa along the plane of occlusion of the maxillary and mandibular teeth
- Asymptomatic, smooth-surfaced, firm solitary papule or nodule (Fig. 8-2)
- Diameter may vary from 1 to 2 cm
- Ulceration due to repeated trauma may occur

DIAGNOSIS
- Shave biopsy

MANAGEMENT
- Shave biopsy, which often results in diagnosis and may lead to ultimate resolution (see Appendix B)
- Excision, if recurrent

Verruca Vulgaris

A **verruca vulgaris** (wart) can occur anywhere in the mouth, including the tongue. Seen in children and young adults, warts often have different clinical features than those that appear on the cutaneous surface.

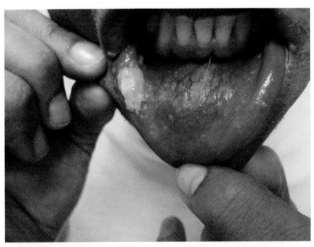

Figure 8-3 This patient has had a liver transplantation and is HIV positive.

DISTINGUISHING FEATURES
- Lesions are softer and more whitish than on the skin
- They may be typical papillomatosis lesions or smooth papules (Fig. 8-3)

DIAGNOSIS
- Clinical
- A shave biopsy, if the diagnosis is in doubt

MANAGEMENT
- Electrodesiccation, cryosurgery with LN_2, and/or laser (see Appendix B)
- Conservative: wait-and-see attitude, because many of the usual wart treatments are difficult to use in this location

☞ ALSO CONSIDER
- Squamous cell carcinoma
- Giant cell fibroma
- Neurofibroma
- Benign and malignant salivary gland tumors

RARELY
- Peripheral giant cell granuloma
- Oral florid papillomatosis

Aphthous Ulcers vs Primary Herpes Gingivostomatitis vs Erythema Multiforme

Aphthous Ulcers

Aphthous ulcers (aphthous stomatitis), commonly known as "canker sores," are very common, recurrent, painful erosions or ulcers of the mucous membranes of the mouth. They occur in children and adults and appear to be more common in women than men. They have no known cause, but an immune mechanism is considered the most likely contributory factor. Patients often ascribe recurrences to psychological stress or local trauma. Women may correlate them with their menstrual cycle. Most cases heal spontaneously, only to recur unexpectedly.

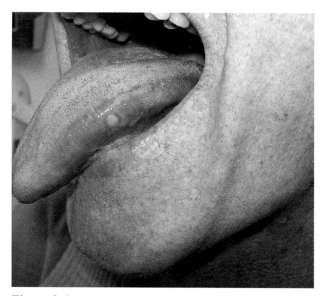

Figure 8-4 Aphthous ulceration.

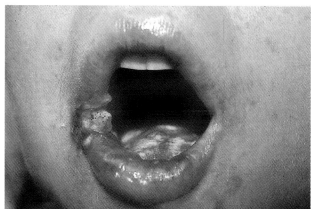

Figure 8-5 Aphthous ulcerations, Behçet disease. (From Goodheart HP. *Goodheart's Photoguide to Common Skin Disorders: Diagnosis and Management.* 3rd ed. Philadelphia, PA: Lippincott Williams & Wilkins; 2009.)

DISTINGUISHING FEATURES
- Painful lesions may be seen on the buccal, labial, and gingival mucosa, as well as on the tongue (Fig. 8-4)
- Single or multiple small (2 to 5 mm) round or oval, shallow, well-demarcated, punched-out erosions covered with gray or yellowish exudate and surrounded by a ring of erythema (halo)
- Begin as vesicobullous lesions that rarely remain intact and unruptured; instead, such lesions usually become erosions or ulcers by the time clinicians see them.
- Tend to heal in 4 to 14 days, without scarring, a duration similar to that of HSV lesions

⚠ **ALERT: Persistent or large painful, persistent aphthae may be seen in Behçet disease, inflammatory bowel disease, and human immunodeficiency virus (HIV)/AIDS (Fig. 8-5)**

✔ **TIP: Because recurrent aphthous stomatitis has a clinical appearance and course similar to those of recurrent herpes labialis (see following discussion), the two conditions are often confused by patient and clinician alike. Herpes simplex virus lesions, particularly recurrent ones, very infrequently occur inside the mouth.**

DIAGNOSIS
- Clinical

MANAGEMENT (see Appendix A)
- Symptomatic therapy with topical anesthetic viscous lidocaine (**Xylocaine**)
- Superpotent (class 1) topical steroid ointments applied directly to lesions and held there by pressure with one's finger
- Tetracycline suspension (250 mg/tsp)—"swish and swallow"
- Diphenhydramine (**Benadryl**) suspension—"gargle and spit"

- Tacrolimus ointment (**Protopic**) 0.1% applied at bedtime may accelerate healing
- Silver nitrate applied directly to lesions also can promote healing
- Intralesional corticosteroid injections or a brief course of systemic corticosteroids are effective in reducing pain and healing; particularly useful in patients with large, persistent, painful ulcers
- In severe cases, consider oral colchicine, dapsone and thalidomide

Primary Herpes Gingivostomatosis

In **primary herpes gingivostomatosis** (see Chapter 7, Lips and Perioral Area), oral erosions that are often indistinguishable from aphthous stomatitis sometimes appear. The virus is shed in saliva and is spread by direct contact with infected secretions. It can also be passed on from individuals without symptoms. Primary herpes gingivostomatosis occurs mainly in infants and young children, often subclinically. Most often the primary infection is mild and unnoticed, but can be severe, although less severe than recurrences. Herpes simplex virus type 1 is most commonly associated with oral-facial involvement.

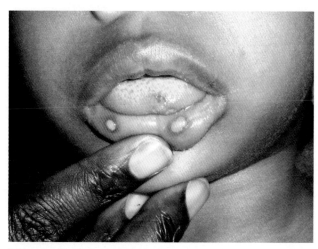

Figure 8-6 Herpes simplex viral stomatitis. Lesions are visible on the tongue and labial mucosa. (Courtesy of Paul S. Matz, MD.)

DISTINGUISHING FEATURES
- Most occur in children between 1 and 5 years of age
- Fever, which may be high, with malaise, restlessness, and excessive drooling

- Gums may become edematous and erythematous and bleed easily (Fig. 8-6)
- Vesicles occur in white patches on the tongue, throat, palate, and insides of the cheeks; they evolve into ulcers with a yellowish coating
- Regional tender lymphadenopathy
- Fever subsides after 3 to 5 days, and recovery is usually complete within 2 weeks

DIAGNOSIS
- Clinical, usually based on clinical appearance and history
- A Tzanck smear (see Appendix B) is the fastest and easiest test to help make the diagnosis
- When necessary, fresh viral culture from intact vesicles or direct florescent antibody testing
- Polymerase chain reaction for HSV DNA detection

MANAGEMENT
- Supportive
- If necessary, oral antiviral therapy (acyclovir, valacyclovir, or famciclovir) is given within 72 hours to reduce pain, viral shedding, and time to healing
- Treatment is discussed in Chapter 7, Lips and Perioral Area, and Appendix A

Erythema Multiforme

Erythema multiforme (EM) minor is a self-limited eruption characterized by symmetrically distributed erythematous macules or papules, which develop into the characteristic target-like lesions (see Chapter 13, Hands, Palmar Surface). Erythema multiforme minor is generally limited to one mucosal surface, with the lips, palate, and gingiva most often affected. The disorder is considered to be a type IV hypersensitivity reaction. It is often idiopathic, but the most common precipitating cause is recurrent labial HSV infections. Also, it may be associated with other underlying causes such as drug reactions, contact dermatitis, mycoplasma infections, and histoplasmosis.

   Erythema multiforme major (Stevens-Johnson syndrome) is the more serious variant of EM. It has much more extensive mucous membrane involvement, systemic symptoms, and widespread lesions. Precipitating factors include drugs (sulfonamides, penicillin, hydantoins, barbiturates, allopurinol, nonsteroidal anti-inflammatory drugs), mycoplasma infection, pregnancy, streptococcus infection, hepatitis A and B, coccidioidomycosis, and Epstein-Barr virus infection.

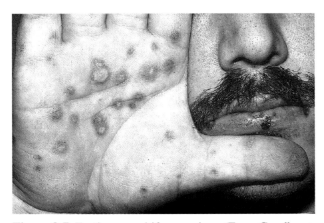

Figure 8-7 Erythema multiforme minor. (From Goodheart HP. *Goodheart's Photoguide to Common Skin Disorders: Diagnosis and Management.* 3rd ed. Philadelphia, PA: Lippincott Williams & Wilkins; 2009.)

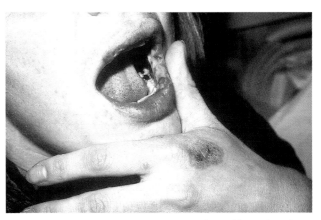

Figure 8-8 Erythema multiforme major. This patient has multiple intraoral lesions as well as vaginal erosions.

DISTINGUISHING FEATURES

Erythema Multiforme Minor

- Most commonly seen in late adolescence and in young adulthood
- Patients are generally well with, at most, mild systemic symptoms
- When present, mucous membrane lesions are limited to the mouth and lips
- The eruption is acute, relatively mild, self-limited, and often recurrent
- An active vesicle or a crusted lesion of recurrent HSV may be present on the vermillion border of the lip during an outbreak or the patient may have a history of recurrent HSV (Fig. 8-7)
- When HSV is the cause, EM minor tends to recur with every bout of cold sores. The viral infection may be subclinical (i.e., visible cold sores may be absent at the time of the reaction)

✔ **TIP: The gums are rarely involved by lesions of EM.**

Erythema Multiforme Major

- Severe, extensive, painful mucous membrane involvement; may be located in multiple sites, including the mouth, pharynx, eyes, and genitalia
- Often accompanied by symptoms of fever, malaise, and myalgias
- At least two mucosal surfaces are seen in EM major and are characterized by hemorrhagic crusting of the lips and ulceration of the mucosa (Fig. 8-8). Occasionally, there are few or no skin lesions
- Erosions of the oral mucosa may result in difficulty in eating and drinking
- Conjunctival involvement may cause lacrimation and photophobia

DIAGNOSIS

- Typical target lesions may be present
- If indicated: complete blood count, erythrocyte sedimentation rate, liver function tests, blood urea nitrogen, creatinine, urinalysis, electrolytes, and blood, urine, or sputum cultures
- Skin and/or mucous membrane biopsy may be necessary

MANAGEMENT (see Appendix A)

- If known, the precipitating cause (e.g., suspected etiologic drug) should be eliminated or discontinued
- Empiric treatment with suppressive doses of oral acyclovir, famciclovir **(Famvir),** or valacyclovir **(Valtrex)** may prevent or mitigate recurrences if erythema multiforme is due to HSV (see Chapter 7, Lips and Perioral Area)
- Most cases of EM minor subside completely within 2 to 3 weeks without any complications
- **ALERT: In life-threatening situations, such as may be seen in EM major, hospitalization is often essential. The use of systemic steroids in such severe cases is controversial, and their effectiveness has not been established. Cyclosporin, intravenous immunoglobulin, hemodialysis, and plasmapheresis have been documented as beneficial in some case reports.**

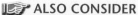 **ALSO CONSIDER**
- Hand-foot-mouth disease
- Herpangina
- Systemic lupus erythematosus
- Erosive oral lichen planus

RARELY
- Cyclic neutropenia
- Pemphigus vulgaris

Oral Candidiasis

Most oral fungal infections are caused by *Candida albicans*, a harmless commensal organism inhabiting the mouths of almost 50% of the world's population. Under suitable circumstances, it can become an opportunistic pathogen. In infants, acute pseudomembranous candidiasis (thrush) may be observed in healthy neonates or in people in whom antibiotics, corticosteroids, or xerostomia (dry mouth) disturb the oral microflora. Oral candidiasis is most prevalent in people with immunosuppressive conditions (HIV-associated oral candidiasis) and diabetes as well as those on long-term broad-spectrum antibiotics and systemic and aerosolized corticosteroids. Xerostomia (as in Sjögren syndrome) and radiotherapy to the head and neck also predispose individuals to oral yeast infections.

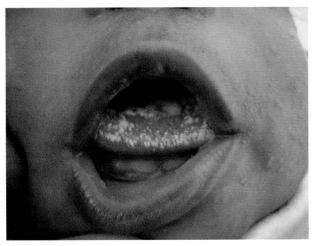

Figure 8-9 Oral thrush. An infant with numerous whitish tongue plaques. (Courtesy of Paul S. Matz, MD.)

DISTINGUISHING FEATURES
Thrush (Acute Pseudomembranous Candidiasis)
- White patches on the surface of the buccal mucosa, palate, or tongue
- Lesions develop into confluent plaques that resemble milk curds and can be wiped off to reveal an erythematous base (Fig. 8-9)

Erythematous Candidiasis
- Erythematous areas found generally on the dorsum of the tongue, palate, or buccal mucosa
- Lesions on the dorsum of the tongue present as depapillated areas
- An associated angular stomatitis (perlèche) (see Chapter 7, Lips and Perioral Area) may be present

HIV-Associated Oral Candidiasis
- Candidiasis ("thrush") is also seen in immunocompromised patients
- Curdlike or erosive lesions can easily be removed with gauze or a tongue blade; such erosive patches often are seen on the palate, the dorsal aspect of the tongue, oropharynx, angles of mouth (perlèche) and buccal mucosa

DIAGNOSIS
- Microscopy and culture of skin swabs and scrapings aid in the diagnosis of candidal infections

MANAGEMENT (see Appendix A)
- Intermittent or prolonged topical or oral antifungal treatment is usually necessary
- Meticulous dental hygiene and an oral rinse containing 0.12% chlorhexidine may be effective
- Nystatin or imidazole lozenges
- Oral therapy with fluconazole (**Diflucan**) produces remission within approximately 1 week. Fluconazole 100 mg daily is more effective than nystatin 500,000 U 4 times a day or clotrimazole troche 10 mg 5 times per day

Oral Lichen Planus

Oral lichen planus (LP) often accompanies cutaneous lichen planus (see Chapter 12, Arms; Chapter 21, Legs), an inflammatory skin condition that predominantly occurs in adults older than 40 years. It is less common in younger adults and rare in children. The cause of LP appears to be autoimmune in nature. Some studies suggest an association between LP and chronic hepatitis C virus infection, chronic active hepatitis, and primary biliary cirrhosis. Oral LP lesions may also be part of the spectrum of chronic graft-versus-host disease that appears after bone marrow transplantation. Other associations include drugs (lichenoid drug reactions), most often biologics, sun exposure (LP actinicus), and contact allergens in dental restorative materials or toothpastes.

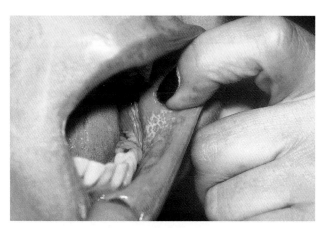

Figure 8-10 Oral lichen planus.

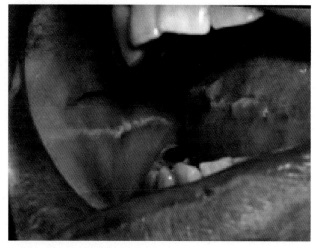

Figure 8-11 Normal bite line.

DISTINGUISHING FEATURES
- Classically manifested as bilateral white striations in a lacelike network (reticular pattern) on buccal mucosa, tongue, or gingivae
- Such reticular lesions are often asymptomatic and the patient is unaware of them (Fig. 8-10)
- Less often, lesions may be erosive or ulcerative and can be very painful and may persist for many years with periods of exacerbation and quiescence

DIAGNOSIS
- Clinical, especially when cutaneous lesions of lichen planus are also present
- Biopsy, if necessary

MANAGEMENT (see Appendix A)
- Identify and remove any potential agent that might have caused a lichenoid reaction, such as drugs that have been started in recent months and contact allergens identified by the history or by patch testing

- Suggest that patient stop smoking
- Topical steroids or a topical calcineurin inhibitor such as tacrolimus ointment (**Protopic** 1%) applied directly to the ulcerations
- Nonsteroidal anti-inflammatory drugs s, sulfonylureas, antimalarials, beta-blockers, and some angiotensin-converting enzyme inhibitors
- Intralesional steroid injections (intralesional triamcinolone)
- In severe cases, systemic corticosteroids or cyclosporin may be used
- Thalidomide

⚠ **ALERT: Although the risk is small, oral, erosive LP may rarely lead to squamous cell carcinoma (SCC). Persistent ulcers and enlarging nodules should undergo biopsy, particularly in patients who are immunosuppressed.**

✔ **TIP: Alternative therapy: Curcumin (tumeric) 100 mg capsules has been reported to be effective for oral, symptomatic LP.**

☞ ALSO CONSIDER
- Normal bite line (image) (Fig. 8-11)
- Squamous cell carcinoma (particularly in ulcerative lesions)
- Aphthous ulcers
- Oral hairy leukoplakia (tongue)
- Herpetic stomatitis
- Secondary syphilis
- Leukoplakia

RARELY
- Chronic mucocutaneous candidiasis, pemphigus vulgaris, bullous pemphigoid, and Behçet disease

Leukoplakia

Leukoplakia is not a diagnosis; rather, it is a descriptive clinical term reserved for white patches or plaques that occur on mucosal surfaces pending definitive diagnosis. The term simply refers to a white patch on a mucous membrane that does not rub off. "Leukoplakia" is often misused to indicate a premalignant lesion; however, fewer than 5% of lesions have been reported to develop into squamous cell carcinoma. Smoking, chewing tobacco, mucosal trauma, and alcohol abuse are all contributing factors.

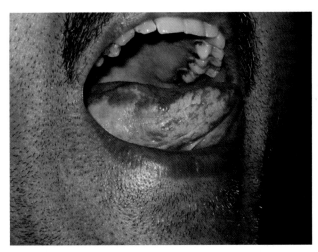

Figure 8-12 Leukoplakia. (Image courtesy of Ashit Marwah, MD.)

DISTINGUISHING FEATURES
- Most commonly occurs in elderly men
- White, adherent mucosal patches or plaques that do not rub off (this definition generally excludes candidiasis, which usually can be rubbed off). The white color is caused by moist hyperkeratosis (Fig. 8-12)
- Lesions occur on the tongue, buccal mucosa, hard palate, and gums

DIAGNOSIS
- Exclusion of trauma (normal bite line) or specific diseases or that may cause similar white lesions such as candidiasis, lichen planus
- Biopsy, if necessary, to rule out SCC or other diagnoses

MANAGEMENT
- The patient should have regular dental examinations
- Treatment mainly involves avoidance of predisposing factors such as smoking, tobacco, betel chewing, alcohol, and removal of chronic irritants like sharp edges of teeth
- If the white patch is caused by irritation, it will disappear within weeks after the source of the irritation is removed
- **ALERT: If the lesion does not resolve, it should be surgically removed and biopsied. Repeat biopsies may be necessary in some cases in which there is a significant risk of cancer or changes in the size, color, or texture.**

Squamous Cell Carcinoma

Most oral cancers are **squamous cell carcinomas (SCCs).** Risk factors include:
- Smoking: 75% of people diagnosed with oral cancer are tobacco users. The higher the tar yield, the greater the risk
- Alcohol consumption: tobacco and heavy drinking act together to significantly increase the risk
- Poor oral health
- Infective agents, particularly the wart virus human papillomavirus types 16 and 18, have been implicated in some oral cancers

Squamous cell carcinoma appears to occur most frequently in persons in developing countries, particularly India, Pakistan, and Bangladesh. In fact, in some parts of India, oral cancer accounts for more than 50% of all cancers.

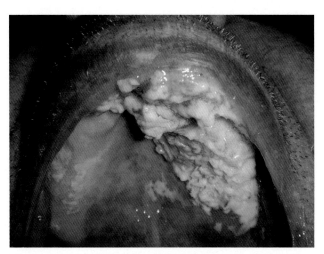

Figure 8-13 Oral florid papillomatosis (squamous cell carcinoma). Image courtesy of Omid Zargari, MD.)

DISTINGUISHING FEATURES
- Oral SCC is twice as common in men as in women
- The most common sites of oral cancer are the lower lip, tongue, and the floor of the mouth, although any part of the mouth may be affected
- May present as *oral florid papillomatosis,* a type of verrucous carcinoma that resembles a cauliflower (Fig. 8-13)

- Many patients with oral SCC also have metastases in the cervical lymph nodes at presentation. At a later stage, cancer may spread to other lymph nodes, lungs, liver, or bones

DIAGNOSIS
- Biopsy and determining the cancer's stage is an important factor because it directs treatment planning

MANAGEMENT
⚠ **ALERT: Early recognition of signs and symptoms of oral cancer is very important.**
- One such sign includes a white patch (leukoplakia), a red/white patch (erythroleukoplakia) on the gums, tongue, or lining of the mouth (see previous discussion)
- Other signs and symptoms are:
  - A small erosion or indurated ulcer that looks like a common aphthous ulcer that fails to heal
  - A papule or nodule that can be felt on the lip or in the mouth or throat
  - Unusual bleeding, pain, or numbness in the mouth
  - Difficulty or pain with chewing or swallowing
  - A change in the voice or hoarseness that lasts for a long time
- Oral SCC is generally treated by surgery and/or radiation therapy. Chemotherapy may also be used in patients with confirmed metastases

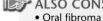
ALSO CONSIDER
- Oral fibroma

Note: A multitude of benign and malignant neoplasms, both relatively common and rare, can appear in the oral cavity. They are too numerous to list in this book.

Geographic Tongue *vs* Mucous Patches of Secondary Syphilis

Geographic Tongue

Geographic tongue, or benign migratory glossitis, is an idiopathic finding. Reports have suggested an association of geographic tongue with psoriasis; however, its 2% incidence in patients with psoriasis is no greater than would be expected in an otherwise healthy population. Variation with the menstrual cycle suggests hormonal factors as having an influence on its appearance.

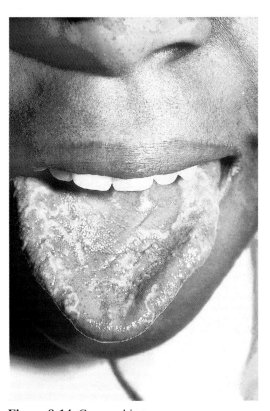

Figure 8-14 Geographic tongue.

DISTINGUISHING FEATURES
- The lesions are areas that are shiny, red, and devoid of papillae (Fig. 8-14) and resemble mucous patches (see following discussion)
- Lesions seem to move about on the surface of the tongue and change configurations from one day to the next; thus, the designation *benign migratory glossitis*
- Appears more commonly in females than males

DIAGNOSIS
- Clinical

MANAGEMENT
- Generally, no treatment is necessary
- Discomfort may be treated with a mouth gargle or rinse containing antiseptic and anesthetic agents

Mucous Patches of Secondary Syphilis

The lesions of secondary syphilis on the tongue are known as *mucous patches*. They are the most infectious manifestation of syphilis.

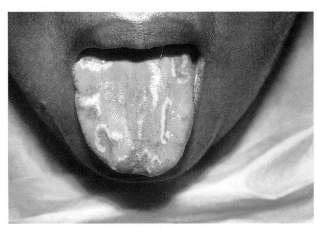

Figure 8-15 Secondary syphilis (mucous patches).

DISTINGUISHING FEATURES
- Asymptomatic round or oval eroded lesions or papules that are devoid of epithelium (Fig. 8-15)
- Alternatively, may be slightly raised grayish-white patches with erythematous halos

DIAGNOSIS
- Lesions teem with spirochetes
- Venereal Disease Research Laboratory (VDRL) and rapid plasma reagin (RPR) tests are reactive

MANAGEMENT (see also Chapter 18, Genital Area)
Non–Penicillin-Allergic Patients
- Benzathine penicillin G (2.4 million units intramuscularly in a single dose)

Penicillin-Allergic Nonpregnant Patients
- Doxycycline (100 mg orally twice daily for 2 weeks) *or*
- Tetracycline (500 mg 4 times daily for 2 weeks)

Penicillin-Allergic Pregnant Patients
- Desensitization to penicillin
- Subsequent treatment with benzathine penicillin G (2.4 million units intramuscularly, with a second dose 1 week later)

HIV-Infected Patients
- Benzathine penicillin G (2.4 million units intramuscularly in one dose)
- Some experts recommend repeated treatment

ORAL CAVITY AND TONGUE

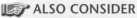 **ALSO CONSIDER**
- Avitaminosis
- Median rhomboid glossitis
- Glossitis (other)/glossodynia

RARELY
- Amyloidosis

Oral Hairy Leukoplakia

Oral hairy leukoplakia (OHL) is associated with the Epstein-Barr virus. It is seen in patients with HIV infection, particularly in those with advanced immunosuppression, and in transplant recipients. It is rarely seen in patients receiving highly active antiretroviral therapy. Oral LP and candidiasis are described earlier in this chapter.

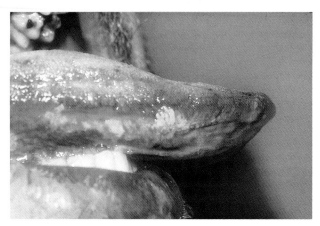

Figure 8-16 Oral hairy leukoplakia.

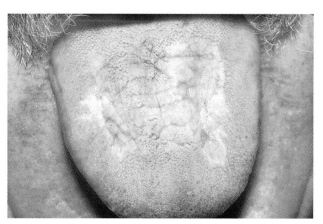

Figure 8-17 Lichen planus.

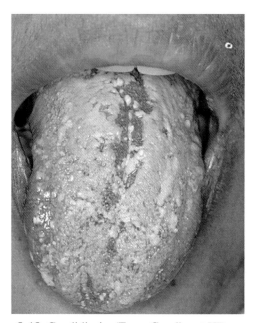

Figure 8-18 Candidiasis. (From Goodheart HP. *Goodheart's Photoguide to Common Skin Disorders: Diagnosis and Management.* 3rd ed. Philadelphia, PA: Lippincott Williams & Wilkins; 2009.)

DISTINGUISHING FEATURES
- Oral hairy leukoplakia appears as unilateral or bilateral white plaques or papillary lesions on the lateral, dorsal, or ventral surfaces of the tongue or on buccal mucosa. The lesions may vary in appearance from smooth, flat, small lesions to irregular, "hairy" or "verrucous" lesions with prominent vertical folds or projections (Fig. 8-16). Figs. 8-17 and 8-18 show LP and candidiasis of the tongue
- Filiform papules on lateral aspects of the tongue that resemble white hairs
- Lesions are white plaques resembling "corrugated cardboard" that are fixed to the mucosa; they are not friable, as in candidiasis (see previous discussion)
- Usually asymptomatic, patients occasionally complain of a burning sensation

DIAGNOSIS
- Clinical
- Definitive diagnosis requires biopsy and demonstration of Epstein-Barr virus

MANAGEMENT

- Treatment necessary only when symptomatic
- Highly active antiretroviral therapy
- Surgical excision is reserved for severe symptomatic cases
- Acyclovir (3.2 g per day) is given with recurrence of lesions on cessation of treatment Famciclovir and valacyclovir may also be considered

- Topical tretinoin (**Retin-A**) 0.05% solution may be applied for 15 minutes once daily using a gauze sponge
- Podophyllin 25% solution is applied sparingly to one side of the tongue at a time and is allowed to air dry. This is repeated once weekly

ORAL CAVITY AND TONGUE

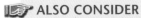 **ALSO CONSIDER**
- Leukoplakia/small cell carcinoma (see previous discussion)

RARELY
- White sponge nevus

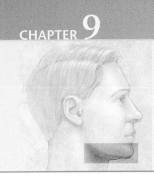

CHAPTER 9

Chin and Mandibular Area

In women, the chin and the mandibular area are common places for adult-onset acne to appear. Folliculitis barbae (shaving bumps) and acne frequently present problems for men in the beard area. Pseudofolliculitis barbae is especially noted in black men. The chin, beard area, and neck are also subject to bacterial (staphylococcal folliculi-tis), and less commonly, fungal (sycosis barbae) and viral folliculitis (herpetic folliculitis) infections.

The beard is a common site for alopecia areata to appear in men. Benign growths such as nevi, flat warts, as well as malignant neoplasms basal cell carcinomas all may appear on the chin and jawline.

IN THIS CHAPTER
- Adult-Onset acne *vs* folliculitis *vs* pseudofolliculitis barbae

Adult-Onset Acne *vs* Folliculitis *vs* Pseudofolliculitis Barbae

Adult-Onset Acne

Adult-onset acne is overwhelmingly a condition of females (see also Chapter 2, Forehead and Temples; Chapter 5, Nose and Perinasal Area; Chapter 6, Cheeks; Chapter 7, Lips and Perioral Area).

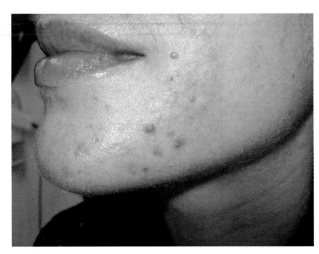

Figure 9-1 Adult-onset acne.

DISTINGUISHING FEATURES
- Affects women much more often than men
- Evanescent, inflammatory red papules and/or pustules
- Lesions occur along the jawline or on the chin; also may arise in the perioral area, the hairline, neck, and upper trunk (Fig. 9-1)
- Relatively or totally comedo-free
- In general, lesions tend to be few in number
- Premenstrual or (less commonly) midcycle flares
- Lesions last for several days; sometimes they persist for a month or longer; sometimes occur without any pattern

DIAGNOSIS
- Clinical

MANAGEMENT
- See Chapter 6, Cheeks, and Appendix C
- ✔ **TIP: Every female acne patient should be questioned about her menstrual history**
- ⚠ **ALERT: A hormonal and gynecologic evaluation is appropriate for a small number of acne patients, particularly women in their mid-20s or older who have treatment-resistant acne, a sudden onset of severe acne, virilizing signs or symptoms, irregular menstrual periods, or hirsutism**

Folliculitis

Folliculitis is a superficial or deep infection or inflammation of hair follicles. If it involves the deeper part of the follicle, it may result in a **furuncle** (boil). Lesions occur on hair-bearing areas—the face, scalp, thighs, and body folds (see also Chapter 1, Hair and Scalp; Chapter 10, Neck). Folliculitis has multiple causes: various infections, physical or chemical irritation, occlusive dressings, or the use of topical or systemic steroids. Nonbacterial, or sterile, folliculitis can arise from physical or chemical irritation. Such irritants include waxing, shaving, depilatories, electrolysis, occlusive dressings, and hair plucking. In bacterial folliculitis, coagulase-positive *Staphylococcus aureus* most often is the responsible pathogenic bacterium. It is more commonly found in patients who are diabetic, obese, or immunocompromised.

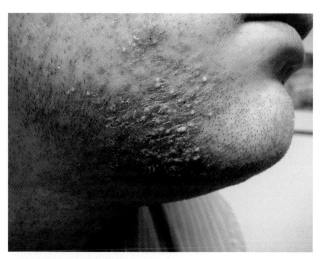

Figure 9-2 Folliculitis.

DISTINGUISHING FEATURES
- Superficial pustule or papule with a central hair (may not always be visible)
- Lesions often polymorphic, displaying a mixture of papules and pustules (Fig. 9-2)
- Comedo-free
- In darkly pigmented patients, primary lesions may consist of obvious papules or pustules; alternatively, only secondary, hyperpigmented lesions may be all that is clinically visible

DIAGNOSIS
- Clinical
- Bacterial culture and sensitivity

MANAGEMENT
Nonbacterial
- Discontinuance or removal of external causes and irritants (e.g., topical steroids waxing, shaving)

Bacterial (see Appendix A)
- **Mild cases** of bacterial folliculitis can sometimes be prevented or controlled with antibacterial soaps
- Topical antibiotics such as clindamycin (**Cleocin**) 1% solution or gel may be applied twice daily
- For chronic, resistant, or recurrent cases, the patient and, if necessary, the patient's family members may require a nasal culture and treatment
- If staphylococcal colonization is present, mupirocin 2% (**Bactroban**) ointment should be applied to the nasal vestibule twice a day for 5 days to eliminate the *S. aureus* carrier state. A systemic antibiotic is often needed for coverage of *S. aureus* because it is the most common pathogen. Dicloxacillin or a cephalosporin such as cephalexin is generally the first choice. Family members may be treated similarly, if necessary; rifampin (600 mg per day for 10 to 14 days) may also eliminate the carrier state

⚠ **ALERT: Herpes virus infections and impetigo due to staphylococci may be clinically indistinguishable from bacterial folliculitis, especially when it occurs in the beard area in men.**

Pseudofolliculitis Barbae

Pseudofolliculitis barbae (PFB) ("shaving bumps") is a very common problem in men of African American, African Caribbean, and Hispanic origin who have tightly curled beard hair that emerge from curved hair follicles. The process of blade shaving can cut the hair at an angle, making it a sharp tip that curls back and punctures the skin and becomes ingrown (reentry phenomenon). Alternatively, the sharpened hair may grow parallel to the skin and penetrate the dermis. Furthermore, newly erupting hairs from below may pierce and aggravate areas that are already inflamed. Thus, growing hairs act as traumatic vehicles that produce an inflammatory foreign body–like reaction.

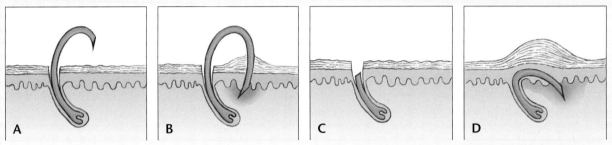

Illustration 9-1. Pseudofolliculitis barbae, or "razor bumps," showing extrafollicular and transfollicular penetration. **A:** A curly hair grows from a sharply curved hair root. When shaved, the hair is left with a sharp point. As this hair grows, the sharp tip curves back and pierces the skin. **B:** The sharpened hair penetrates the skin. **C** and **D:** When hairs are cut too closely, they can penetrate the side of the hair root. Both types of follicular reentry cause a foreign body–like reaction (papule). (Modified from Crutchfield CE III. The causes and treatment of pseudofolliculitis barbae. *CUTIS* 1998;61:351–356, with permission.)

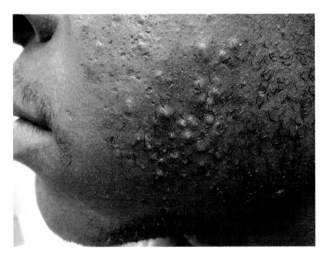

Figure 9-3 Pseudofolliculitis barbae.

DISTINGUISHING FEATURES
- On close inspection, tight, curly hairs that have been sharpened by shaving penetrate the skin are noted
- Inflammatory papules and possibly pustules (Fig. 9-3)
- Lesions are seen on the beard, particularly on the anterior neck and the submental areas
- Ultimately, persistent flesh-colored papules that represent hypertrophic scars
- Postinflammatory hyperpigmentation

DIAGNOSIS
- Clinical

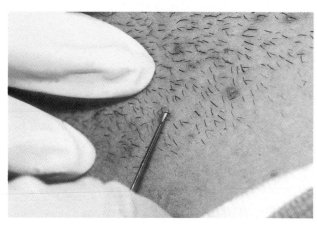

Figure 9-4 Pseudofolliculitis barbae (a curled hair is lifted with a fine needle).

MANAGEMENT

Preventive Measures

- Discontinuance of shaving; however, this is generally not a desired choice
- Hairs may be lifted with a fine needle or a toothpick before they penetrate the skin (Fig. 9-4)
- Shaving should be performed in the direction of the follicle
- Avoidance of close shaving, use of "**PFB Bump Fighter**" razor, or electric razor
- Electric hair clippers that leaves the cut hairs long
- No plucking

Treatment (see Appendix A)

- Used once daily, **BenzaClin, Duac,** or **Benzamycin gel** to reduce inflammation
- Systemic antibiotics such as minocycline and other tetracycline derivatives are helpful when marked inflammation and pustulation are present
- Chemical depilatories such as **Magic Shave** and **Royal Crown** powders are effective in removing and softening hairs; however, they can be irritating and they have an unpleasant odor
- Hair destruction using an extended pulse-width laser has been shown to be effective
- Electrolysis is difficult to use on inflammatory foci, but it can be partially effective as an adjunctive treatment method

 ALSO CONSIDER

- Overuse of topical steroids
- Acne vulgaris
- Endocrinopathic acne
- Physically induced and occupational acne
- Demadex folliculitis
- Pityrosporum folliculitis (*Malassezia furfur*)
- Herpetic folliculitis (viral folliculitis may be seen in patients with human immunodeficiency virus infection)
- Sycosis barbae (tinea barbae)

RARELY

- Actinomycosis
- Gram-negative folliculitis

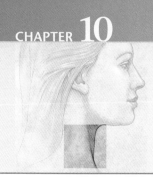

CHAPTER 10

Neck

Many of the conditions seen on the neck represent an extension of disorders noted on the face, scalp, or trunk. Acne, folliculitis, and pityriasis rosea are common examples. There are, however, certain disorders that are found primarily on the neck and beard area: pseudofolliculitis barbae, "razor bumps" (see Chapter 9, Chin and Mandibular Area), and photosensitivity reactions such as polymorphous light eruption and poikiloderma of Civatte. Dermatoheliosis (sun damage) and photosensitivity reactions similarly are noted in a photodistribution—the sun-exposed and the open-collar "V" regions of the neck—neither of which are continually protected by hair or clothing.

Conversely, the area under the chin (anatomically sun-protected) and other shaded areas, such as those covered by long hair, are shielded from chronic sun exposure and are generally spared from sun-related disorders and malignant neoplasms. Basal cell carcinomas and squamous cell carcinomas, when they do arise on the neck, mostly occur in men in areas that are chronically sun-exposed (the nape, "V," and lateral neck).

Acne keloidalis, a disorder that appears most often in black men, is noted on the posterior neck and occipital area. The posterior neck is also often a focus for chronic pruritus, lichen simplex chronicus, and folliculitis.

Benign neoplasms that are often hereditary, such as skin tags, small seborrheic keratoses, and nevi, are very frequently seen on the neck. The neck and the axillary areas are a common location for acanthosis nigricans (see Fig. 10-15).

IN THIS CHAPTER

- Poikiloderma of Civatte *vs* solar elastosis (dermatoheliosis)
- Polymorphous light eruption *vs* systemic lupus erythematosus *vs* dermatomyositis
- Lichen simplex chronicus *vs* atopic dermatitis *vs* contact dermatitis
- Acne keloidalis nuchae *vs* folliculitis/furunculosis
- Skin tags *vs* seborrheic keratoses

Poikiloderma of Civatte

Poikiloderma of Civatte is a common condition that occurs primarily in middle-aged, fair-skinned, women. It affects the skin of the sides and front of the neck. It characteristically spares the area under the chin and other shaded areas such as those covered by long hair. Contributing factors include fair skin, accumulated sun exposure, photosensitizing components of cosmetics and toiletries, especially perfumes, and hormonal changes related to menopause.

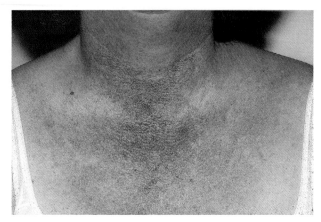

Figure 10-1 Poikiloderma of Civatte.

DISTINGUISHING FEATURES
- Most patients are middle-aged or elderly women
- Erythema associated with a mottled hyperpigmentation located on the sides, and "V" of the neck (sun-exposed areas) (Fig. 10-1)
- The term *poikiloderma* refers to a change in the skin where there is thinning, increased pigmentation, and dilation of the fine blood vessels (telangiectasia)
- Photodistribution; the sparing of the shaded submental and submandibular areas support chronic sunlight exposure as the apparent of cause of this condition

DIAGNOSIS
- Clinical

MANAGEMENT
- It is mainly a cosmetic concern to patients
- The patient should be advised about avoiding sun exposure and the proper use of sunscreens to prevent further skin involvement
- Avoid all perfumes on or near the affected area
- Although there is no totally effective medical treatment, the pulsed-dye laser has been noted to decrease the redness of this condition and intense pulsed light treatments help to reduce the telangiectasia and pigmentation

Solar Elastosis (Dermatoheliosis)

Solar elastosis (dermatoheliosis, actinic elastosis, cutis rhomboidalis nuchae, farmer's neck) is due to chronic sun exposure and results from breakage and clumping of the elastic fibers in the skin and thickening of the epidermis.

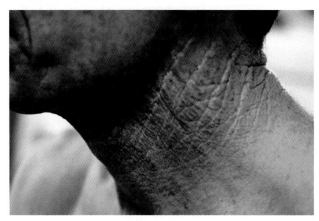

Figure 10-2 Solar elastosis (dermatoheliosis).

DISTINGUISHING FEATURES
- The skin has a yellowish hue with irregular, firm papules that produces a chicken skin–like appearance (Fig. 10-2)
- Photodistribution
- As in poikiloderma of Civatte (see previous discussion), the sparing of the shaded submental and submandibular are evidence that chronic sunlight exposure is the cause
- Deep furrows (*cutis rhomboidalis nuchae*)

DIAGNOSIS
- Clinical

MANAGEMENT
- The patient should be advised about avoiding further sun damage and the proper use of sunscreens
- Chemical peels and lasers

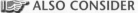 **ALSO CONSIDER**
- Systemic lupus erythematosus
- Dermatomyositis

RARELY
- Papular mucinosis
- Pseudoxanthoma elasticum
- Poikiloderma atrophicans vasculare
- Riehl's melanosis

Polymorphous Light Eruption

Besides sunburn, **polymorphous light eruption (PMLE)** is the most frequently seen acute skin reaction caused by ultraviolet (UV) exposure. It generally occurs in adult women age 20 to 40 and is more common in those who are fair-skinned. Polymorphous light eruption is thought to be caused by an immune reaction to a compound in the skin that is altered by exposure to UV radiation. It is usually provoked not only by short-wavelength UVB but also longer wavelength UVA. In fact, the rash can occur even when the sunlight is coming through window glass that does not shield out UVA.

The term *polymorphous* stems from the wide spectrum of clinical lesions that occur in various patients ("different patterns in different patients"); however, the lesions in any one patient tend to be relatively uniform. Polymorphous light eruption is usually most prominent following the first sun exposure in the spring or during a winter trip to sunny climates. The rash appears hours to days after exposure, lasts for several days, and resolves spontaneously. There is often some degree of "hardening" over the summer, and more sun can be tolerated without a rash; however, recurrences are to be expected.

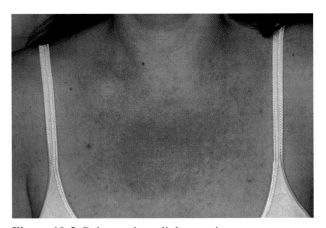

Figure 10-3 Polymorphous light eruption.

DISTINGUISHING FEATURES
- Female sex
- On different patients, lesions may be papules (most common), papulovesicles, erythematous plaques, erythema multiforme-like, or purpuric
- The rash appears within hours to days of exposure, and it subsides over the next 1 to 7 days
- The areas of greatest involvement are the "V" areas of the neck and chest (Fig. 10-3) and particularly the extensor surfaces of the arms (see Chapter 12, Arms). Curiously, the face is usually spared

- Most patients have associated pruritus, but some patients describe stinging and pain
- Typically, the lesions of PMLE first erupt at the onset of a vacation in a sunny place or at a high altitude and disappear by the time the patient returns home, and it decreases in severity as the summer progresses
- Usually only one morphology dominates in a given individual

DIAGNOSIS
- Based on the history and clinical picture
  The recognition of PMLE and other photosensitivity disorders resides in their photodistribution
- Skin biopsy; if necessary (see Appendix B)
- Normal titers of antinuclear antibodies (ANAs), as well as normal urine, stool, and blood porphyrin levels, help support the diagnosis
- Provocative photo testing when indicated

MANAGEMENT (see Appendix A)
- Broad-spectrum sunscreens and sun protective clothing
- Topical steroids
- Short, tapering course of oral steroids
- Beta carotene
- Hydroxychloroquine for difficult cases
- Controlled gradual exposure to UVB or psoralens and UVA light (PUVA) can harden skin and increase tolerance

Systemic Lupus Erythematosus

Besides the classic malar "butterfly" rash (see Chapter 6, Cheeks), photosensitivity is one of the eleven American College of Rheumatology criteria for **systemic lupus erythematosus (SLE).** According to the American College of Rheumatology, a person has SLE if four or more of the following criteria are present:

1. "Butterfly" rash
2. Lesions of chronic cutaneous lupus erythematosus such as discoid lupus erythematosus
3. Photosensitivity
4. Oral or pharyngeal ulcers
5. Arthritis in two or more joints
6. Serositis: pleuritis or pericarditis
7. Renal disorder
8. Neurologic disorder
9. Hematologic disorder
10. Immunologic disorder: anti-DNA, anti-Smith antibody, or a false-positive syphilis serologic result
11. ANAs

DISTINGUISHING FEATURES

- Marked female predominance; more common in blacks and Hispanics
- Macular erythematous or violaceous rash
- When involved, the eruption on the neck is in a photodistribution
- Less commonly, acute SLE presents as a generalized photosensitive eruption
- Photosensitivity may be the initial symptom of SLE
- Fatigue, fever, arthralgias, and malaise may be the presenting nonspecific symptoms
- Other cutaneous features of SLE may be present (e.g., "butterfly rash" [see Chapter 6, Cheeks], discoid lesions [see Chapter 1, Hair and Scalp], alopecia, nailfold changes)
- Major organ systems (renal, cardiac, neuropsychiatric)

DIAGNOSIS

- ANA titers are positive in 95% of patients (most often in a peripheral rim pattern)
- Anti-ds DNA (antibody to native double-stranded DNA) is present in 60% to 80% of patients and is more specific for SLE
- Anti-Sm antibody has a strong specificity for SLE. This is particularly relevant in patients in whom anti-dsDNA results are negative and may help exclude underlying systemic involvement

- Antiphospholipid antibodies are present in 25% of patients
- The erythrocyte sedimentation rate is usually elevated
- Hypocomplementemia occurs in 70% of patients and is noted especially when there is renal involvement in active SLE

MANAGEMENT

- Sun exposure should be avoided
- Prednisone is the mainstay of therapy
- Oral antimalarials hydroxychloroquine (**Plaquenil**) and chloroquine (**Aralen**) are sometimes used as first-line therapy
- Other therapeutic agents include:
  - Dapsone, gold, oral retinoids such as isotretinoin, and immunosuppressive drugs such as azathioprine (**Imuran**) and cyclophosphamide (**Cytoxan**) and methotrexate may be helpful. Such agents are used as adjuvant therapy because of their steroid-sparing effects
- Mycophenolate (**CellCept**) as well as interferon alfa-2a and alfa-2b (**Roferon** and **Intron A**) may also be used.
- Thalidomide and intravenous gamma-globulin are used in controlling recalcitrant cases

Dermatomyositis

Dermatomyositis is an inflammatory skin and muscle disease that is related to polymyositis; in fact, both conditions are considered to be the same disease except for the presence or absence of the rash. Cutaneous manifestations without detectable muscle disease are known as *amyopathic dermatomyositis*. An autoimmune origin has been proposed as a possible cause of dermatomyositis. As a result, antibodies that attack the skin and muscle are produced.

⚠ **ALERT: Adults with dermatomyositis appear to have an increased risk of internal malignant diseases. The skin disease often follows the clinical course of exacerbations and remissions of the cancer. Most are the common cancers (e.g., colon and breast cancer).**

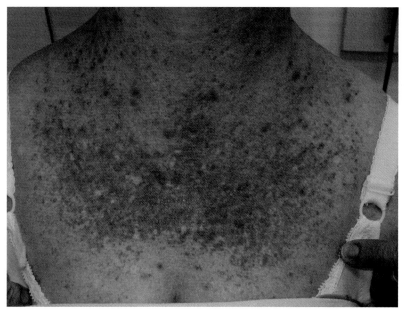

Figure 10-4 Dermatomyositis ("shawl" sign). (Image courtesy of Benjamin Barankin, MD.)

DISTINGUISHING FEATURES
- The female-to-male ratio is 2:1
- Poikiloderma is a characteristic rash of dermatomyositis, consisting of telangiectasia, atrophy, hyperpigmentation, and hypopigmentation. When it occurs on the "V" of the neck and upper back, it is referred to as the "shawl" sign (Fig. 10-4). It is also seen on the extensor (sun-exposed) forearms.
- Photosensitivity in areas of poikiloderma
- The heliotrope rash consists of red or violaceous coloration around the eyes and periorbital edema
- Gottron's papules are erythematous or violaceous, flat-topped papules on the dorsal knuckles and periungual telangiectasias and nail dystrophy (see Chapter 13, Hands and Fingers)
- Atrophic lesions may occur on the knees and elbows
- Proximal muscle weakness, arthralgias, pulmonary fibrosis, dysphagia, myocardial disease, and vasculitis, may occur
- Calcinosis cutis is seen in the juvenile form of dermatomyositis

DIAGNOSIS (see Appendix B)
- Skin biopsy findings are often nonspecific, but generally are suggestive of a connective tissue disease
- Elevation of creatine phosphokinase levels is often a reliable indicator of muscle involvement
- Aldolase levels may be increased
- Electromyography may aid in the diagnosis
- Muscle biopsy may aid in the diagnosis as well• Autoantibodies, such as anti-DNA, anti-RNP, and anti-Ro, may be found. Anti-M-1 antibody is highly specific for dermatomyositis (seen in only 25% of patients)
- An overlap syndrome with scleroderma or lupus (mixed connective tissue disease) is characterized by the presence of antiribonucleoprotein (anti-RNP) antibodies

✔ **TIP: ANA results are less likely to be positive in dermatomyositis, which mimics lupus erythematosus both clinically and histologically.**

MANAGEMENT (see Appendix A)

- For skin:
  - Sun exposure should be avoided; UV radiation may also exacerbate the underlying disease process itself
  - Antimalarial drugs: hydroxychloroquine **(Plaquenil),** low-dose oral methotrexate
- For systemic issues:
  - Systemic steroids (when used for systemic symptoms, may also improve skin conditions)
- Low-dose oral methotrexate
- Cyclosporine
- Cyclophosphamide
- Azathioprine
- Plasmapheresis
- Interferon
- Intravenous high-dose gamma-globulin
- Physical therapy, if necessary

ALSO CONSIDER
- Other photosensitivity/photodermatoses:
  - Photocontact dermatitis
  - Photodrug reaction
  - Solar urticaria
- Mixed connective tissue disease or overlap syndrome

RARELY
- Actinic prurigo
- Hydroa vacciniforme
- Chronic actinic dermatitis
- Erythropoietic porphyria

Lichen Simplex Chronicus *vs* Atopic Dermatitis *vs* Contact Dermatitis

Lichen Simplex Chronicus

Lichen simplex chronicus (LSC), also known as *neurodermatitis*, is a common, chronic, often solitary, pruritic eczematous eruption caused by repetitive rubbing and scratching. It is most often noted in adults, particularly in patients with other atopic manifestations such as asthma and allergic rhinitis. The neck, wrists, extensor forearms, ankles, pretibial areas, and inner thighs are common sites. Lichen simplex chronicus may also involve the vulva, scrotum, intragluteal area, and perianal area (see Chapter 12, Arms and Wrists; Chapter 18, Genital Area; Chapter 21, Legs).

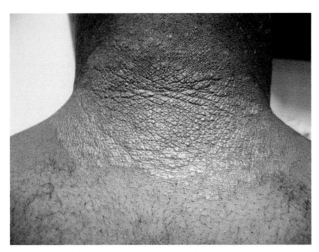

Figure 10-5 Lichen simplex chronicus.

DISTINGUISHING FEATURES
- Focal lichenified plaque or multiple plaques, most often on the nape of the neck (Fig. 10-5)
- Thick, leathery skin, due to constant scratching and rubbing results in the epidermis becoming hypertrophied and results in thickening of the skin and exaggeration of the normal skin markings, giving the skin a tree bark–like appearance
- Chronic or paroxysmal pruritus is the primary symptom

DIAGNOSIS
- Atopic history often noted
- The diagnosis is readily apparent and is made on clinical grounds
- No history of contactant (e.g., hair dye, cosmetics, perfume)

MANAGEMENT (see Appendix A)
- The most important aspect of therapy is the elimination of scratching and rubbing
- May be treated with an intermediate-strength (class 3 or 4) topical corticosteroid. If necessary, a high-potency (class 1) topical corticosteroid can be used
- Oral antihistamines may be helpful at bedtime because of their sedative effect

Atopic Dermatitis

Atopic dermatitis (atopic eczema) often starts in early infancy. By age one, lesions begin to occur in the flexural creases and diaper area (see Chapter 18, Genital Area). For a more complete discussion, see Chapter 3, Eyelids and Periorbital Area.

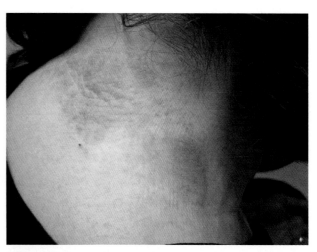

Figure 10-7 Atopic dermatitis.

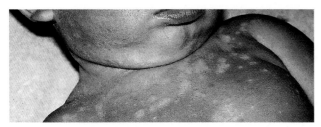

Figure 10-6 Atopic dermatitis, infant.

DISTINGUISHING FEATURES
- In infants, red, glazed, sometimes scaly, pruritic eczematous plaques in neck flexures (Fig. 10-6)
- Children and adults tend to have lichenified plaques (Fig. 10-7)

DIAGNOSIS
- Clinical
- Atopic diathesis in family (in first- or second-degree relative)
- Eczematous lesions are often present elsewhere on the body

MANAGEMENT (see Appendix A)
- Low-potency topical steroids; higher potency in adults
- Tacrolimus (**Protopic ointment**) 1%, 0.03%, pimecrolimus cream (**Elidel**)
- Emollients, barrier creams/lotions such as **CeraVe** and **EpiCeram**

Contact Dermatitis

There are two types of **contact dermatitis (CD):** irritant contact dermatitis **(ICD)**, caused by excessive contact with water, soaps, and makeup, and **allergic contact dermatitis (ACD),** which involves a true allergic reaction to material in contact with the skin (see also Chapter 6, Cheeks). Hair dye, makeup, and perfumes are potential causes of CD in women, and aftershave products and cologne are causes in men. Chemicals in the air may produce an airborne ICD or ACD; for example, insecticide sprays or from the burning residue of *Rhus* (poison ivy or poison oak), which causes rhus dermatitis. In infants, ICD tends to occur most often in the diaper area (diaper rash, napkin dermatitis).

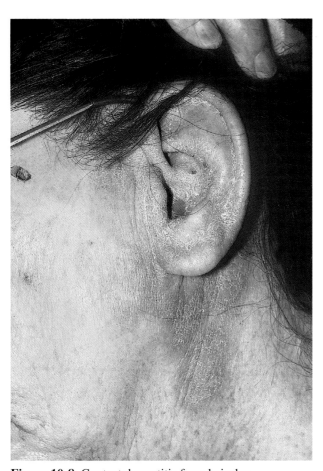

Figure 10-8 Contact dermatitis from hair dye.

INFANT/CHILD

DISTINGUISHING FEATURES
- Neck folds and diaper area (see Chapter 18, Genital Area)
- Affects males and females equally
- Generally non–immune-mediated condition (ICD)

DIAGNOSIS
- History

MANAGEMENT (see Appendix A)
- Avoidance of contactant
- Low-potency topical steroids
- Petrolatum, **DESITIN Rapid Relief Cream** (13% zinc oxide, aloe, and vitamin E), barrier creams/lotions such as **CeraVe** and **EpiCeram**

ADULT

DISTINGUISHING FEATURES

- Affects females more than males
- History of contactant (e.g., hair dye, cosmetics, perfume)
- Pattern and distribution of the eruption often suggests the cause (Fig. 10-8)
- Immune-mediated condition (ACD) or non–immune mediated condition (ICD)

DIAGNOSIS

- History
- Patch testing (see Appendix B), if necessary

MANAGEMENT

- Avoidance of contactant
- Low- to high-potency topical steroids

ALSO CONSIDER
- Infant/child
  - Seborrheic dermatitis
  - Fungal infections

RARELY
- Histiocytosis X (Langerhans cell histiocytosis)
- Adult
  - Seborrheic dermatitis
  - Psoriasis
  - Berlock dermatitis

RARELY
- Cutaneous T-cell lymphoma (mycosis fungoides)

Acne Keloidalis Nuchae *vs* Folliculitis/Furunculosis

Acne Keloidalis

Acne keloidalis nuchae (folliculitis keloidalis) is a condition affecting the nape of the neck. The name *acne keloidalis* is actually a misnomer. It has nothing to do with acne; it is actually a type of folliculitis, although keloids may result. The pathogenesis of acne keloidalis is similar to that of pseudofolliculitis barbae (see Chapter 9, Chin and Mandibular Area), in which coiled hairs produce a reentry phenomenon and the ingrown hairs irritate the wall of the hair follicle and result in inflammation. As in pseudofolliculitis barbae, acne keloidalis nuchae it most frequently affects adult African American, African Caribbean, and Hispanic men. The condition may persist for many years.

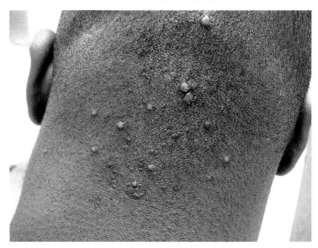

Figure 10-9 Acne keloidalis nuchae.

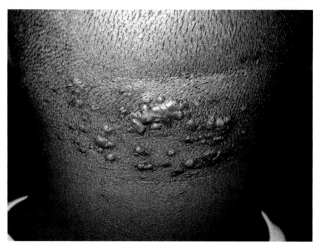

Figure 10-10 Acne keloidalis nuchae with scarring. (Image courtesy of Benjamin Barankin, MD.)

DISTINGUISHING FEATURES
- Affects males much more than females
- Characteristically seen in the lower occipital area, but it can extend to the adjacent nape of the neck or the entire scalp and thus may be indistinguishable from folliculitis decalvans (see Chapter 1, Hair and Scalp)
- Initially, inflammatory papules and pustules are noted (folliculitis) in young black men
- Ultimately, small scars form characterized by flesh-colored papules (Fig. 10-9)
- Hypertrophic scarring alopecia and, ultimately, keloid formation may occur (Fig. 10-10)

DIAGNOSIS
- Clinical

MANAGEMENT (see Appendix A)
- Avoidance of close clipper shaves and haircuts
- Potent topical or intralesional steroids (5 to 10 mg/mL) help decrease itching and inflammation (see Appendix B)
- **Topical antibiotics** are used when papules and pustules are present
- A systemic antibiotic such as minocycline seems to be helpful because of its anti-inflammatory effect
- Oral isotretinoin (**Accutane**)
- Surgical treatment is not without risk. It is reserved for extreme cases and may result in keloidal scarring
- Laser excision or vaporization

Folliculitis/Furunculosis

Folliculitis is defined as a superficial or deep infection or inflammation of hair follicles. If it involves the deeper part of the follicle, it may result in a **furuncle** (boil). Individual furuncles can cluster together and form an interconnected network of furuncles called **carbuncles.** Lesions occur on hair-bearing areas (see also Chapter 1, Hair and Scalp; Chapter 9, Chin and Mandibular Area; Chapter 11, Axillae; Chapter 21, Legs). Folliculitis has multiple causes: various infections, physical or chemical irritation, occlusive dressings, or the use of topical or systemic steroids. Bacterial folliculitis, most often, coagulase-positive *Staphylococcus aureus* is the responsible pathogenic bacterium more commonly found in patients who are diabetic, obese, or immunocompromised.

DISTINGUISHING FEATURES
- Folliculitis consists of superficial pustules or papules with a central hair (may not always be visible)
- Lesions often polymorphic, displaying a mixture of papules and pustules (Fig. 10-11)
- A furuncle is a deep form of folliculitis that is often quite tender

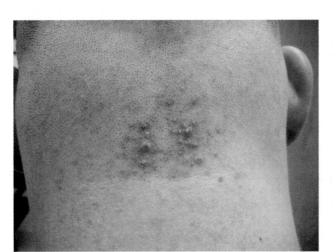

Figure 10-11 Folliculitis.

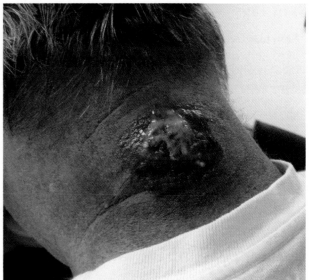

Figure 10-12 Carbuncle.

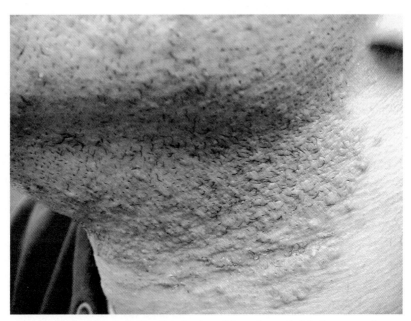

Figure 10-13 Pseudofolliculitis barbae. Note the curled hairs reentering the skin and the acnelike papules.

- Carbuncles are furuncles with "multiple heads" (Fig. 10-12)

DIAGNOSIS
- Clinical
- Bacterial culture and sensitivity

MANAGEMENT
- See Chapter 9, Chin and Mandibular Area
- **Furuncle**
  - Warm compresses
  - Incision and drainage when fluctuant
  - Oral antibiotics are often unnecessary after an incision and drainage is performed

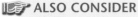 **ALSO CONSIDER**
- Acne
- Folliculitis decalvans
- Pseudofolliculitis barbae (Fig. 10-13)

Skin Tags *vs* Seborrheic Keratoses

Skin Tags

Skin tags (acrochordons, fibroepithelial polyps, fibroepitheliomas) are extremely common benign skin lesions; when large, they are referred to as soft fibromas or pedunculated lipofibromas. Skin tags are often seen in the body folds (neck, axillae, eyelids, and groin) and tend to be more numerous in persons who are obese. Larger lesions (fibroepitheliomas) can be up to 5 cm in diameter are often noted in the inguinal area. A family history of skin tags often exists and an association with type 2 diabetes mellitus has been observed (see also Chapter 3, Eyelids and Periorbital Area and Chapter 20, Inguinal Area).

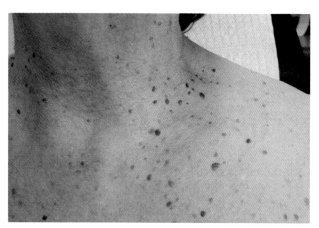

Figure 10-14 Skin tags and seborrheic keratoses.

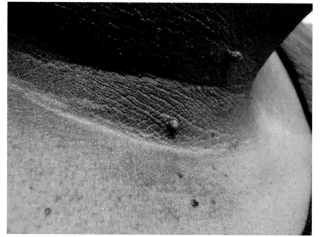

Figure 10-15 Acanthosis nigricans and skin tags. (Image courtesy of Rebecca Kleinerman, MD.)

DISTINGUISHING FEATURES
- Pedunculated, sessile, or filiform, flesh-colored or brown 1 to 10 mm round, soft, papules on the sides of the neck
- Often seen in association with acanthosis nigricans and in pregnant women (Figs. 10-14 and 10-15)
- **TIP:** Appear primarily in adults
- Primarily of cosmetic concern; however, they may become a nuisance from irritation of necklaces or catching on collars

DIAGNOSIS
- Skin tags are easy to recognize; a skin biopsy is rarely necessary

MANAGEMENT
- Small skin tags are easily removed by snipping them off at their base using an iris scissors, with or without prior local anesthesia
- Occasionally, they may spontaneously self-destruct, become necrotic, and autoamputate
- ✔ **TIP: A rapid and painless treatment for small skin tags is to dip a "mosquito" forceps into liquid nitrogen (LN$_2$) for 10 to 15 seconds and then gently grasp each skin tag for about 5 to 10 seconds. There is little or no collateral damage, just a narrow rim of erythema occurs. Multiple lesions can be treated by this method. The frozen skin tag will be shed in approximately 10 days. This is a good approach for small skin tags on the eyelids and neck (see also Appendix B).**

Seborrheic Keratoses

A **seborrheic keratosis (SK)** is an extremely common benign, harmless, lesion. It is the most common neoplasm in the elderly (see Chapter 2, Forehead and Temples). Some cases are inherited through an autosomal dominant mode.

DISTINGUISHING FEATURES
- Affects males as much as females
- Appearance of lesions on the neck tends to be indistinguishable from small pigmented skin tags (see previous discussion) (see Fig. 10-14)
- Color ranges from tan to dark brown to black
- As with skin tags, SK may itch and rub or catch on clothing, thus becoming inflamed
- Mainly a cosmetic concern, SK also serves as a daily reminder of aging and may have negative psychological connotations

DIAGNOSIS
- Easily recognized
- If necessary, a shave or scissor snip biopsy may be performed for histologic confirmation

MANAGEMENT (see Appendix B)
- Cryosurgery is performed with LN$_2$ spray or cotton swab
- Light electrocautery and curettage

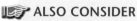
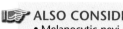

ALSO CONSIDER
- Melanocytic nevi
- Warts
- Neurofibroma

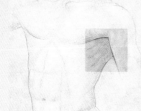

Axillae

Intertriginous areas such as the axillae, inframammary area, toe webs, and groin represent two opposing surfaces that are continually in intimate contact due to repeated friction. In addition, such warm, moist environments provide an excellent setting for potential fungal as well as bacterial infections.

The axillary areas are subject to a host of irritants, such as underarm shaving, deodorants, and antiperspirants, as well as a venue for a variety of inflammatory dermatoses such as atopic dermatitis, psoriasis, seborrheic dermatitis, and intertrigo. The sun-shaded axillae are not likely to absorb much in the way of ultraviolet exposure and are generally spared many skin cancers, although various benign skin growths such as skin tags, melanocytic nevi, and seborrheic keratoses are commonly found here (see Chapter 10, Neck).

IN THIS CHAPTER

- Intertrigo *vs* contact dermatitis *vs* atopic dermatitis
- Inverse psoriasis *vs* cutaneous candidiasis
- Hidradenitis suppurativa *vs* folliculitis/furuncle

Intertrigo vs Contact Dermatitis vs Atopic Dermatitis

Intertrigo

Intertrigo is a very common superficial inflammatory process that occurs in places where opposing skin surfaces rub against each other: the axillae, creases of the lips (see Chapter 7, Lips and Perioral Area), inguinal and intragluteal creases (see Chapter 19, Buttocks and Perineal Area, Gluteal Cleft), under the breasts (see Chapter 16, Breasts and Inframammary Area), and the abdominal folds. Intertrigo may also affect other similar areas (folds of the neck creases, antecubital fossae, umbilicus, and finger web spaces).

Such restricted areas are prone to inflammatory rashes because of the relatively high skin temperature, moisture from insensible water loss, and sweat that is prevented from evaporating. Furthermore, friction from movement of adjacent skin results in maceration and chafing. Complicating factors may include atopy, hyperhidrosis, diabetes, and obesity as well as colonization by secondary infection such as *Candida albicans* (see later discussion) and certain bacteria that normally reside on the skin without any problems.

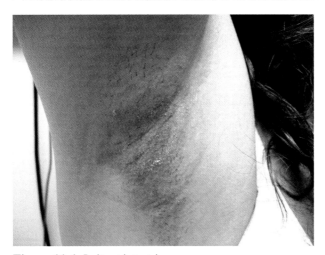

Figure 11-1 Irritant intertrigo.

DISTINGUISHING FEATURES
- It begins as a mild erythema followed by erythematous well-demarcated patches or plaques that oppose each other on either side of the skinfolds (mirror image) (Fig. 11-1)
- Often pruritic; may progress to erosions, oozing, exudation, and painful fissures within the plaques
- Particularly common in those who are obese
- Secondary overgrowth with *Candida* species, tinea, and bacteria, should be considered

DIAGNOSIS
- Clinical
- Exclusion of other diagnoses (e.g., contact dermatitis, psoriasis, seborrheic dermatitis, as well as bacterial or fungal infection (negative potassium hydroxide [KOH] and/or fungal culture), although such infections may be may be secondary phenomena)

MANAGEMENT
Prevention
- Promote drying, aeration, and skin-to-skin friction (e.g., air conditioning, fans, hair dryer with heat off)
- Nonrestrictive clothing
- Weight loss, if necessary
- Gentle underarm shaving techniques
- Avoid oily or irritant ointments or cosmetics
- **Zeasorb** powder

Treatment (see Appendix A)
- Burow's solution compresses to exudative, oozing areas
- The lowest-potency nonfluorinated topical steroids are used to avoid atrophy and striae. To achieve rapid improvement, treatment may be initiated with a higher-potency (class 5) steroid that is used for several days before it is changed to a lower-potency (class 6 or 7) agent
- ⚠ **ALERT: Intertriginous areas are inherently moist and occluded; therefore, the penetration and potency of topical agents are increased in these regions; consequently, topical steroids are more likely to produce striae (linear atrophy), and, possibly ulcers**
- For longer term use:
  - Tacrolimus (**Protopic**) ointment 0.03% or 0.1% once or twice daily
  - Pimecrolimus (**Elidel**) cream 1% once or twice daily

Contact Dermatitis

Contact dermatitis, both **nonallergic contact dermatitis (irritant contact dermatitis [ICD])** and **allergic contact dermatitis (ACD),** occur in the axillary vault. Examples of irritants include various soaps, underarm shaving, and deodorants/antiperspirants that can irritate and damage the skin after repeated contact. Patients who have atopic dermatitis are more likely to develop ICD as a result of their inherent skin sensitivity and defective barrier function. ACD in this area may be the result of an allergy to dry cleaning solvents (formaldehyde), topical medications, as well as deodorants and antiperspirants. For a more complete discussion, see Chapter 3, Eyelids and Periorbital Area.

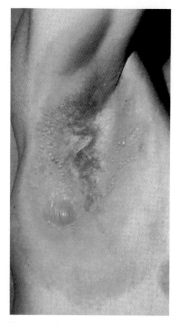

Figure 11-2 Contact dermatitis due to formaldehyde in dry cleaning fluid (note sparing of axillary vault). (Image courtesy of Vincent S. Beltrani, MD.)

DISTINGUISHING FEATURES

- Mild erythema initially, followed by erythematous, well-demarcated plaques
- Pruritus

DIAGNOSIS

- History of contactant (e.g., deodorants/antiperspirants or dry cleaning solvents) (Fig. 11-2)
- Exclusion of other diagnoses such as atopic dermatitis (see previous discussion)
- Patch testing (see Appendix B), if necessary, is used to confirm ACD and identify potential allergen(s).
- ⚠ **ALERT: Topical steroid contact dermatitis should be suspected if the dermatitis worsens with steroid applications. The allergen may be the steroid itself or in the vehicle of the topical preparation**

MANAGEMENT

- Patients should be told to avoid the offending agent or to minimize contact with it
- Low- to high- (short-term) potency topical steroids (see Appendix A)

Atopic Dermatitis

Often an intertriginous eruption is a variant of **atopic dermatitis** (Fig. 11-3). An atopic history is frequently elicited.

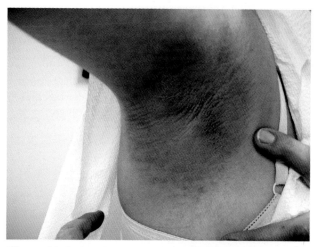

Figure 11-3 Atopic dermatitis (note lichenification).

DIAGNOSIS/MANAGEMENT

- See Chapter 18, Genital Area

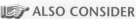

ALSO CONSIDER
- Tinea corporis
- Cutaneous candidiasis
- Inverse psoriasis (see following discussion)
- Intertriginous seborrheic dermatitis

RARELY
- Erythrasma
- Fox Fordyce disease
- Hailey-Hailey disease

Inverse Psoriasis vs Cutaneous Candidiasis

Inverse psoriasis

Inverse psoriasis occurs when psoriatic lesions occur primarily in the intertriginous areas such as the axillae, inframammary, perineal, and inguinal creases (see also Chapter 16, Breasts and Inframammary Area; Chapter 17, Umbilicus; Chapter 19, Buttocks and Perineal Area, Gluteal Cleft; Chapter 20, Inguinal Area). Because of the moist nature of the skinfolds, the appearance of the psoriatic plaques is slightly different than that seen on the elbows and knees—they generally do not have the typical silvery scale; rather, they are characteristically shiny and smooth. There also may be fissuring in the depth of the skin creases. Flexural psoriasis is often difficult to tell apart from atopic dermatitis, seborrheic dermatitis, intertrigo, and candidiasis.

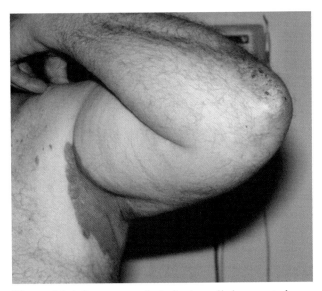

Figure 11-4 Inverse psoriasis (note well-demarcated plaque).

DISTINGUISHING FEATURES
- The deep pink to red color and well-defined borders characteristic of psoriasis may be obvious; however, lesions generally lack scale (constant rubbing of two apposing surfaces does not allow scale to build up) (Fig. 11-4)
- May be pruritic
- Fissures may occur

DIAGNOSIS
- Clinical
- Psoriasis may be present elsewhere on the body
- Negative KOH and/or fungal culture

MANAGEMENT (see Appendix A)
- Low-potency, nonfluorinated topical steroids (class 6 or 7) or, if necessary, a higher-potency (class 5) steroid that is used for several days before it is changed to a lower-potency agent
- Stronger topical steroids need to be used with care and only for a few days at a time. If the psoriasis has cleared, the application of the steroid cream should be discontinued; however, it may be used again short-term when the condition recurs
- Systemic agents are rarely required for limited flexural psoriasis, and phototherapy is ineffective because the skinfolds are hidden from ultraviolet light exposure
- Vitamin D-like compounds such as calcipotriol **Dovonex** and **Vectical** cream or ointment may be used primarily or in rotation with a mild topical steroid
- Calcineurin inhibitors, tacrolimus (**Protopic**) ointment 1%, or pimecrolimus (**Elidel**) cream 1% are applied once or twice daily for longer-term use
- Different topical medications are used together or in rotation for best effect or to minimize side effects

☑ **TIP: Inverse psoriasis is commonly misdiagnosed by those who are not dermatologists as tinea or candidiasis. Accordingly, it is often incorrectly treated with topical antifungal agents.**

⚠ **ALERT: Overuse and/or continuous application of topical steroids may cause stretch marks and marked thinning of the skin, and it can result in aggravation (rebound) of psoriasis (tachyphylaxis).**

Cutaneous Candidiasis

Cutaneous candidiasis (see also Chapter 16, Breasts and Inframammary Area; Chapter 17, Umbilicus; Chapter 19, Buttocks and Perineal Area, Gluteal Cleft; Chapter 20, Inguinal Area) is characterized by infection with *Candida* species. *Candida* species are a common secondary and sometimes primary cause of intertrigo in both elderly, diabetic, and immunocompromised patients. Most cases occur in skinfolds, where occlusion by clothing produces warm, moist conditions. Candidal infection of the skin under the breasts occurs when such areas become macerated under pendulous breasts.

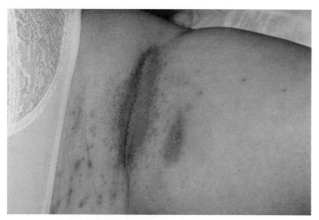

Figure 11-5 Candidiasis (note satellite pustules).

DISTINGUISHING FEATURES
- "Beefy red" lesions
- Satellite pustules may be seen beyond the border of the plaques (Fig. 11-5)
- Maceration and fissures may be present
- Soreness and/or pruritus

DIAGNOSIS
- Positive KOH examination for budding yeast or positive culture for *Candida* species

MANAGEMENT (see Appendix A)
- The skin should be patted dry or dried with a hair dryer (no heat)
- Topical ketoconazole, clotrimazole, or miconazole twice daily
- Patients with extensive infection may require the addition of fluconazole (**Diflucan**) or itraconazole (**Sporanox**) or ketoconazole
- For acute candidal intertrigo, apply **Burow's solution** compresses to exudative, oozing areas

ALSO CONSIDER
- Tinea corporis
- Atopic dermatitis
- Intertrigo
- Contact dermatitis
- Intertriginous seborrheic dermatitis

RARELY
- Erythrasma
- Fox Fordyce disease
- Hailey-Hailey disease

Hidradenitis Suppurativa

Hidradenitis suppurativa (HS), referred to as *acne inversa* in Europe, is a chronic, recurrent, scarring, autosomal dominant, inflammatory disease that affects the skin-bearing apocrine sweat glands of the axillae, inguinal folds, suprapubic area, anogenital area, buttocks, areola, and submammary areas. Lesions may also be seen on the perineum, submammary areas, and the buttocks. HS tends to have a higher incidence and be more severe in black women. The cause is unknown. Bacterial involvement is considered a secondary pathogenic event. In its early stages, HS is most often confused with chronic furunculosis. Remissions may occur more frequently as the patient ages or as more scar tissue develops; however, total spontaneous resolution is rare. HS tends to decline in severity at, or after, menopause.

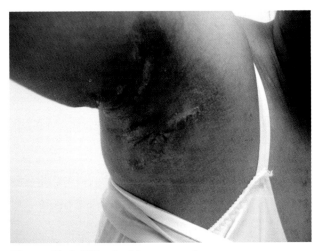

Figure 11-6 Hidradenitis suppurativa.

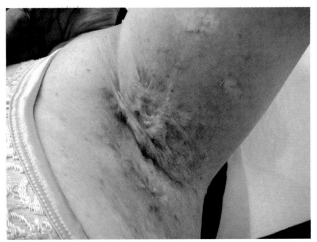

Figure 11-7 Hidradenitis suppurativa.

DISTINGUISHING FEATURES
- Seen almost exclusively in women and only rarely before puberty
- Similar to acne, HS is related to androgen excess and often flares with menstruation
- Frequently improves during pregnancy, only to flare during the postpartum period
- Initially, HS presents with nodules and abscesses that may be indistinguishable from furuncles or common "boils" (see following discussion)
- Lesions are painful and tender, and they often become infected secondarily and exude a serosanguineous or foul-smelling purulent material that may stain clothing (Fig. 11-6)
- Lesions recur, new lesions crop up, and old lesions scar in a frustrating, unrelenting process
- Chronic HS is indicated by the appearance of sinus tract and fistula formation, ulcerations, and eventually, hypertrophic, ropelike linear bands of scars and contractures (Fig. 11-7)
- Characteristic multiple open comedones ("blackheads") develop in long-standing cases

DIAGNOSIS
- The multiple lesions that scar and form sinus tracts should be easily distinguishable from other conditions

MANAGEMENT
General Measures
- Actively discharging lesions should be cultured
- Hidradenitis suppurativa is a difficult, frustrating condition to control
- Weight loss
- Use of ventilated cotton clothing

Treatment
- **Topical therapy**
  - Limited and very early disease may be helped somewhat by the daily use of topical antibiotics such as clindamycin or erythromycin
- **Systemic therapy** (see Appendix A and B)
  - Long-term administration of an antibiotic, such as minocycline that also has an anti-inflammatory action, can be used to prevent episodic flares. Lower doses may effective for maintenance once control is established. Alternative antibiotics include erythromycin, ciprofloxacin, cephalexin, and dicloxacillin
  - A tapering course of prednisone over 2 to 3 weeks for acute flares/or intralesional corticosteroid injections triamcinolone acetonide (**Kenalog,** 2.5 to 10 mg/mL)
  - Oral contraceptives and oral antiandrogens do not seem to work as well as they do with acne

- Systemic retinoids, such as oral isotretinoin (**Accutane**), have been used with limited benefit
- Infliximab (**Remicade**) and adalimumab (**Humira**) are monoclonal antibodies that target tumor necrosis factor-alpha have been anecdotally reported to be effective in some severe cases of HS

- **Surgical therapy**
  - Incision and drainage of large, painful cysts
  - Early radical excision of severe refractory HS may produce a definitive cure
  - Narrow excisions may help temporarily, but this method has a high recurrence rate
  - Ablation techniques using a carbon dioxide laser that spares normal tissue have been tried successfully

Folliculitis/Furunculosis

Axillary **folliculitis** is often due to irritation from underarm shaving (see also Chapter 9, Chin and Mandibular Area; Chapter 10, Neck). Lesions occur on hair-bearing areas—the face, scalp, thighs, and body folds (see also Chapter 1, Hair and Scalp; Chapter 21, Legs). Axillary folliculitis has multiple causes: various infections, physical or chemical irritation, and occlusive dressings. Nonbacterial, or sterile, folliculitis can arise from physical or chemical irritation. Such irritants include waxing, shaving, depilatories, and electrolysis. Bacterial folliculitis, most often coagulase-positive *Staphylococcus aureus,* is the responsible pathogenic bacterium. If folliculitis involves the deeper part of the follicle, it may result in a **furuncle.**

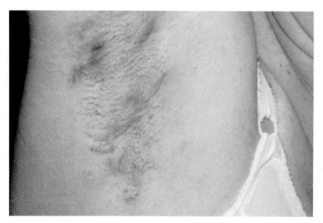

Figure 11-8 Chronic folliculitis/furunculosis.

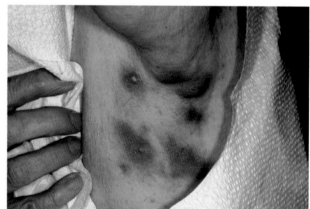

Figure 11-9 Furunculosis.

DISTINGUISHING FEATURES
- **Bacterial folliculitis** (usually *S. aureus*)
  - Red, follicular papules and pustules displaying a mixture of papules and pustules may be present in one or both axillae (Fig. 11-8)
- **Furuncle**
  - An acute, tender, inflamed nodule(s)
  - After a few days, the surface may thin, become fluctuant, and rupture spontaneously

DIAGNOSIS
- Clinical
- Pustules or draining furuncles may be cultured (bacterial culture and sensitivity)

MANAGEMENT
- **Folliculitis:** for further discussion, see Chapter 9, Chin and Mandibular Area
- **Furuncle/furunculosis:** for further discussion, see Chapter 10, Neck (Fig. 11-9)

ALSO CONSIDER
- Abscess
- Lymphadenitis
- Cat-scratch disease

RARELY
- Sinus tracts and fistulas associated with ulcerative colitis and regional enteritis
- Hailey-Hailey disease

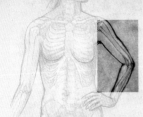

CHAPTER 12

Arms

The upper arms and forearms have two contrasting aspects—the sun-exposed extensor surface and the sun-protected flexor surface. Different conditions affect each side. Predictably, the sun-exposed arm is subject to sun damage (dermatoheliosis), photoeruptions (polymorphous light eruption), systemic lupus erythematosus, dermatomyositis, solar keratoses, squamous cell carcinomas (SCCs), keratoacanthoma, solar lentigines, and melanoma. In contrast, the inner, sun-protected flexural areas (e.g., antecubital and popliteal fossae) are common settings for atopic dermatitis (AD) and not sun-induced dermatoses. The elbows and knees are the primary sites for psoriasis, and the flexor wrists and extensor legs are primary sites for lichen planus and scabies.

IN THIS CHAPTER

Upper Arms
- Keratosis pilaris *vs* acne vulgaris
- Melanoma *vs* benign nevus

Elbows
- Localized plaque psoriasis *vs* lichen simplex chronicus
- Granuloma annulare *vs* eruptive and tuberous xanthomas

Extensor Surface
- Polymorphous light eruption *vs* drug-induced photosensitivity
- Solar keratosis *vs* squamous cell carcinoma *vs* keratoacanthoma

Antecubital Fossae, Flexor Forearms, and Wrists
- Atopic dermatitis *vs* rhus dermatitis (poison ivy, poison oak) *vs* scabies *vs* lichen planus

Keratosis Pilaris

Keratosis pilaris (KP), an inherited disorder of keratinization, is a very common condition in which there are numerous rough follicular papules that most often arise on the outer aspect of the upper arms. Keratosis pilaris may also appear on the cheeks (see also Chapter 6, Cheeks, Fig. 6-3), thighs, and less often on the forearms, upper back, and buttocks. It is most obvious during the teenage years, but may also be present in infants and persist into adult life. Keratosis pilaris is uncommon in the elderly; however, it is particularly prevalent in those who have atopic dermatitis and/or ichthyosis vulgaris.

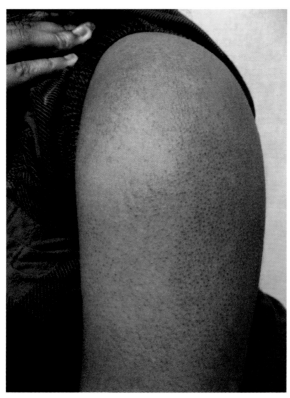

Figure 12-1 Keratosis pilaris.

DISTINGUISHING FEATURES
- Tiny, rough, whitish, red, or tan spiny bumps distributed in a gridlike pattern (Fig. 12-1)
- "Goose flesh," "sandpaperlike" appearance and texture when palpated
- When erythematous and inflamed, KP resembles, and is often mistaken for, acne
- Usually worse during the winter months
- In children, the lateral sides of the cheeks are frequently involved

DIAGNOSIS
- Clinical, often made by simple inspection and palpation of the affected skin

MANAGEMENT (see Appendix A)
- There is no cure or very effective treatment; however, the roughness can be lessened temporarily by applying certain moisturizers, exfoliating or barrier creams, or lotions such as ammonium lactate 10% **(Lac-Hydrin),** available in a cream or lotion, reduces roughness and softens the keratin plugs. However, it does not lessen the redness caused by the condition. Urea-containing products such as **Carmol** and **Keralac** moisturize and soften dry, rough skin. They also help loosen and remove the dead skin cells
- Topical retinoids may be an effective temporary treatment, but they can cause bothersome skin irritations, such as severe dryness, redness, and exfoliation. Tretinoin **(Retin-A Micro, Avita)** and tazarotene **(Tazorac)** are examples of topical retinoids

Acne Vulgaris

Acne vulgaris frequently involves the upper arms, shoulders, and trunk (see also Chapter 2, Forehead and Temples; Chapter 6, Cheeks; Chapter 15, Trunk). Besides typical teenage acne, performance-enhancement supplements have been implicated in acnelike lesions on the arms and trunk.

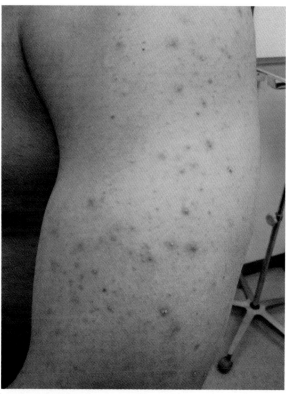

Figure 12-2 Acne.

DISTINGUISHING FEATURES
- Acneiform lesions, papules, and pustules (Fig. 12-2)
- Small lesions may be difficult to distinguish from KP

DIAGNOSIS
- Clinical

MANAGEMENT (see Appendix C)

ALSO CONSIDER
- Ichthyosis vulgaris (see Chapter 21, Legs)
- Follicular eczema

RARELY
- X-linked ichthyosis

Melanoma *vs* Benign Nevus

Melanoma

Melanoma (see also Chapter 15, Trunk; Chapter 21, Legs), a cancer of melanocytes, generally occurs in the skin and, much less commonly, in the eyes, ears, gastrointestinal tract, leptomeninges of the central nervous system, and oral and genital mucous membranes. It is the most common cancer in women 25 to 29 years of age. Melanoma is also commonly seen in patients with defects of DNA repair such as *xeroderma pigmentosum* and in patients with *familial atypical mole syndrome*. Uncommon in blacks and Asians, it is also more often seen in patients who have an abundance of melanocytic nevi. Although basal cell and squamous cell carcinoma (nonmelanoma skin cancers) are associated with long-term exposure to sunlight, melanoma is more likely to occur with infrequent but strong exposures that result in sunburns. Melanomas are more likely to occur on areas that are less often exposed and frequently burned, specifically the backs of men and the legs of women. Risk factors include:

- Light complexion, an inability to tan, and a history of sunburns
- Moles that are numerous, changing, or atypical such as **dysplastic nevi** (see Chapter 15, Trunk)
- A personal or family history of melanoma (first-degree relatives)
- A personal or family history of basal or squamous cell carcinoma

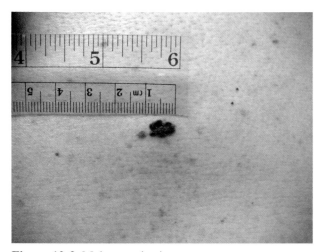

Figure 12-3 Melanoma in situ.

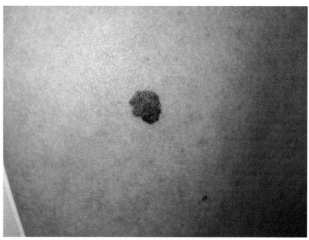

Figure 12-4 Superficial spreading melanoma. Note asymmetry, notched border, variegated color, and more than 6 mm in diameter.

DISTINGUISHING FEATURES

- Warning signs: symptomatic moles (e.g., moles that itch, burn, or are painful)
- Superficial spreading melanoma (SSM), by far the most common type, may arise de novo or in a pre-existing nevus. An initial in situ slow horizontal growth phase (Fig. 12-3), if left untreated, is followed in months or years by a vertical growth phase (lesions that extend vertically in the skin), which indicates invasive disease and potential metastasis. White coloration may indicate regression or scarring

- The lesions of SSM may conform to some (or all) of the "ABCDE" criteria for melanoma, in which the primary lesion is a macular lesion or an elevated plaque that displays the following (Fig. 12-4):
  - **Asymmetry:** if the lesion "folded" on itself, the halves do not match
  - **Border:** irregular or jagged (like a jigsaw puzzle)
  - **Color:** varied or having different shades (may have brown, black, pink, blue-gray, white, or admixtures of these colors)

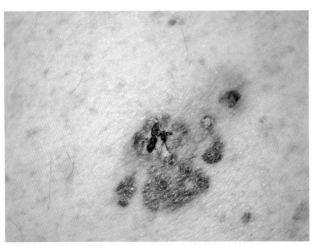

Figure 12-5 Invasive melanoma. Note asymmetry, notched border, variegated color, more than 6 mm diameter, and crusting. (Image courtesy of Benjamin Barankin, MD.)

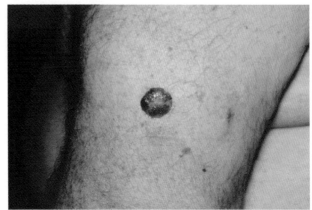

Figure 12-6 Nodular melanoma.

- **Diameter:** greater than 6 mm (the size of a pencil eraser) but may be smaller when first detected
- **Evolution** (or change in a pre-existing lesion): in size, color, elevation, or any new symptom such as bleeding, itching, or crusting (Fig 12-5)
- **Clinical variants**
  - Nodular melanoma
    - The lesion arises de novo as a nodule or plaque. It occurs in 15% to 20% of patients (Fig. 12-6)
    - Because of their rapid vertical growth phase, lesions invade early
    - Lesions are blue, blue-black, or nonpigmented (as in amelanotic melanoma); color is generally more uniform than that of SSM
    - May ulcerate and bleed with minor trauma
    - Occur more commonly on the legs and trunk
  - Lentigo maligna/lentigo maligna melanoma (see Chapter 6, Cheeks)
  - Acral lentiginous melanoma (see Chapter 14, Fingernails; Chapter 22, Feet)

DIAGNOSIS
- Dermoscopy, also referred to as *dermatoscopy* (see Appendix B). is a noninvasive method that allows the evaluation of colors and microstructures of the epidermis. Diagnostic patterns related to the distribution of colors and structures can better suggest a malignant or benign lesion
- Excisional biopsy that includes as much of the pigmented lesion as possible

MANAGEMENT
- Elliptical excision should include the entire visible lesion down to the subcutaneous fat
- Surgical margins of 5 mm currently are recommended for melanoma in situ
- For lesions with a thickness of less than 1 mm, a 1-cm margin of normal skin is usually adequate
- For thicker lesions, the margin should be more than 1 cm. The margin size is based on the histologic type and anatomic location of the lesion
- Elective lymph node dissection is not recommended for lesions that are less than 1 mm thick, unless lymph nodes are palpable. The decision whether to perform elective lymph node dissection on thicker lesions (1 to 4 mm) is controversial
- Sentinel lymph node biopsy, the dissection and evaluation of the lymph node closest to the site of the primary melanoma), may allow for a less dramatic lymph node ablation. The use of sentinel lymph node biopsy is also a controversial issue (see Appendix B)
- In more advanced stages of malignant melanoma, chemotherapy and radiation therapy have not been very effective at achieving remission of metastatic disease
- Vaccines, interleukin-2, arterial limb perfusion, and immunotherapy are more promising adjuncts to surgery

Melanoma *vs* Benign Nevus (*Continued*)

Long-Term Management

- Patients who have had malignant melanoma should be followed every 3 months for the first 2 years and annually thereafter
- At each visit, the patient's skin (all over) and lymph nodes should be examined
- Patients with invasive disease require annual chest x-ray film, complete blood count, and liver function studies

PROGNOSIS

- Five-year survival is based on the thickness of the tumor

Table 12-1 BRESLOW'S MEASUREMENT

Tumor Thickness (mm)	5-Year Survival (%)
<0.75	98–99
0.76–1.50	94
1.51–2.25	83
2.26–3.00	72–77
>3.00	<50

- Table 12-1 gives the prognosis in terms of lesion thickness. This is known as Breslow's measurement

Benign Nevus

In contrast to a melanoma, a **benign melanocytic nevus** (plural, nevi), a mole or "beauty mark," most often is, as its name suggests, a benign proliferation of nevus cells that are derived from melanocytes. Congenital nevi may be present at birth or in the neonatal period. During childhood and adolescence, acquired nevi appear. Congenital and acquired nevi are much more often seen in patients with light or fair skin than in blacks or Asians. Large congenital nevi have a low but real risk for malignant transformation and the development of melanoma. Benign nevi are generally asymptomatic, unless they are inflamed.

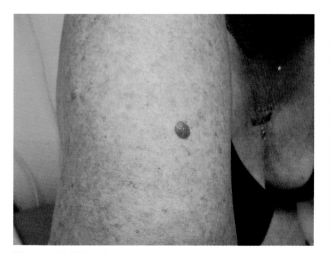

Figure 12-7 Benign compound melanocytic nevus.

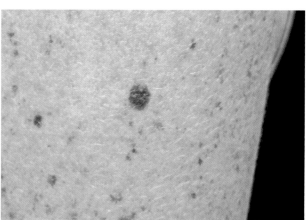

Figure 12-8 Benign junctional melanocytic nevus.

DISTINGUISHING FEATURES

Compound Melanocytic Nevus

- Seen most often on the face (see Figs. 2-8 and 5-3), arms, legs, and trunk
- Elevated, dome-shaped, papillomatous, wartlike papules or nodules that are uniformly brown to dark brown and may contain hairs (Fig. 12-7)

Dermal Melanocytic Nevus

- Most arise on the face and neck
- They are elevated, dome-shaped, wartlike, or pedunculated
- Tan or brown, or dappled with pigmentation
- With age, they often become skin-colored (see Fig. 5-4)

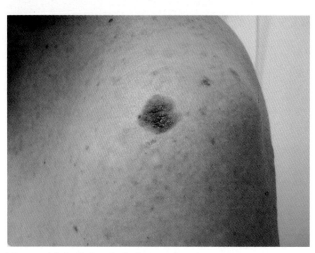

Figure 12-9 Seborrheic keratosis.

Junctional Melanocytic Nevus
- Acquired or congenital, junctional nevi are most prevalent on the face, arms, legs, trunk, genitalia, palms, and soles
- Small, flat, frecklelike; uniform in color; vary from brown to dark brown to black

DIAGNOSIS (see Appendix B)
- Based on clinical appearance or, if necessary, a histopathologic evaluation after removal
- Dermoscopy
- Shave removal/shave biopsy, if indicated
- **TIP: The 5 S's suggest a benign lesion (Fig. 12-8):**
  - **Symmetrical, the halves will match if the lesion is "folded" on itself**
  - **Smooth, unnotched, nonblurry border**
  - **Same uniform color**
  - **Smaller than the diameter of a pencil eraser (<6 mm)**
  - **Stable, unchanging over time**

MANAGEMENT
- Removed most often for cosmetic purposes
- Shave removal/biopsy
- Less commonly, an elliptical excision is performed with the intent of removing lesions completely, including hairs
- **ALERT: All melanocytic nevi should be carefully examined and considered for biopsy, particularly if there is any suggestion of clinical atypia**

ALSO CONSIDER
- Seborrheic keratosis (see Fig. 12-9)
- Lentigo

ALERT: Pyogenic granuloma (may be indistinguishable from a nodular melanoma)
- Spindle cell nevus

Localized Plaque Psoriasis

Localized plaque psoriasis (see also Chapter 21, Legs, *Knees*) is the most common presentation of psoriasis; it may remain limited and localized, or it may become unstable and become widespread. Lesions of psoriasis result from an increase in epidermal cell turnover. The cell's transit time from the basal layer of the epidermis to the stratum corneum is decreased from the normal 28 days to 3 or 4 days. This "turned-on" epidermis, with its rapid accumulation of cells, accounts for the characteristic lesion of psoriasis: a red papule or plaque. It also explains the accumulation of white or silvery (micaceous) scale that the great increase in cellular kinetics prevents time for shedding.

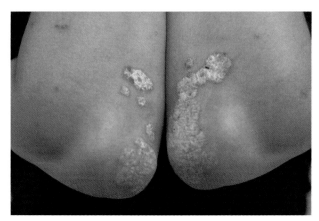

Figure 12-10 Localized plaque psoriasis.

DISTINGUISHING FEATURES
- In its mildest manifestation, psoriasis is an incidental finding and consists of mildly erythematous, well-demarcated, whitish or silvery plaques on the elbows and/or knees (Fig. 12-10)
- Usually not pruritic (compare lichen simplex chronicus, later)
- Tends to be symmetric

DIAGNOSIS
- Clinical
- Skin biopsy if the diagnosis is in doubt

MANAGEMENT (see Appendix A)
Initial
- The use of a potent (class 1) topical steroid for a limited period, followed by a less-potent topical steroid for maintenance
- Occlusion of topical steroids (see Appendix B) of a medium- or high-potency agent is applied and then covered with polyethylene wrap (e.g., **Saran Wrap**) for several hours or overnight, or the application of **Cordran tape**

Maintenance
- Less-potent topical steroids can be used for maintenance (e.g., triamcinolone ointment 0.1%) twice daily
- Intralesional steroids (Appendix B)
- Topical calcitriol **(Vectical)** ointment
- ✔ TIP: Rotational therapy. This strategy decreases cumulative side effects and drug tolerance (tachyphylaxis), and it often allows for lower dosages and shorter durations of therapy for each agent. For example, the use of a superpotent (class 1) topical steroid, such as clobetasol, may be applied for 2 weeks, discontinued for 1 or 2 weeks, and then restarted. Alternatively, clobetasol may be used on weekends only and Vectical ointment can be used during the week
- Topical calcipotriene vitamin D_3 **(Dovonex)** cream
- Topical vitamin D_3–potent steroid combination **(Taclonex** ointment)
- If tolerated, natural sun exposure should be encouraged when available

Lichen Simplex Chronicus

Lichen simplex chronicus, also called *neurodermatitis*, is a common, chronic, often solitary, pruritic eczematous eruption exacerbated and caused by repetitive rubbing and scratching. When it appears on the elbows, it is commonly mistaken for psoriasis. It is most often noted in adults, particularly in patients with other atopic manifestations, such as asthma, allergic rhinitis, and atopic dermatitis. The neck, wrists, extensor and flexor forearms, ankles, pretibial areas, or inner thighs are common sites. Lichen simplex chronicus may also involve the vulvae, scrotum, intragluteal area, and perianal area (see also Chapter 10, Neck; Chapter 18, Genital Area, Scrotum, Vulva; Chapter 21, Legs, Lower Legs).

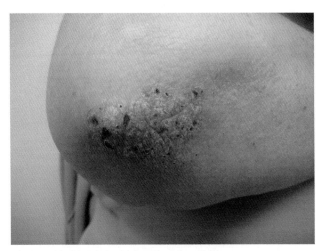

Figure 12-11 Lichen simplex chronicus.

DISTINGUISHING FEATURES
- Atopic history often present
- Focal lichenified (thickened skin with accentuated skin lines) plaques usually on both elbows (Fig. 12-11)
- Pruritic; crusts and excoriations may be seen
- Lesions are poorly demarcated; they blend gradually into normal surrounding skin

DIAGNOSIS
- Readily apparent and is made on clinical grounds

MANAGEMENT (see Appendix A)
- An intermediate-strength (class 3 or 4) topical corticosteroid is applied. If necessary, a high-potency (class 1 to 2) topical corticosteroid can be used
- Occlusion of topical steroids enhances effectiveness (see Appendix B)
- **Cordran tape** is helpful because it protects the affected area from scratching as well as providing the delivery of a potent topical steroid

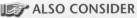

ALSO CONSIDER
- Acquired and congenital hyperkeratosis
- Frictional lichenoid dermatitis in children

Granuloma Annulare

Granuloma annulare is an idiopathic, generally asymptomatic, ring-shaped grouping of dermal papules. The papules are composed of focal granulomas. Granuloma annulare on the elbows is seen most frequently in adult women who most often have typical annulare lesions elsewhere on the body. Proposed pathogenic mechanisms include cell-mediated immunity (type IV), immune complex vasculitis, and an abnormality of tissue monocytes. None of these theories have convincing evidence to support them.

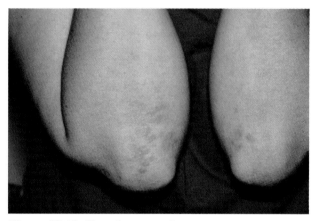

Figure 12-12 Granuloma annulare.

DISTINGUISHING FEATURES

- Lesions appear as skin-colored or red firm dermal papules on one or both elbows and/or knees (Fig. 12-12)
- Lesions are most often noted on dorsal surfaces of hands, fingers (see Chapter 13, Hands and Fingers, *Dorsal Surface*) and feet
- Occasionally, granuloma annulare may present as subcutaneous nodules that are similar to rheumatoid nodules
- In the generalized form, multiple small, skin-colored, erythematous or violaceous lesions appear in a symmetrical fashion on the trunk and, to a lesser extent, on the limbs, and the distinctive annular pattern is not always present

DIAGNOSIS

- Most often made on clinical grounds and evidence of lesions elsewhere on the body
- Skin biopsy, if diagnosis is in doubt

MANAGEMENT (see Appendix A)

- Potent topical steroids, if desired, may be used alone under polyethylene occlusion, or **cordran tape**
- Intralesional triamcinolone acetonide **(Kenalog)** in a dosage of 2 to 4 mg/mL is injected directly into the elevated border of the lesions with a 30-gauge needle (see Appendix B)

Eruptive and Tuberous Xanthomas

Xanthomas are lesions characterized by accumulations of lipid-laden macrophages. They can develop in the setting of altered systemic lipid metabolism or as a result of local cell dysfunction.

Eruptive xanthomas most commonly arise over the buttocks, the shoulders, and the extensor surfaces of the extremities. They are seen as skin markers for various types of hyperlipidemias, hypothyroidism, chronic renal failure, or secondary to diabetes. High circulating levels of various lipoproteins can result in deposition of cholesterol and other lipids in the skin, tendons, and other organs. Eruptive xanthomas are associated with hypertriglyceridemia, particularly that associated with types I, IV, and V (high concentrations of very low density lipoproteins and chylomicrons). **Tuberous xanthomas** usually develop in pressure areas, such as the extensor surfaces of the knees, the elbows, and the buttocks. They are associated with hypercholesterolemia and increased levels of low-density lipoprotein cholesterol, as well as familial dysbetalipoproteinemia and familial hypercholesterolemia. They may be present in some of the secondary hyperlipidemias (e.g., nephrotic syndrome, hypothyroidism).

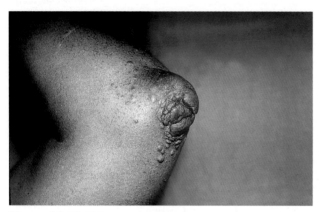

Figure 12-13 Tuberous xanthomas.

DISTINGUISHING FEATURES
Eruptive Xanthomas
- Lesions typically erupt as crops of small, red-yellow papules on an erythematous base, and they may spontaneously resolve over weeks
- Pruritus is common, and the lesions may be tender
- Firm, yellow papulonodules that are painless. The lesions can coalesce to form multilobated tumors
- Often widespread

Tuberous Xanthomas
- Usually develop in pressure areas, such as the extensor surfaces of the knees, the elbows (Fig. 12-13), and the buttocks

DIAGNOSIS
- Clinical
- Shave or punch biopsy (see Appendix B)

MANAGEMENT
- Referral for evaluation and treatment of lipid abnormality, etc.

ALSO CONSIDER
- Cutaneous sarcoidosis
- Rheumatoid nodules
- Gouty tophi

ARMS

Polymorphous Light Eruption *vs* Drug-induced Photosensitivity

Polymorphous Light Eruption

Polymorphous light eruption (PMLE) is seen most often in fair-skinned women 20 to 40 years of age. Caused by ultraviolet exposure, PMLE is usually most prominent following the first sun exposure in the spring or during a winter trip to sunny climates. (For a more complete discussion, see Chapter 10, Neck.)

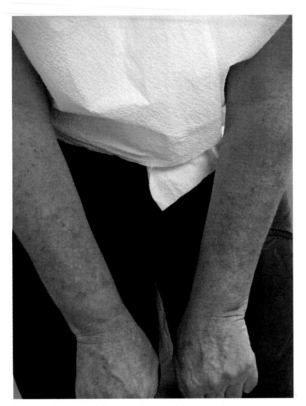

Figure 12-14 Polymorphous light eruption.

DISTINGUISHING FEATURES
- Female sex
- On different patients, lesions may be papules (most common), papulovesicles, erythematous plaques, erythema multiforme—like, or purpuric
- The rash appears within hours to days of exposure, and it subsides over the next 1 to 7 days
- The areas of greatest involvement are the "V" areas of the neck and chest (see Fig. 10-3) and particularly the extensor surfaces of the arms (Fig. 12-14)

DIAGNOSIS
- Usually based on the history and clinical picture; the recognition of PMLE and other photosensitivity disorders resides in their photodistribution
- Skin biopsy, if necessary (see Appendix B)
- Normal titers of antinuclear antibodies, as well as normal urine, stool, and blood porphyrin levels, help support the diagnosis
- Provocative photo testing when indicated

MANAGEMENT
- See Appendix A and Chapter 10, Neck

Drug-Induced Photosensitivity

Drug-induced photosensitivity refers to the development of a cutaneous eruption as a result of the combined effects of a drug and light exposure. These include phototoxic and photoallergic reactions. Photosensitivity reactions may result from systemic medications as well as topically applied medications. Photoallergic reactions are cell-mediated immune responses, whereas phototoxic reactions result from direct damage to tissue caused by a photoactivated compound. Photosensitizing drugs may also cause a lichen planus–like eruption in sun-exposed areas.

Acute phototoxicity often begins as an exaggerated sunburn reaction with erythema and edema that occurs within minutes to hours of light exposure. Both phototoxic and photoallergic reactions occur in sun-exposed areas of skin, including the face, "V" of the neck, and dorsa of the hands and forearms. The hair-bearing scalp, postauricular and periorbital areas, and submental portion of the chin are usually spared.

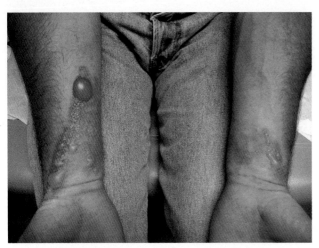

Figure 12-15 Drug-induced photosensitivity Topical drug-induced (8-methoxy psoralen) phototoxic eruption.

DISTINGUISHING FEATURES

- **Phototoxic reactions** develop in most individuals if they are exposed to sufficient amounts of light and drug. They are much more common than photoallergic reactions
  - Typically appear as an exaggerated sunburn response (erythema, edema, vesicles, and/or bullae) and generally occur within minutes or hours (Fig. 12-15)
  - Causal drugs most often reported: tetracyclines (demeclocycline, doxycycline), fluoroquinolones, hypoglycemics (tolbutamide, glipizide, glyburide), griseofulvin, phenothiazines (chlorpromazine), amiodarone, diuretics (furosemide, chlorothiazide), nonsteroidal anti-inflammatory drugs (naproxen, piroxicam)

- **Photoallergic reactions** typically develop in sensitized individuals 24 to 48 hours after exposure
  - The reaction usually manifests as a pruritic eczematous eruption similar to allergic contact dermatitis (see Chapter 3, Eyelids and Periorbital Area; Chapter 6, Cheeks; Chapter 7, Lips and Perioral Area)
  - Photoallergic reactions can be caused by either topical or systemic administration of a drug. Most often, reported causes are:
    - Topical: sunscreens (para-aminobenzoic acid, benzophenones), musk ambrette
    - Systemic: sulfonamides (trimethoprim-sulfamethoxazole)

DIAGNOSIS

- History of sun exposure and systemic or oral photosensitizer
- Patch testing and photopatch testing

MANAGEMENT

- Discontinue/avoid responsible photosensitizer
- **Phototoxic reactions**
  - As with acute sunburns, sun protection/avoidance, topical steroids, if necessary
  - If severe, cool wet dressings, infection prophylaxis, systemic steroids
- **Photoallergic reactions**
  - Sun protection/avoidance and topical steroids/systemic steroids, if necessary
  - See "Rhus Dermatitis" later in this chapter and Chapter 3, Eyelids and Periorbital Area, for the treatment of contact dermatitis
  - In severe or persistent cases, immunosuppression with azathioprine or cyclosporine may be necessary

ALSO CONSIDER
- Porphyria cutanea tarda (see Chapter 13, Hands and Fingers)
- Lichen planus–like photo drug eruption
- Lupuslike drug reaction
- Systemic lupus erythematosus
- Subacute cutaneous lupus erythematosus

RARELY
- Persistent light reaction (chronic actinic dermatitis)
- Lichen planus actinicus
- Pseudoporphyria

Solar Keratosis

Solar keratoses (see Chapter 1, Hair and Scalp; Chapter 2, Forehead and Temples; Chapter 4, Ears; Chapter 5, Nose and Perinasal Area; Chapter 6, Cheeks) are extremely common on the sun-exposed extensor forearms and hands (see Chapter 13, Hands and Fingers, *Dorsal Surface*) of elderly, fair-complexioned individuals.

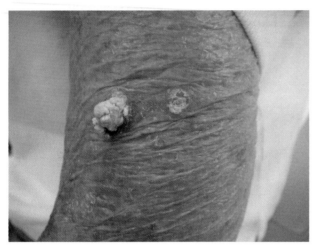

Figure 12-16 Hypertrophic solar keratosis (cutaneous horn) and smaller solar keratosis.

DISTINGUISHING FEATURES
- Men are affected more than women (increasing incidence in women)
- Elderly whites most often affected
- Single or multiple elevated scaly papules with an erythematous base covered by a white, yellowish, or brown scale (hyperkeratosis)
- May evolve into *hypertrophic solar keratosis* or a *cutaneous horn* (see also Chapter 4, Ears; Chapter 6, Cheeks) (Fig. 12-16)
- A small percentage progress to SCC (see later discussion)

DIAGNOSIS
- Clinical
- A shave biopsy when diagnosis in doubt or to rule out an SCC

MANAGEMENT
- See Chapter 1, Hair and Scalp, and Appendix B

Squamous Cell Carcinoma

Most cutaneous **squamous cell carcinomas** arise in solar keratoses (see previous discussion). As seen in solar keratoses, the forearms are common sites for these lesions to appear on the sun-exposed extensor forearms and hands.

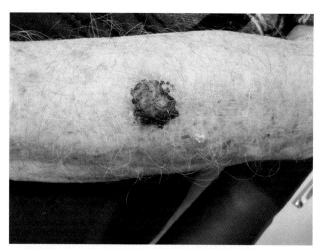

Figure 12-17 Squamous cell carcinoma.

⚠ **ALERT: Metastases are much more likely to arise from lesions that appear de novo without a preceding solar keratosis. Lesions that are softer, nonkeratinizing, or ulcerated also carry a greater risk. Poorly differentiated, large (>2 cm) lesions are more likely to spread. This is especially a concern in the immunocompromised patient.**

DISTINGUISHING FEATURES
- Males are affected more than females (increasing incidence)
- Elderly whites; fair skin
  - Scaly papule, plaque, or nodule with a smooth or thick hyperkeratotic surface
  - Ulceration may be the only finding (Fig. 12-17)
- Clinical variants include SCC in situ (Bowen disease) (Fig. 12-18)
  - As with solar keratoses (see previous discussion), an SCC, as well as an SCC in situ, may also produce a cutaneous horn on its surface
  - Often indistinguishable from a hypertrophic solar keratosis

DIAGNOSIS
- Shave or excisional biopsy
  An isolated lesion or lesions of SCC in situ (Bowen disease [Fig. 12-18]) may be indistinguishable from localized patch/plaque psoriasis.

MANAGEMENT
- See Chapter 1, Hair and Scalp, and Appendix B

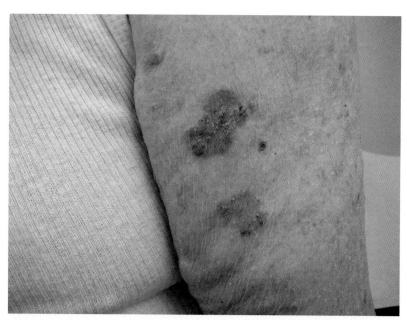

Figure 12-18 Squamous cell carcinoma in situ (Bowen disease; lesions resemble psoriatic plaques).

Keratoacanthoma

As with solar keratoses and SCC, a **keratoacanthoma** is found on the sun-exposed extensor forearms of elderly, fair-complexioned individuals. There is controversy about the benign versus malignant nature of this lesion. A keratoacanthoma resembles an SCC histologically and is considered by some dermatologists and dermatopathologists to be a low-grade variant of an SCC.

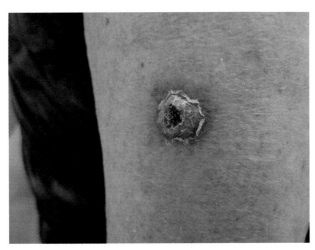

Figure 12-19 Keratoacanthoma.

DISTINGUISHING FEATURES

- Males are affected more than females
- Age over 65
- Occurs on the sun-exposed forearms, dorsa of hands, face, ears, and neck (see also Chapter 4, Ears; Chapter 5, Nose and Perinasal Area)
- Rapidly growing, usually taking 3 to 4 weeks to appear
- Arises as a single dome-shaped erythematous or skin-colored nodule plus a central keratin core (crater) with an overlying crust (Fig. 12-19)
- May attain a diameter of 1.0 to 2.5 cm
- Often clinically indistinguishable from an SCC and a hypertrophic solar keratosis

DIAGNOSIS

- An excisional or incisional biopsy is often recommended so that the complete architecture of the lesion can be evaluated histologically (a deep shave biopsy is often adequate to obtain sufficient tissue)

MANAGEMENT (see Appendix B)

- Excision
- Electrodesiccation and curettage
- Intralesional 5-fluorouracil
- Micrographic (Mohs) surgery for recurrences

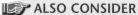

ALSO CONSIDER
- Seborrheic keratosis
- Basal cell carcinoma
- Wart
- Localized patch/plaque psoriasis

- Solar lentigines
- Melasma
- Lentigo maligna/lentigo maligna melanoma

Atopic Dermatitis

Atopic dermatitis (AD) commonly presents on the flexor creases (antecubital and popliteal fossae) in children 2 through 12 years of age. Lesions tend to become lichenified and excoriated because of repeated rubbing and scratching. Atopic dermatitis and lichen simplex chronicus also appear on the extensor as well as flexor wrists. Atopic dermatitis may become widespread and secondarily infected (impetiginized).

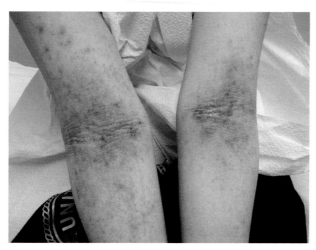

Figure 12-20 Atopic dermatitis.

DISTINGUISHING FEATURES

- Lesions tend to occur symmetrically on the antecubital fossae as well as the extensor and flexor wrists
- Lichenified plaques are generally prominent and tend to blend into surrounding normal skin (Fig. 12-20)
- Crusts and excoriations often evident
- Postinflammatory hyperpigmentation and hypopigmentation often follow in the wake of the eruption and may last a lifetime

DIAGNOSIS
- Clinical

MANAGEMENT (see Appendix A)
- Topical steroid therapy
    - The application of a potent class 1 to 4 topical steroid usually results in prompt improvement in most patients
    - Topical steroids should be used only as short-term therapy, if possible, and only against active disease (i.e., with itching and erythema)
    - They should not be used for prevention of future lesions or for cosmetic concerns, such as postinflammatory hyperpigmentation
    - "Stronger" is often preferable to "longer" because long-term application is more often associated with side effects
    - When the condition is under control, the frequency of application and the potency of the topical steroids are reduced ("downward titration") or discontinued
- For long-term application:
    - Tacrolimus ointment 1% (**Protopic**) and pimecrolimus cream 1% (**Elidel**)
    - Emollients or barrier creams/lotions such as **CeraVE** and **EpiCeram**
- ✔ TIP: For severe or widespread eczema, "soak and smear" and "bleach baths" are quickly effective (see Appendix B)

Rhus Dermatitis (Poison Ivy, Poison Oak)

Rhus dermatitis, a type of allergic contact dermatitis, frequently occurs on flexor as well as extensor surfaces of the arms. In the United States, rhus dermatitis is commonly referred to as "poison ivy," "poison oak," and "poison sumac." Poison ivy is found throughout the country; poison oak is more commonly found in the western United States; and poison sumac is found only in woody, swampy areas. The plants' invisible oils may reach the skin not only through direct contact but also through indirect contact (garden tools, pet fur, golf clubs) or the smoke of a burning plant. Identical or related antigens are found in the resin of the Japanese lacquer tree, ginkgo trees, cashew nut shells, the dye of the India marking nut (used as a clothing dye in India), and the skin of mangoes. All cause similar skin rashes in sensitized people. In the eastern United States, rhus dermatitis occurs mainly in the spring and summer. In the western and southeastern United States, where outdoor activity is common all year, rhus dermatitis may occur in any season. Approximately 85% of the population develops a reaction on exposure to one of the plants.

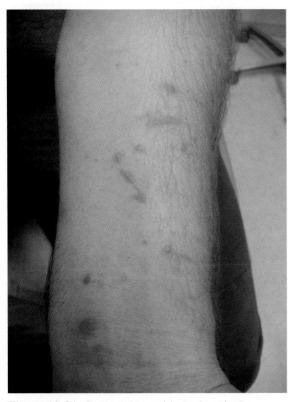

Figure 12-21 Contact dermatitis (poison ivy).

DISTINGUISHING FEATURES
- The characteristic eruption consists of intensely pruritic linear streaks of erythematous papules, vesicles, and blisters (Fig. 12-21)
- The rash typically occurs 2 days after contact with the plant
- Generally, exposed areas of the body are affected first. The rash may later involve covered areas that have come into contact with the plant oil

DIAGNOSIS
- The diagnosis is based on history of exposure to the antigen and the characteristic distribution of the lesions
- ⚠ **ALERT: Further dissemination (autoeczematization) is believed to occur through hematogenous spread and subsequent immune-complex deposition in the skin. This spread may occur within 5 to 7 days after the initial office exposure, and the resulting rash may last for 3 weeks or more**

MANAGEMENT
- Advice on how to avoid the offending plant ("leaves of three, let them be")
- A limited eruption and mild itching may be relieved by the following:
  - "Soak and smear" (see Appendix B) with potent or superpotent topical corticosteroids (class 1), such as clobetasol ointment 0.05%
  - Cool compresses of Burow's solution help dry vesicles and bullae and prevent secondary bacterial infection
- More severe eruptions may be treated with:
  - Systemic corticosteroids. Prednisone is commonly used, in a tapering dosage schedule that often starts at 1 mg/kg and decreases by 5 mg every 2 days for at least 2 weeks and for as long as 3 weeks. The dosage may be increased again if flares occur during the tapering regimen. Prednisone tablets should be taken with meals
- ✔ **TIP: Intramuscular corticosteroids. Triamcinolone diacetate or hexacetonide may be used if the patient has gastrointestinal intolerance to oral corticosteroids**
- ✔ **TIP: In patients with severe rhus dermatitis, it is important to continue prednisone for 2 to 3 weeks because a shorter course may allow a rebound of the condition**
- Contrary to common belief, the fluid in blisters does not transfer the rash to others or cause the rash to spread on the affected person

Scabies

Scabies is a skin infestation caused by the mite *Sarcoptes scabiei*. It is usually spread by skin-to-skin contact, most frequently among family members and by sexual contact in young adults. Transmission by means of underwear or bed linen is rare. Occasionally, epidemics occur in nursing homes and similar extended-care institutions such as college dormitories. The diagnosis can be easily overlooked, and treatment is often delayed for long periods. Black and African Caribbean individuals infrequently acquire scabies; the reason is unknown. Pathogenesis involves a fertilized female mite excavating a burow in the stratum corneum, laying her eggs, and depositing fecal pellets (scybala) behind her as she advances. The egg-laying scybala, or other secretions, act as irritants or allergens, which may account for the itching and subsequent delayed type IV hypersensitivity reaction.

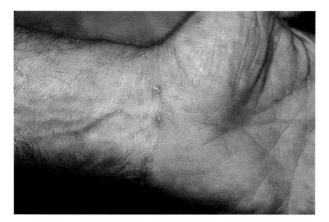

Figure 12-22 Scabies. Note whitish burows.

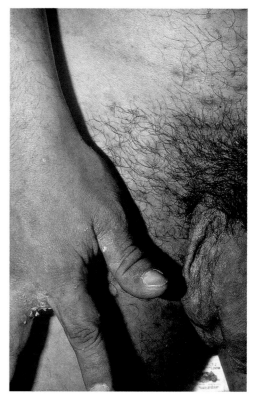

Figure 12-23 Scabies in typical locations. Note scrotal nodules.

DISTINGUISHING FEATURES

- The initial lesions include tiny pinpoint vesicles and erythematous papules that may evolve into *burows*, the classic telltale lesions of scabies. The burows (linear or S-shaped excavations) are easiest to find on the hands (see Chapter 13, Hands and Fingers, *Sides of Web Spaces and Fingers*)
- Lesions are most often located on the flexor wrists (Fig. 12-22), interdigital finger webs, sides of the hands, areolae of the breasts, feet, umbilicus, waistband area, penis, axillae, ankles, buttocks, and groin
- Pruritic scrotal or penile nodules are virtually pathognomonic (Fig. 12-23)
- Children and adults rarely have lesions above the neck, an important diagnostic sign
- Infants tend to have more widespread involvement, including the face and scalp and especially the palms and soles
- Immunocompromised patients also tend to have a widespread distribution of lesions (Norwegian or crusted scabies)
- Itching (nocturnal pruritus) has traditionally been considered a symptom that is characteristic of scabies; however, pruritus that occurs in many other skin conditions also tends to be more severe during the nighttime hours when people are inclined to be less distracted by their daytime routines

- A generalized distribution of lesions is probably the result of a hypersensitivity reaction

DIAGNOSIS

- Considered when an individual complains of intractable, persistent pruritus, especially when other family members, consorts, or fellow inhabitants of an institution have similar symptoms
- A conclusive diagnosis is made by finding scabies mites, eggs, or feces. This is where the mites may be found
- A therapeutic trial with scabicides
- Infants: frequently, intact vesicles are seen on the palms and soles
- Elderly patients: particularly in an institutional setting, they can have intense pruritus and few papular lesions, excoriations, or simply dry, scaly skin

MANAGEMENT (see Appendix A)

- If scabies is strongly suspected on clinical grounds, scabicidal treatment should be initiated
  - The prescription scabicides, **Elimite** and **Acticin** both contain permethrin cream 5%; they are safe and effective and are currently considered the treatment of choice. They have not been proven to be safe in infants younger than 2 months or in pregnant and nursing women
  - Gamma benzene hexachloride (**Lindane, Kwell, Scabene**) should only be used in patients who cannot tolerate or have failed first-line treatment with safer medications

⚠ **ALERT: Seizures and deaths have been reported following Lindane Lotion use with repeat or prolonged application**

- Precipitated sulfur ointment (6%) in infants younger than 2 months or in pregnant and nursing women
  - Ivermectin (**Stromectol**) is an effective oral treatment (see Appendix A for dosage)
  - Laundering of all bed linen and clothes is often suggested shortly after the initial treatment

✔ **TIP: Contacts should be treated simultaneously to avoid "ping-ponging" (reinfection)**

✔ **TIP: Treatment failure may result from noncompliance (i.e., treating lesions only) or reinfection**

✔ **TIP: Symptoms may persist after appropriate treatment (lesions tend to be eczematous)**

Lichen Planus

Lichen planus (LP) is a pruritic, idiopathic eruption with characteristic shiny, flat-topped (Latin: planus, "flat") purple papules on the skin, often accompanied by mucous membrane lesions (see Chapter 8, Oral Cavity and Tongue). It is an inflammatory condition that predominantly occurs in adults over 40; it is less common in younger adults and rare in children.

Mucous membrane involvement is common (in both sexes) and genital involvement is common in men with cutaneous disease (see Chapter 18, Genital Area *Penis*). The cause of LP appears to be autoimmune in nature. Some studies suggest an association between LP and chronic hepatitis C virus infection, chronic active hepatitis, and primary biliary cirrhosis. Lichen planus lesions may also be part of the spectrum of chronic graft-versus-host disease that appears after bone marrow transplantation. Other associations include drugs (lichenoid drug reactions) and sun exposure.

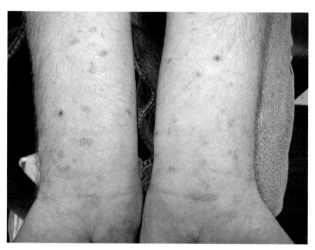

Figure 12-24 Lichen planus (note the purple, planar, polygonal, and pleomorphic papules).

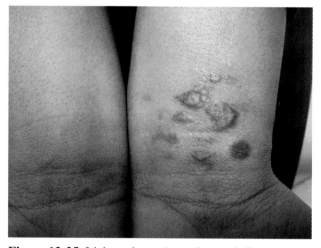

Figure 12-25 Lichen planus (note the postinflammatory hyperpigmentation and the Köebner phenomenon (isomorphic response) due to scratching.

DISTINGUISHING FEATURES
- Lichen planus is most commonly found on extremities, particularly the flexor areas such as the wrists, and pretibial shafts (see Chapter 21, Legs, Lower Legs)
- May become widespread and chronic
- The **"Seven P's"** (Figs. 12-24 and 12-25)
  1. Lesions are often **pruritic** but may be asymptomatic
  2. Lesions are often **purple** (actually violaceous) in color
  3. Lesions tend to be **planar** (flat-topped)
  4. Lesions form **papules** or **plaques**
  5. Lesions may be **polygonal**
  6. Lesions may be **pleomorphic** in shape and configuration (i.e., oval, annular, linear, confluent (plaquelike), large and small, even on the same person)
  7. Lesions tend to heal with residual **postinflammatory hyperpigmentation**

- **Other clinical phenomena associated with LP:**
  - The **Köebner phenomenon** (isomorphic response) is seen as a reaction to trauma such as scratching (Fig. 12-25) in which LP lesions appear at sites of scratching and rubbing injury or other traumas to the skin
  - **Wickham's striae** are characteristic white streaks that are best visualized on the surface of lesions after mineral oil is applied
  - **Mucous membrane lesions** characterized by white lacy streaks in a netlike pattern, or atrophic erosions or ulcers may be found without skin involvement (see Chapter 8, Oral Cavity and Tongue)
  - **Nail lesions** that may exhibit a mild dystrophy to a total loss of the nails
  - **Scalp lesions** that result in a scarring follicular alopecia (lichen planopilaris [see Chapter 1, Hair and Scalp])

DIAGNOSIS

- Lichen planus is often diagnosed by its appearance
- Skin biopsy is performed if necessary (see Appendix B)

⚠ **ALERT: Underlying diseases such as hepatitis C or drugs associated with a lichenoid reaction should be ruled out**

MANAGEMENT (See Appendix A)

- The first-line treatments of cutaneous LP are potent topical or intralesional steroids
- More severe cases, especially those with scalp, nail, and mucous membrane involvement, may require systemic therapy
- Systemic steroids in short, tapering courses may be necessary for symptom control and possibly more rapid resolution
- Oral metronidazole, griseofulvin, psoralen with ultraviolet A, and narrowband ultraviolet B may be useful
- Oral acitretin (**Soriatane**) and isotretinoin
- Immunosuppressive agents, including cyclosporine, mycophenolate mofetil, and azathioprine have been used with some success for severe and refractory cases

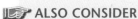 **ALSO CONSIDER**

- Atopic dermatitis or dyshidrotic eczema
- Pityriasis rosea
- Lichen simplex chronicus
- Lichenoid (lichen planus–like) eruptions
- Guttate psoriasis
- Tinea corporis
- Insect bites, such as flea bites
- Systemic drug reactions
- Pruritus associated with systemic diseases, such as renal disease, hepatic disease, lymphomas, AIDS, leukemias, and Hodgkin disease
- Drug eruptions and other itchy rashes, including urticaria, tinea, and xerosis
- Reactions to meadow grass and other plants may cause contact dermatitis
- Herpes zoster

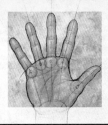

CHAPTER 13

Hands and Fingers

The hands and fingers are the workhorses of the body, constantly in contact with, and exposed regularly to the external environment in all seasons. Sun exposure, soaps, and other harsh contactants are daily insults and irritants. The palmar surfaces are adapted with a thick stratum corneum that is a much more resilient barrier than the stratum corneum on the dorsal surfaces; thus, the palmar surfaces experience less frequent episodes of irritant and allergic contact dermatitis.

IN THIS CHAPTER

Dorsal Surface
- Granuloma annulare *vs* tinea corporis
- Solar lentigines *vs* seborrheic keratoses
- Solar keratosis *vs* squamous cell carcinoma

Palmar Surface
- Hand eczema (acute and chronic hand dermatitis) *vs* palmar psoriasis *vs* tinea manuum

Hands and Fingers
- *Dorsal* Contact dermatitis *vs* atopic hand dermatitis *vs* porphyria cutanea tarda
- *Palmar* Erythema multiforme *vs* acute urticaria

Sides and Web Spaces of Fingers
- Dyshidrotic eczema *vs* scabies *vs* erosio interdigitalis blastomycetica (interdigital candidosis)

Fingers and Periungual Area
- Verrucae vulgaris (common warts) *vs* pyogenic granuloma
- Herpetic whitlow *vs* digital mucous cyst
- Systemic lupus erythematosus *vs* dermatomyositis *vs* scleroderma
- Acute paronychia *vs* chronic paronychia

Granuloma Annulare

Granuloma annulare (GA) is an idiopathic, generally asymptomatic, ring-shaped grouping of dermal papules (see also Chapter 12, Arms, Elbows). The papules are composed of focal granulomas that coalesce to form curious circles or semicircular plaques which are often misdiagnosed as "ringworm". GA is seen most frequently in very young children in whom it is most often self-limiting. It also appears in adult women (female-to-male ratio is 2.5:1). In adults, GA tends to be more chronic. There is also an adult form of disseminated GA, which may be associated with diabetes. Proposed pathogenic mechanisms include cell-mediated immunity (type IV), immune complex vasculitis, and an abnormality of tissue monocytes.

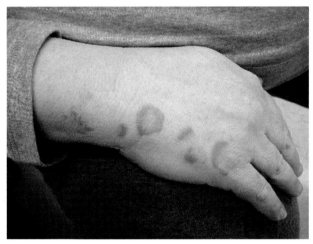

Figure 13-1 Granuloma annulare.

DISTINGUISHING FEATURES
- Lesions are red or skin-colored firm dermal papules that most often arise on the dorsal surfaces of hands, fingers, and feet, as well as on the extensor aspects of the arms and legs
- May be individual, isolated papules or joined in annular or semiannular (arciform) plaques with central clearing (Fig. 13-1)
- Lesions have no epidermal change (i.e., scale; compare "Tinea Corporis," later)
- Centers of lesions may be slightly hyperpigmented and depressed relative to their borders
- Generally asymptomatic; primarily a cosmetic concern

- In adults, GA may also be found on the elbows (see Chapter 12, Arms, Elbows), trunk, legs, and neck
- Subcutaneous nodules similar to rheumatoid nodules may be seen on arms and legs
- In the generalized form, multiple small, skin-colored, erythematous or violaceous lesions appear on the trunk and, to a lesser extent, on the limbs, and the distinctive annular pattern is not always present
- **ALERT: Diabetes mellitus may be associated with the generalized form of GA.**

DIAGNOSIS
- Most often made on clinical grounds
- Skin biopsy, if the diagnosis is in doubt. Granuloma annulare has a characteristic histopathology consisting of foci of altered collagen and mucin surrounded by granulomatous inflammation of histicytic and lymphocytic cells. The degenerative collagen is referred to histopathologically as *necrobiosis*

MANAGEMENT (see Appendices A and B)
- The patient should be reassured of the benign nature of the condition
- Localized lesions in very young children are often best left untreated
- Generalized forms of GA are more difficult to treat and are less likely to resolve spontaneously
- Potent topical steroids, if desired, used may be used alone or under polyethylene occlusion
- Intralesional triamcinolone acetonide **(Kenalog)** in a dosage of 2 to 5 mg/mL is injected directly into the elevated border of the lesions with a 30-gauge needle
- Light therapy (psoralen plus topical ultraviolet A [PUVA]) may be used in severe cases of generalized GA

Tinea Corporis

Tinea corporis (see also Chapter 6, Cheeks; Chapter 15, Trunk; Chapter 19, Buttocks and Perineal Area; Chapter 21, Legs) is commonly referred to as "ringworm", a term used by lay persons, and frequently by many in the health care community, to describe practically *any* annular or ringlike eruption on the body. Tinea corporis is most often acquired by contact with an infected animal, usually a kitten and occasionally a dog. It may also spread from other infected humans, or it may be autoinoculated from other areas of the body infected by tinea such as tinea pedis, tinea cruris, or tinea capitis. Another common method of transmission of tinea corporis is noted in wrestlers (tinea gladiatorum). *Microsporum canis*, *Trichophyton rubrum*, and *Trichophyton mentagrophytes* are usually the causal pathogens in tinea corporis.

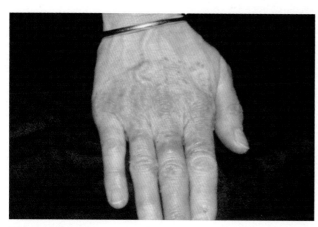

Figure 13-2 Tinea corporis.

DISTINGUISHING FEATURES
- Lesions are often annular, with peripheral enlargement and central clearing; however, a non-ringlike, confluent scaly patch with a typical scaly, "active border" is usually seen on the dorsal hands (Fig. 13-2)
- May be pruritic or asymptomatic

DIAGNOSIS
- Diagnosis is confirmed by a positive potassium hydroxide (KOH) examination or fungal culture (it is especially easy to find hyphae in those patients who have been previously treated with topical steroids ["tinea incognito"])
- A history of a newly adopted kitten or association with another infected contact is helpful in making the diagnosis

MANAGEMENT (see Appendix A)
- Topical antifungal agents such as 2% ketoconazole and clotrimazole 1% cream may be curative if the infection is limited
- Systemic antifungal agents such as griseofulvin, terbinafine (**Lamisil**), or itraconazole (**Sporanox**) are sometimes necessary when multiple lesions are present, or in those patients who are unresponsive to topical therapy
- If pets appear to be the source of infection, they may also need antifungal treatment after evaluation by a veterinarian

 ALSO CONSIDER
- Eczematous dermatitis (atopic/contact)
- Erythema migrans rash of Lyme disease
- Urticaria
- Erythema multiforme
- Lichen planus
- Annular cutaneous sarcoidosis
- Cutaneous candidiasis

RARELY
- Subacute cutaneous lupus erythematosus
- Erythema elevatum diutinum

Solar Lentigines *vs* Seborrheic Keratoses

Solar Lentigines

Solar lentigines (singular, lentigo), or "liver spots," are small, acquired, tan macules that appear on the sun-exposed extensor arms, dorsal hands, and anterior legs, as well as on the face. This is discussed more extensively in Chapter 2, Forehead and Temples; and Chapter 6, Cheeks.

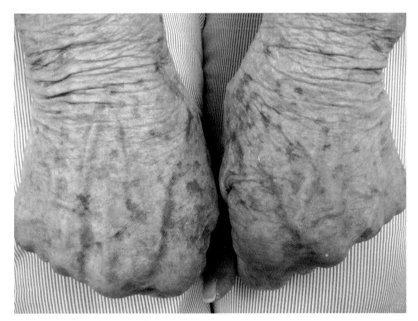

Figure 13-3 Solar lentigines.

DISTINGUISHING FEATURES
- Arise in fair-complexioned, older adults
- Sharply circumscribed tan to dark brown macules (Fig. 13-3)
- Uniformly pigmented oval to geometric shape

DIAGNOSIS
- Clinical
- Biopsy, if diagnosis is in doubt

MANAGEMENT
- See Chapter 2, Forehead and Temples, as well as Appendix B

Seborrheic Keratosis

Seborrheic keratoses are very common benign lesions with no malignant potential. They are often located on the back, chest (see Chapter 15, Trunk), legs (see Chapter 21, Legs), and face, particularly along the frontal hairline (Chapter 2, Forehead and Temples) and scalp (see Chapter 1, Hair and Scalp).

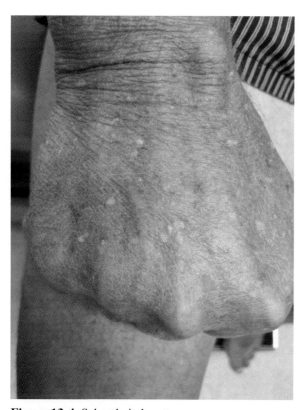

Figure 13-4 Seborrheic keratoses.

DISTINGUISHING FEATURES
- Typically, seborrheic keratoses have a warty, "stuck-on" appearance
- Relatively flat or almost flat lesions (Fig. 13-4) tend to occur on the dorsal hands and are often indistinguishable from solar keratoses, solar lentigines, and flat warts
- Seborrheic keratoses are mainly a cosmetic concern, except when they are inflamed or irritated

DIAGNOSIS
- A biopsy (generally a shave biopsy) is performed if necessary to confirm the diagnosis

MANAGEMENT
- See Chapter 2, Forehead and Temples, as well as Appendix B
- Treatment methods include:
  - Cryosurgery is performed with liquid nitrogen (LN_2) spray or cotton swab
  - Light electrocautery and curettage

HANDS AND FINGERS

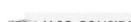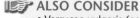 **ALSO CONSIDER**
- Verrucae vulgaris (common warts)
- Verrucae planae (flat warts)
- Pigmented solar keratoses
- Melanocytic nevi

Solar Keratosis *vs* Squamous Cell Carcinoma

Solar Keratosis

Solar keratoses (see Chapter 1, Hair and Scalp; Chapter 2, Forehead and Temples; Chapter 4, Ears; Chapter 5, Nose and Perinasal Area; Chapter 6, Cheeks) are extremely common on the sun-exposed extensor forearms and hands of elderly, fair-complexioned individuals.

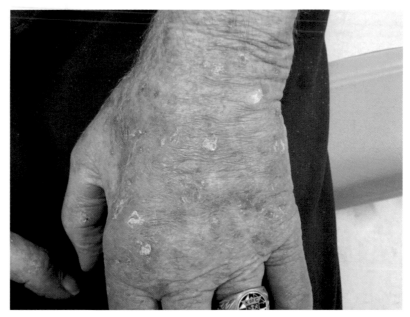

Figure 13-5 Solar keratoses.

DISTINGUISHING FEATURES
- Males are affected more than females; however, the incidence is increasing in females
- Elderly whites, with fair skin
- Single or multiple elevated scaly papules with an erythematous base covered by a white, yellowish, or brown scale (hyperkeratosis) (Fig. 13-5)
- May evolve into hypertrophic solar keratosis or a cutaneous horn (see Chapter 4, Ears)
- A very small percentage progress to squamous cell carcinoma (SCC) (see later discussion)

DIAGNOSIS
- Clinical
- A shave biopsy when diagnosis in doubt or to rule out an SCC

MANAGEMENT
- See Chapter 1, Hair and Scalp, as well as Appendix B

Squamous Cell Carcinoma

Squamous cell carcinomas (SCC) most often arise in solar keratoses and are seen in the identical clinical context as solar keratoses on the sun-exposed dorsum of the hands.

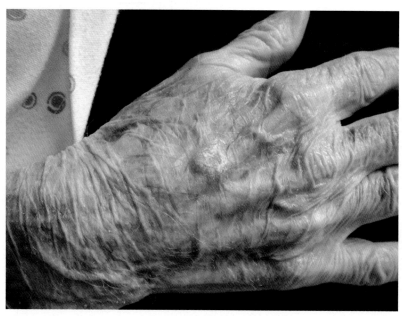

Figure 13-6 Squamous cell carcinoma.

DISTINGUISHING FEATURES
- Males are affected more than females (as with solar keratoses, the incidence is increasing in females)
- Elderly whites, with fair skin
- Scaly papule, plaque, or nodule with a smooth or thick hyperkeratotic surface (Fig. 13-6)

DIAGNOSIS
- Shave or excisional biopsy

MANAGEMENT
- See Chapter 1, Hair and Scalp, as well as Appendix B

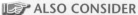 **ALSO CONSIDER**
- Melanocytic nevus
- Verruca vulgaris
- Seborrheic keratosis

Hand Eczema (Acute and Chronic Hand Dermatitis)

Hand eczema (acute and chronic hand dermatitis) may be caused and exacerbated by a contactant or may be due to atopy. As suggested by its name, chronic hand dermatitis often runs a relapsing and remitting course. *Dyshidrotic eczema* is a type of eczema affecting the hands and fingers and sometimes the feet. It is also known as *pompholyx*, particularly when there are large vesicles on the palms and/or soles. Acute hand dermatitis due to a contactant or irritant is less commonly seen on the palmar surfaces because they are protected by a much thicker stratum corneum than the dorsal hands. Nevertheless, a diligent history must be taken to rule out contactant etiology.

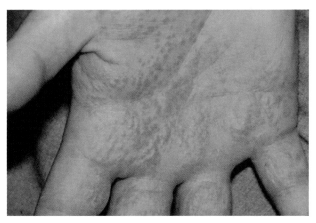

Figure 13-7 Hand eczema: pompholyx ("wet type").

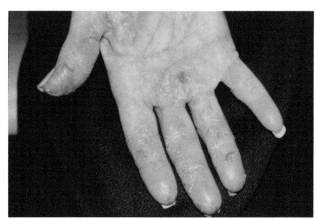

Figure 13-8 Hand eczema ("dry type").

DISTINGUISHING FEATURES
"Wet" Type
Dyshidrotic eczema, the wet type (Fig. 13-7), or *pompholyx* (the Greek word for bubble), is characterized by the following:
- Itchy, clear vesicles that are typically located on the sides of the fingers (see "Fingers"), but they can also occur on the palms and, less commonly, on the soles of the feet and the lateral aspects of the toes
- Initially, the vesicles are very small and clear and resemble little bubbles
- Later, as they dry and resolve without rupturing, they turn golden brown ("sago grain" vesicles)

☑ **TIP: On occasion, contact allergy to nickel has been shown to cause dyshidrotic eczema**

"Dry" Type
Nondyshidrotic hand eczema, the dry, scaly type (Fig. 13-8), is characterized by the following:
- Scale and erythema
- The skin surface often loses its flexibility and develops painful fissures
- Hyperkeratotic, lichenified plaques may arise.
- Palms and fingers may become dry, wrinkled, red, and fragile, with resultant fissures (see Fig. 13-20) and erosions

Features Common to Both Types
- Oozing and secondary bacterial infection ("honey-crusted" skin) can occur

☑ **TIP: It is also common for both exogenous (contact) and endogenous (atopic) factors to be at work in the same patient**

DIAGNOSIS
- Atopic history often elicited
- Patch testing with putative allergens may be performed if a contact dermatitis is suspected (see Appendix B)

MANAGEMENT (see Appendix A)

- Protective cotton-lined gloves are used for washing dishes or other similar tasks
- The regular use of hand emollients and avoidance of frequent contact with irritants such as water, soap, solvents, and detergents are the mainstays of therapy
- The application of emollient barrier creams and protective gloves in dry winter months
- Mild cleansers or soap substitutes are recommended
- For oozing and infected lesions, compresses with Burow solution and/or mupirocin cream or ointment
- Class 1 to 3 topical corticosteroids are the mainstay of treatment. Used under occlusion or "soak and smear" therapy (see Appendix B), they can be very effective
- ⚠ **ALERT: Potent topical corticosteroids applied under occlusion should be used only intermittently and for short periods, because they increase the risk of atrophy.**

- Ointments penetrate skin better than creams, but patients may prefer to use creams during the daytime. Lower strength (class 4 or 5) corticosteroids may sometimes be applied for long-term maintenance
- Alternative treatments:
  - Tacrolimus ointment (**Protopic**) 1% or pimecrolimus (**Elidel**) 1% cream applied twice daily may be helpful
  - For severe or refractory cases, the short-term use of systemic corticosteroids, acitretin (**Soriatane**), PUVA, broad band and narrow band ultraviolet B (UVB), oral cyclosporine, azathioprine, mycophenolate mofetil (**CellCept**) and low-dose methotrexate may be tried

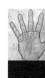

HANDS AND FINGERS

Palmar Psoriasis

Psoriasis may involve the palms and/or soles (palmoplantar psoriasis) alone, or these areas may be a part of more extensive psoriasis that is also present elsewhere on the body. The palmar location of these lesions often presents additional problems to the patients such as pain, impairment of function, fissuring, bleeding, and embarrassment. As with chronic hand eczema, this condition runs a chronic course and is sometimes very difficult to manage.

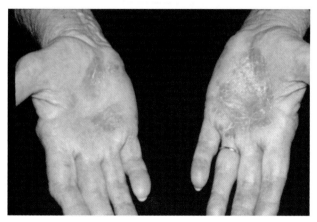

Figure 13-9 Palmar psoriasis.

DISTINGUISHING FEATURES
- Well-defined plaques, with or without thick scales (Fig. 13-9)
- Pustular variant is much less common
- Psoriasis may be seen elsewhere on body
- Less likely to itch than eczema
- Nails may show characteristic changes (see Chapter 14, Fingernails)
- Positive family history of psoriasis (50%)

DIAGNOSIS
- Clinical

MANAGEMENT (see Chapter 15, Trunk, as well as Appendix A)
Initial Treatment
- If necessary, a salicylic acid preparations such as 6% salicylic acid (**Salex, Cream** or **Lotion**) or **Keralyt gel** (see Appendix B) may be used to remove thick scale prior to the application of:
  - Potent (class 1) topical steroids for a limited period, followed by a less-potent topical steroid for maintenance
  - Occlusion of topical steroids of a medium- or high-potency agent is applied and then covered with vinyl or rubber gloves overnight

Maintenance Treatment
- Less potent topical steroids can be used for maintenance (e.g., triamcinolone ointment or cream 0.1%)twice daily
- Topical calcitriol (**Vectical**) ointment
- Topical calcipotriene vitamin D_3 (**Dovonex**) cream
- Topical vitamin D_3–potent steroid combination (**Taclonex** ointment)

Severe, Refractory Cases
- PUVA, broad band and narrow band UVB, excimer laser
- Systemic therapies:
  - Oral cyclosporine, azathioprine, mycophenolate mofetil (**CellCept**), low-dose methotrexate, acitretin (**Soriatane**)
  - Tumor necrosis factor-alpha inhibitors and monoclonal antibody agents ("biologics") that are immunologically directed, such as etanercept (**Enbrel**), infliximab (**Remicade**), adalimumab (**Humira**), and ustekinumab (**Stelara**)

Tinea Manuum

Tinea (see "Tinea Corporis") can present on one or both palms (tinea manuum). See also Chapter 22, Feet.

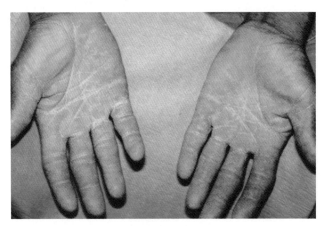

Figure 13-10 Tinea manuum.

DISTINGUISHING FEATURES
- Fine scale with minimal or no inflammation (Fig. 13-10)
- Usually asymptomatic, unless fissured

✔ **TIP: Often there is coexisting tinea pedis—"two feet, one hand" and onychomycosis (Fig. 13-11) (see Chapter 14, Fingernails; Chapter 22, Feet), which is pathognomonic for tinea. Thus, involvement of the hands should always prompt inspection of the feet and vice versa**

DIAGNOSIS
- Positive KOH or fungal culture

MANAGEMENT (see Appendix A)
- Oral antifungal agents such as:
  - Terbinafine (**Lamisil**) 250 mg daily every day for 14 days or longer
  - Itraconazole (**Sporanox**) 200 mg daily every day for 14 days or longer
  - Fluconazole (**Diflucan**) 150 to 200 mg every day for 4 to 6 weeks
- Application of concomitant topical antifungal agents such as ketoconazole 2% and clotrimazole 1% are used as adjunctive treatment

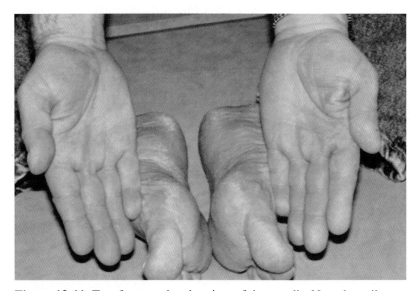

Figure 13-11 Two feet, one hand variant of tinea pedis. Note the nail involvement.

 ALSO CONSIDER
- Contact dermatitis
- Secondary syphilis
- Erythema multiforme
- Hyperkeratosis palmaris

RARELY
- Epidermolytic hyperkeratosis
- Pachyonychia congenita
- Pityriasis rubra pilaris
- Palmoplantar pustulosis
- Pellagra

Contact Dermatitis

Contact dermatitis frequently occurs on the dorsa of the hands and far less commonly on the palmar surfaces, which are protected by a much thicker stratum corneum. Hand dermatitis is particularly common in individuals working in industries involving cleaning, catering, metalwork, hairdressing, gardening, health care, and mechanical work. Such occupational factors often lead to irritant contact dermatitis. For example, the frequent immersion of the hands in water, particularly if the skin is exposed to detergents and shampoos (e.g., hairdressers and hair care products) and solvents (e.g., painters and turpentine), may strip the skin of its natural protective layer.

Allergic contact dermatitis occurs hours to days after the contact has occurred (see Rhus Dermatitis [poison ivy] in Chapter 12, Arms, Antecubital Fossae, Flexor Forearms, and Wrists); however, it can sometimes be difficult to identify the origin of the rash. Nonoccupational contactants that can cause allergic contact dermatitis include nickel, fragrances, rubber accelerators (gloves), and *p*-phenylenediamine (found in permanent hair dyes).

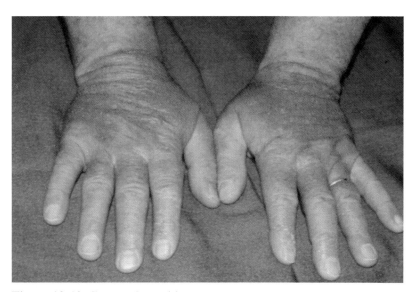

Figure 13-12 Contact dermatitis.

DISTINGUISHING FEATURES

Acute

- Erythema and pruritus (Fig. 13-12; see also Fig. 12-21)
- Pruritic erythematous papules, "juicy" vesicles, and/or blisters (e.g., rhus dermatitis)

Subacute and Chronic

- Crusted, pruritic, eczematous plaques
- Lichenified plaques are generally prominent and tend to blend into surrounding normal skin

DIAGNOSIS

- Clinical
- Historical evidence of occupational and/or daily habitual exposure may be clues to the specific irritant or allergen
- Consider patch testing to identify relevant allergens (see Appendix B)

MANAGEMENT (see also Chapter 12, Arms, Antecubital Fossae, Flexor Forearms, and Wrists)

- Topical steroids (class 1 to 3) are applied once or twice daily (see Appendix A)
- After identification, contact with the causative material must be strictly avoided
- If due to occupational exposure, a few days off work may be helpful; occasionally, a change of occupation is necessary
- Vinyl gloves are less likely to cause allergic reactions than rubber ones
- Frequent application of moisturizers and barrier creams may be effective
- **ALERT: Latex gloves may elicit a contact urticaria, and latex allergy has been reported to have a risk of anaphylaxis.**

Atopic Hand Dermatitis

Atopic hand dermatitis may appear on any area of the hands and is often clinically indistinguishable from acute and chronic contact dermatitis (see previous discussion); however, atopic dermatitis occurs in association with a personal or family history of hay fever, asthma, allergic rhinitis, sinusitis, or atopic dermatitis itself. Also, a history of allergies to pollen, dust, house dust mites, ragweed, dogs, or cats may be uncovered (see also Chapter 3, Eyelids and Periorbital Area; Chapter 12, Arms; Chapter 15, Trunk; Chapter 21, Legs).

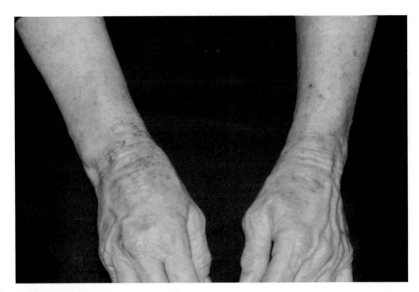

Figure 13-13 Atopic dermatitis.

DISTINGUISHING FEATURES (may be identical to those of contact dermatitis discussed previously)

Acute

- Erythema and pruritus
- Pruritic erythematous papules, "juicy" dyshidrotic vesicles, and/or blisters

Subacute and Chronic

- Crusted, pruritic, eczematous plaques
- Lichenified plaques are generally prominent and tend to blend into surrounding normal skin (Fig. 13-13)

DIAGNOSIS

- Clinical
- Atopic history
- Lack of history of contactant/irritant

MANAGEMENT

- Topical steroids (class 1 to 3) are applied once or twice daily (see Appendix A)
- Frequent application of moisturizers and barrier creams

Porphyria Cutanea Tarda

Porphyria cutanea tarda is a form of porphyria caused by a defective enzyme in the liver, uroporphyrinogen decarboxylase, resulting in hepatic and cutaneous findings. An increase in porphyrins in the skin results in photosensitivity. Characteristically, the urine is darker than usual, with a reddish color. Porphyria cutanea tarda generally begins in middle adulthood after exposure to certain chemicals or diseases that increase the production of porphyrins in the liver. These include alcohol, chronic liver disease, oral contraceptives, iron overload, or polychlorinated aromatic hydrocarbons (e.g., dioxins), as well as certain chronic blood disorders such acquired or hereditary hemochromatosis.

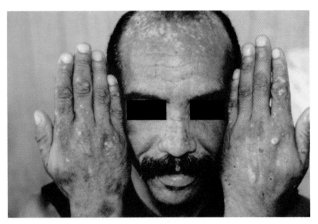

Figure 13-14 Porphyria cutanea tarda (note blisters on hands and frontal forehead; also characteristic excess hair on lateral cheeks).

DISTINGUISHING FEATURES
- Vesicles and bullae and crusts on the backs of the sun-exposed hands (Fig. 13-14)
- Erosions following relatively minor trauma to the skin (increased skin fragility)
- Scattered discrete lesions rather than the more diffuse pattern seen in hand eczema (see previous discussion)
- Increased sensitivity to the sun
- Milia (see Chapter 2, Forehead and Temples) may appear as the blisters heal
- Hypertrichosis on cheeks and temples
- Less commonly, sclerodermoid findings on the neck, face, or chest

DIAGNOSIS
- Clinical findings plus:
  - Skin biopsy to differentiate porphyria cutanea tarda from other blistering diseases such as epidermolysis bullosa acquisita
  - Examination of the urine with a Wood lamp: coral pink fluorescence due to excessive porphyrins occurs
  - Elevated levels of uroporphyrins in the urine and elevated coproporphyrins and uroporphyrins in feces
- Other important tests include complete blood count to assess hemoglobin levels, iron stores, and liver enzymes

MANAGEMENT
- Avoidance of alcohol, estrogens, iron, and contact with polychlorinated aromatic hydrocarbons
- Opaque sun-blocks
- Phlebotomy
- Antimalarials such as low-dose chloroquine or hydroxychloroquine
- Autologous red cell transfusion

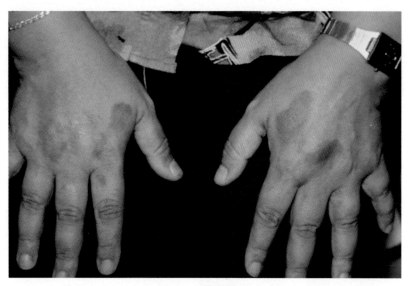

Figure 13-15 Berloque dermatitis: postinflammatory hyperpigmentation (the other "lime" disease). This patient squeezed limes while mixing some alcoholic beverages at a barbecue.

ALSO CONSIDER
- Photodermatitis
- Phytophotodermatitis (Berloque dermatitis): reaction to presence of certain plant materials, such as lime and lemon juice, on skin in combination with ultraviolet light (Fig. 13-15)
- Bullous pemphigoid
- Bullous erythema multiforme

RARELY
- Epidermolysis bullosa acquisita
- Pseudoporphyria

Erythema Multiforme

Erythema multiforme (EM) minor is a self-limited eruption characterized by symmetrically distributed erythematous macules or papules, which develop into targetlike lesions consisting of concentric color changes with a dusky central zone that may become bullous (see also Chapter 8, Oral Cavity and Tongue; Chapter 15, Trunk). Besides the characteristic targetoid skin lesions, EM minor is generally limited to one mucosal surface and is considered to be a type IV hypersensitivity reaction. It is often idiopathic, but the most common precipitating cause of EM minor is recurrent labial herpes simplex virus infections. Also, it may be associated with, and triggered by, multiple underlying causes such as reactions to various drugs, contact dermatitis, and infections (e.g., mycoplasma, histoplasmosis, and certain viruses).

 Erythema multiforme major (Stevens–Johnson syndrome) is the more serious variant of EM. It has much more extensive mucous membrane involvement, systemic symptoms, and widespread lesions. Precipitating factors include drugs (sulfonamides, penicillin, hydantoins, barbiturates, allopurinol, nonsteroidal anti-inflammatory drugs), mycoplasma infection, pregnancy, streptococcus infection, hepatitis A and B, coccidioidomycosis, and Epstein-Barr virus infection.

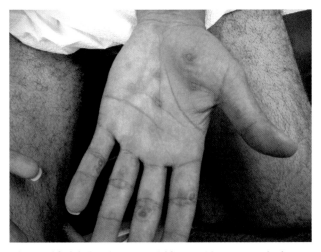

Figure 13-16 Erythema multiforme. Note target lesions on palms.

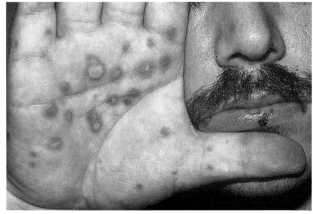

Figure 13-17 Erythema multiforme and recurrent herpes labialis.

DISTINGUISHING FEATURES
- Most commonly seen in late adolescence and in young adulthood
- Lesions begin as round, dull-red macules or urticarial plaques that expand over 24 to 48 hours.
- Some lesions evolve to form targetoid plaques (iris lesions) with a dark center that may become vesicobullous (Fig. 13–16)
- Lesions persist (are "fixed") for at least 1 week; thereafter, erosions and crusts form
- Bilateral and symmetric, lesions are found predominantly on the distal surfaces of the extremities and spread centripetally
- The palms and soles, dorsa of hands and feet, extensor forearms, face, and legs may be affected

Erythema Multiforme Minor
- Acute, self-limited, and often recurrent
- Mucous membrane lesions are limited to the mouth
- Evidence of herpes labialis may be present (Fig. 13-17)
- When herpes simplex virus (HSV) is the cause, EM minor tends to recur with subsequent bouts of cold sores. The viral infection may be subclinical; that is, visible evidence of HSV may be absent at the time of the reaction

Erythema Multiforme Major (Stevens–Johnson Syndrome)

- Longer course than EM minor
- Severe, extensive, painful mucous membrane involvement, affecting at least 2 mucosal surfaces. This form may be located in multiple sites, including the mouth, pharynx, eyes, and genitalia (see Chapter 8, Oral Cavity and Tongue)
- As with EM minor, cutaneous targetoid lesions may be present
- Often accompanied by symptoms of fever, malaise, lymphadenopathy, and myalgias

DIAGNOSIS

- Typical target lesions; mucous membrane lesions
- If indicated: complete blood count, erythrocyte sedimentation rate, liver function tests, blood urea nitrogen, creatinine, urinalysis, electrolytes, and blood, urine, or sputum cultures
- Skin and/or mucous membrane biopsy may be necessary

MANAGEMENT (see Appendix A)

- Wet dressings (e.g., Burow solution) and topical steroids may be applied to oozing lesions
- If known, the precipitating cause should be eliminated (e.g., drug) or treated (e.g., infection)
- Empiric treatment with oral acyclovir, famciclovir (**Famvir**), or valacyclovir (**Valtrex**) may prevent or mitigate recurrences if erythema multiforme is due to HSV (see Chapter 7, Lips and Perioral Area)
- Most cases of EM minor subside completely within 2 to 3 weeks without any complications
- **ALERT: In life-threatening situations, such as may be seen in EM major, hospitalization is often essential. The use of systemic steroids in such severe cases is controversial, and their effectiveness has not been established.**

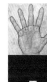

HANDS AND FINGERS

Acute Urticaria

Acute urticaria, commonly known as hives, is a reaction of cutaneous blood vessels that produces a transient dermal edema consisting of papules or plaques of different shapes and sizes. Urticaria may be classified as acute or chronic. By definition, acute urticaria are hives that last for less than 6 weeks and chronic urticaria lasts longer than 6 weeks (see Chapter 15, Trunk, for further discussion of chronic urticaria).

Pathophysiology involves the release of histamine and other compounds by mast cells and basophils. Mast cell activation causes degranulation of intracellular vesicles that contain histamine, leukotriene C4, prostaglandin D2, and other chemotactic mediators that recruit eosinophils and neutrophils into the dermis. Histamine and chemokine release leads to extravasation of fluid into the dermis (edema).

Histamine effects account for many of the clinical and histologic findings of urticaria. Urticaria may be immune-mediated or nonimmune-mediated. Immune, immunoglobulin E (IgE)-mediated causes include certain foods, drugs, acute upper respiratory infection, parasites, and whole blood transfusions. Non–IgE-mediated physical stimuli that can produce hives include dermatographism, cold urticaria, and solar urticaria. Acute urticaria also may be result from physical stimuli such as pressure, cold, sunlight, or exercise.

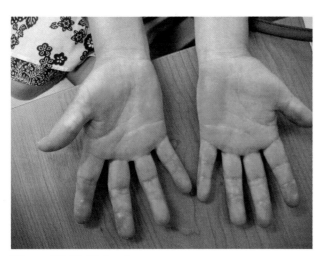

Figure 13-18 Urticaria.

DISTINGUISHING FEATURES

- Wheals are the color of the patient's skin or pale red (Fig. 13-18)
- May be present on the eyelids, lips, legs, and trunk
- Lesions generally itch
- Episodes last for hours to days (generally less than 30 days)
- Individual lesions disappear within 24 hours (evanescent wheals)
- Finger may swell, and rings are difficult to remove
- Lesions may be accompanied by a deeper swelling (angioedema)
- ⚠ **ALERT: Anaphylaxis or an anaphylactoid reaction can occur.**

DIAGNOSIS
- Clinical (history and physical findings)

MANAGEMENT (see also Chapter 15, Trunk)
- If possible, the cause of the hives should be determined and eliminated
- If self-limiting, treatment is symptomatic with antihistamines and cool soaks
- Sedating antihistamines such as histamine H_1 blockers include hydroxyzine (**Atarax**), diphenhydramine (**Benadryl**), and cyproheptadine (**Periactin**)
- Nonsedating antihistamines, such as loratadine (**Claritin**) 10 mg, desloratadine (**Clarinex**) 5 mg, fexofenadine (**Allegra**) 60/180 mg, and cetirizine (**Zyrtec**) 5 to 10 mg may be used during the day, and a more sedating H_1/H_2 blocker such as doxepin (**Sinequan**) may be added at bedtime
- Systemic steroids are sometimes used for a short period
- When individual wheals persist for more than 24 hours, the process is less likely to be urticaria

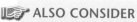 **ALSO CONSIDER**
- Bullous pemphigoid
- Drug reaction/drug-induced bullous disorders
- Graft-versus-host disease in the appropriate clinical setting

RARELY
- Pemphigus vulgaris
- Urticarial vasculitis (when individual wheals persist for more than 24 hours)
- Bullous lupus erythematosus
- Pseudoporphyria
- Behçet disease
- Epidermolysis bullosa acquisita

HANDS AND FINGERS

Dyshidrotic Eczema

Dyshidrotic eczema is a type of dermatitis affecting the hands (see previous discussion) and sometimes the feet. An atopic diathesis is believed to play a role in hand eczema in most cases; however, on occasion, allergy to nickel has been shown to cause it. The term *dyshidrotic* is a misnomer based on the erroneous assumption that the vesicles are caused by *trapped sweat*. We now understand that they result from inflammation and foci of intercellular edema (*spongiosis*), which becomes loculated in the thick stratum corneum in this location.

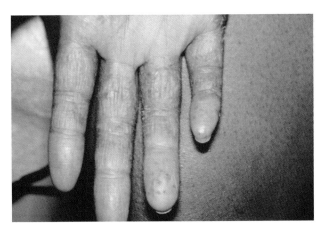

Figure 13-19 Dyshidrotic eczema and lichenified hand eczema. Note dyshidrotic vesicles on fingertips.

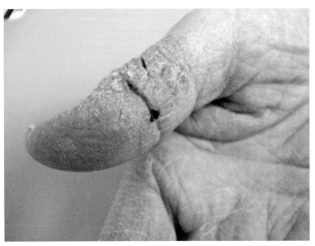

Figure 13-20 Hand eczema with fissuring.

DISTINGUISHING FEATURES
- Itchy, clear vesicles that are typically located on the sides of the fingers, and possibly the lateral aspects of the toes (Fig. 13-19)
- Initially, the vesicles are very small and clear and resemble little bubbles
- Later, as they dry and resolve without rupturing, they turn golden brown
- Over time, fingertips may become dry, scaly, wrinkled, and red, and painful fissures and erosions may develop (Fig. 13-20)

DIAGNOSIS
- Clinical
- Negative KOH or fungal culture

MANAGEMENT
- See Atopic Hand Dermatitis
- ✔ **TIP: Fingertip contact dermatitis from allergy to foods may be seen in cooks; it involves the nondominant hand that holds the food while the dominant hand holds a knife or other implement.**

Scabies

Scabies is frequently noted on the lateral sides of fingers and interdigital finger webs as well as on the flexor wrists (see Chapter 12, Arms, Antecubital Fossae, Flexor Forearms, and Wrists). These locations are important diagnostic features.

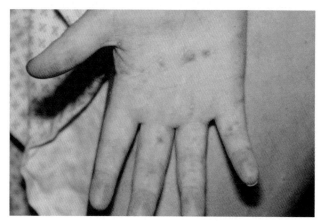

Figure 13-21 Scabies (see also Fig. 12-23).

DISTINGUISHING FEATURES
- Tiny pinpoint vesicles that resemble dyshidrotic vesicles (see previous discussion) and/or erythematous papules that may evolve into burows (Fig. 13-21)
- The burow is a linear or S-shaped excavation that is pinkish white and slightly scaly and ends in the pinpoint vesicle or papule. This is where the mites may be found
- Burows are easiest to find in the finger webs and wrists in adults and on the palms and soles in infants
- Adults, who are more efficient scratchers than children, tend to remove the definitive evidence of scabies (i.e., mite) with their fingernails

✔ **TIP: Because mites are particularly difficult to find in adults, the time and effort spent searching for the mite may be better used by taking a thorough history and counseling the patient and his or her contacts.**

DIAGNOSIS/ MANAGEMENT
- See Chapter 12, Arms, Antecubital Fossae, Flexor Forearms, and Wrists, as well as Appendix A

Erosio Interdigitalis Blastomycetica (Interdigital Candidosis)

Erosio interdigitalis blastomycetica (interdigital candidosis), a variant of intertrigo, typically presents with erythema, fissuring, and maceration in the web spaces of affected fingers.

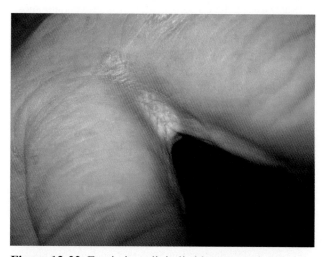

Figure 13-22 Erosio interdigitalis blastomycetica (interdigital candidosis). (Image courtesy of Benjamin Barankin, MD.)

DISTINGUISHING FEATURES
- Superficial interdigital, pruritic, scaly, erythematous erosions or fissures occur in the web spaces of the fingers (Fig. 13-22)

DIAGNOSIS
- Positive KOH ("pseudohyphae") or fungal culture (*Candida* species)

MANAGEMENT (see Appendix A)
- Pat dry area after bathing or washing hands
- Ketoconazole 2% cream twice daily

✔ **TIP: Workup for diabetes or other endocrinopathy is necessary.**

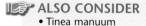 **ALSO CONSIDER**
- Tinea manuum

RARELY
- Acrodermatitis enteropathica

Verrucae Vulgaris (Common Warts)

Verrucae vulgaris (common warts) are benign growths that are confined to the epidermis. All warts are caused by the human papillomavirus. Common warts are most often found at sites subject to frequent trauma, such as the hands and feet. Warts often vary widely in shape, size, and appearance, and the different names for them generally reflect their clinical appearance, location, or both. For example, filiform warts are threadlike, planar warts (see Chapter 2, Forehead and Temples) are flat, and plantar warts are located on the soles of the feet (see Chapter 22, Feet). Common warts are predominantly seen in children and young adults. An estimated 20% of school-aged children will at some time have at least one wart. HIV/AIDS, other immunosuppressive diseases (e.g., lymphomas), immunosuppressive drugs that decrease cell-mediated immunity (e.g., prednisone, cyclosporine, and chemotherapeutic agents), pregnancy, and handling of raw meat or fish in one's occupation (e.g., butchers) are all risk factors for becoming infected. The virus is transmitted primarily through skin-to-skin contact or from the recently shed virus kept intact in a moist, warm environment.

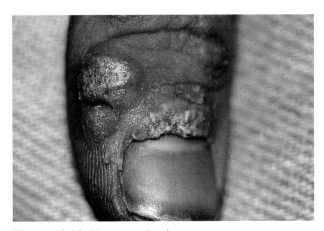

Figure 13-23 Verruca vulgaris.

DISTINGUISHING FEATURES
- Rough-surfaced, hyperkeratotic, papillomatous, raised, skin-colored to tan papules 5 to 10 mm in diameter; may coalesce into a mosaic 1 to 3 cm in diameter (Fig. 13-23)
- Pathognomonic "black dots" (thrombosed dermal capillaries) may be seen (see Chapter 22, Feet; see Fig. 22-14)
- Both common and plantar warts generally demonstrate the following clinical findings:
  - A loss of normal skin markings (dermatoglyphics) such as finger, foot, and hand prints
  - Lesions solitary or multiple; may be in clusters (mosaic warts)
  - Most frequently on hands, knees, and elbows
  - Generally asymmetric distribution

DIAGNOSIS
- Most often made on clinical appearance
- Skin biopsy, if necessary

MANAGEMENT (see Appendix A)
- Benign neglect; most warts tend to regress spontaneously in children

- Method of treatment depends on the age of the patient, the patient's pain threshold, as well as the type of wart and its location
- In many adults and immunocompromised patients, however, warts often prove difficult to eradicate
- Medication (drugs)
  - Self-treatment with over-the-counter keratolytic (peeling) agents such as **Duofilm, Compound W,** primarily containing salicylic or salicylic acid plus lactic acid
  - Office-based and prescription treatment
- Cantharidin in flexible collodion (**Cantharone**) or **Cantharone Plus** with podophyllin and salicylic acid
- Cryotherapy with liquid nitrogen (LN_2) applied with a cotton swab or with a cryotherapy gun (**Cryogun**) is best for warts on hands
- Light electrocautery, with or without curettage, is best for warts on the dorsa of hands. It requires local anesthesia
- The abundance of the following therapeutic modalities is a reflection of the fact that none of these remedies are uniformly effective:
  - Photodynamic therapy
  - CO_2 or pulse-dye laser ablation: expensive and requires local anesthesia
  - Imiquimod (**Aldara**) 5% cream, a local inducer of interferon, is applied at home by the patient or parent
  - Immunotherapy: induction of delayed-type hypersensitivity with diphencyprone, dinitrochlorobenzene (DNCB), and squaric acid dibutylester (SADBE)
  - Intradermal injections of bleomycin, alpha-2 interferon, intralesional mumps or *Candida* antigen, oral high-dose cimetidine, acitretin (**Soriatane**)
  - Other agents, including dichloroacetic acid, trichloroacetic acid, formic acid, 5-fluorouracil, topical or intravenous cidofovir for recalcitrant warts in the setting of HIV/AIDS, have all been used with varying results

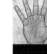

☑ **TIPS:**
- For surgical procedures (e.g., LN$_2$, electrocautery), especially in anxious children, pretreatment with anesthetic cream such as EMLA (emulsion of lidocaine and prilocaine)

- Occlusion: easiest and least expensive. Cover wart with waterproof tape (e.g., duct tape) and leave on for 6 days; then soak, pare with emery board, leave uncovered overnight, then reapply tape cyclically for 8 cycles

Pyogenic Granuloma

Pyogenic granuloma, a vascular hyperplasia that occurs most often in children and young adults, is a benign growth that presents as a shiny red papule or nodule. Pyogenic granuloma arises most frequently on the fingers, an area that is frequently traumatized. Lesions also tend to appear on the head, neck, upper trunk, and the lips (see Chapter 7, Lips and Perioral Area). It may arise during pregnancy (granuloma gravidarum) on the lips, gums, and buccal mucosa and in neonates (umbilical granuloma) (see Chapter 17, Umbilicus). The cause is unknown.

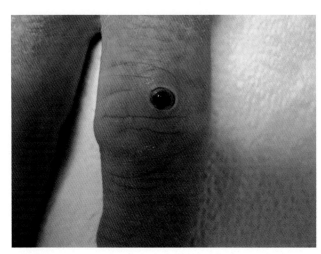

Figure 13-24 Pyogenic granuloma. Note surrounding collarette of skin.

DISTINGUISHING FEATURES
- Generally solitary, a pyogenic granuloma first appears as a small, pinhead-sized red, brownish-red, purple, or blue-black papule that grows rapidly to become 2 mm to 1 cm in diameter
- The base of the lesion is often surrounded by a characteristic collarette of skin (Fig. 13-24)
- Asymptomatic, but they tend to bleed readily even after minor trauma

DIAGNOSIS
- Clinical appearance
- Shave biopsy if there is any doubt about the diagnosis (see Appendix B)

MANAGEMENT
- The lesion is generally destroyed by curettage and electrocautery, and the feeding blood vessel cauterized to reduce the chances of regrowth
- Laser therapy, cryosurgery, or excisional surgery
- Recurrences are not uncommon if the lesion is not completely removed

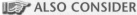 **ALSO CONSIDER**
- Foreign body reaction
- Granulation tissue
- Solar keratosis/squamous cell carcinoma in adults

RARELY
- Amelanotic melanoma
- Kaposi sarcoma
- Glomus tumor

Herpetic Whitlow *vs* Digital Mucous Cyst

Herpetic Whitlow

Herpetic whitlow is a painful lesion that results from the direct inoculation of the HSV on the fingertip. This infection was most commonly due to infection with HSV-1, usually occurring in children who sucked their thumbs. Before the current stringent infection control measures and the widespread use of gloves by health care providers, herpetic whitlow was an occupational hazard in dental and medical health care personnel whose fingertips came in contact with infected oral excretions. Currently, herpes whitlow due to HSV-2 is increasingly recognized and probably due to digital-genital contact in sexually active individuals.

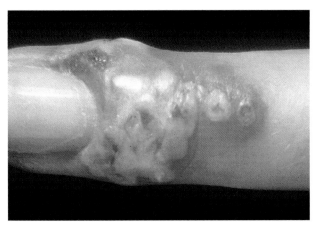

DISTINGUISHING FEATURES
- Painful grouped vesicles on an erythematous base on the distal finger (Fig. 13-25)

DIAGNOSIS/MANAGEMENT
- See Chapter 7, Lips and Perioral Area

Figure 13-25 Herpetic whitlow.

Digital Mucous Cyst

Digital mucous cyst is not a true cyst because it lacks an epidermal lining. It is actually a focal collection of clear, viscous mucin (focal mucinosis) that occurs over the distal interphalangeal joint or, more commonly, at the base of the nail. Some myxoid cysts are believed to be a consequence of osteoarthritis, rather than from trauma.

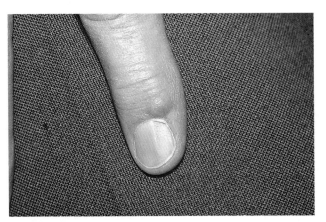

Figure 13-26 Digital mucous cyst (note longitudinal groove in nail).

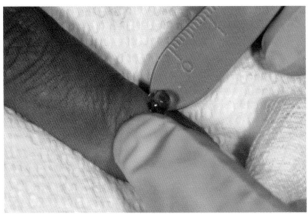

Figure 13-27 Digital mucous cyst (extruded mucoid material).

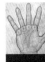

DISTINGUISHING FEATURES

- This rubbery lesion occurs exclusively in adults, particularly in women older than 50 years of age
- Generally painless (compare with herpetic whitlow), solitary, dome-shaped cystic papule, with normal overlying skin
- Pressure from the lesion on the nail matrix (root) often results in a characteristic longitudinal groove in the nail plate (Fig. 13-26)
- Contains a viscous, gelatinous, clear mucoid material (Fig. 13-27)
- When the lesion occurs more proximally, such as over the distal interphalangeal joint, there is no longitudinal groove

DIAGNOSIS

- Generally clinical, especially when longitudinal groove in the nail plate is present
- After incision and drainage, the expressed mucoid contents are noted

MANAGEMENT

- This benign lesion may be treated as follows:
  - It may be ignored, particularly if it is asymptomatic
  - Lesions have reportedly resolved after several weeks to months of daily firm compression
  - Incision and drainage, cryosurgery with LN_2, and intralesional triamcinolone injections have been tried with varying results
  - Surgical excision is reserved for the rarely painful, or otherwise troublesome, lesion

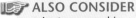 **ALSO CONSIDER**
- Acute paronychia
- Epidermoid cyst

RARELY
- Subcutaneous granuloma annulare
- Giant-cell tendon sheath tumor
- Heberden node
- Gouty tophus

HANDS AND FINGERS

Systemic Lupus Erythematosus *vs* Dermatomyositis *vs* Scleroderma

Systemic Lupus Erythematosus

Systemic lupus erythematosus may present with photosensitivity as well as lesions on the hands and fingers.

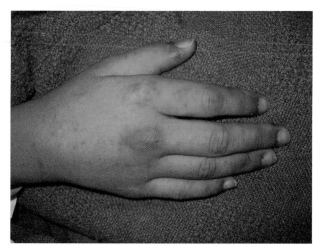

Figure 13-28 Systemic lupus erythematosus (note lesions are located *between* the joints). (Image courtesy of Benjamin Barankin, MD.)

DISTINGUISHING FEATURES
- On the dorsal hands, violaceous plaques that spare the skin overlying the joints are characteristic of systemic lupus erythematosus (Fig. 13-28). Conversely, in dermatomyositis, the joints are affected (see Gottron's papules, later)
- Palmar erythema
- Nailfold telangiectasias and edema of periungual skin may be evident
- Necrotic, painful, vasculitic ulcers may be present on the fingertips
- Erythematous macules or bullous lesions resembling erythema multiforme

DIAGNOSIS/MANAGEMENT
- See Chapter 10, Neck

Dermatomyositis

Dermatomyositis (see Chapter 10, Neck) has several findings on the dorsal hands and fingers, Gottron's papules, and periungual telangiectasias.

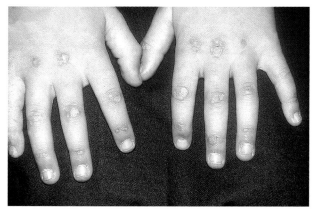

Figure 13-29 Dermatomyositis (Gottron's papules).

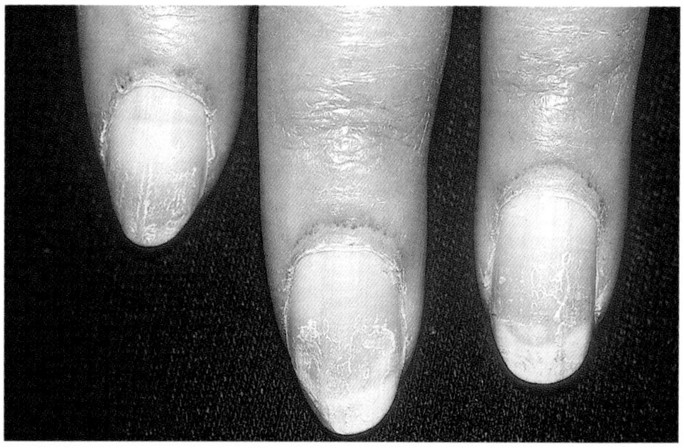

DISTINGUISHING FEATURES
- Gottron's papules consist of erythematous or violaceous, flat-topped papules on the dorsa of the hands Lesions are located *on* the knuckles and interphalangeal joints of the fingers (Fig. 13-29); they begin as papules and later become atrophic and hypopigmented
- Periungual erythema with telangiectasias (Fig. 13-30)
- Cuticles may become dystrophic and ragged

Figure 13-30 Dermatomyositis (periungual telangiectasias).

DIAGNOSIS/MANAGEMENT
- See Chapter 10, Neck

Scleroderma

Scleroderma is an autoimmune connective tissue disease in which excess collagen results from an increase in number and activity of fibroblasts which results in induration and thickening of the skin and subcutaneous tissues. Systemic sclerosis (systemic scleroderma) is a multisystem disease that results in fibrosis and vascular abnormalities. It appears to be 3 to 4 times more common in women than men and is rare in children. The condition leads to a breakdown of the skin, subcutaneous tissue, muscles, and internal organs. Thickening and tightening of the skin that becomes tightly bound to underlying structures is especially seen on the hands and face. *Raynaud phenomenon* is often the first symptom of systemic sclerosis. Patients experience episodes of vasospasm, which causes blood vessels in the fingers and toes to constrict. As less blood is reaching these extremities, the skin changes color to white and the fingers and toes may feel cold and numb. As they warm up, they go blue and then red before returning to normal again. *Morphea*, or localized scleroderma, is limited to the skin and has rarely been reported to progress to systemic scleroderma. *CREST syndrome* (defined later), which accounts for 90% of the cases of systemic sclerosis, is a relatively benign variant with a delayed appearance of visceral involvement.

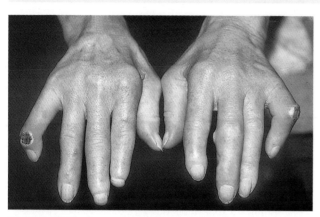

Figure 13-31 Scleroderma with sclerodactyly and vasculitic ulcers.

DISTINGUISHING FEATURES

- Taut, shiny, thickening of the skin of the fingers, followed by atrophy and sclerosis
- Fingers become spindle-shaped (sclerodactyly) (Fig. 13-31)
- Loss of manual dexterity; later, contractures of the hands and shortening of fingers resulting from distal bone resorption
- Gradually, the skin becomes shiny, stiff, waxy, and atrophic
- Painful fingertip ulcers may result from vasculitis (Fig. 13-31)
- In CREST syndrome, the cutaneous involvement is limited to acral areas (hands, feet, face, and forearms)
- **CREST** syndrome consists of the following:
  - **C**alcinosis cutis, most commonly occurring on the palms, fingertips, and bony prominences
  - **R**aynaud phenomenon
  - **E**sophageal dysfunction
  - **S**clerodactyly ("claw deformity")
  - **T**elangiectasia (macular lesions) on the face, lips, palms, back of hands, and trunk

DIAGNOSIS

- The diagnosis of progressive systemic sclerosis and CREST is generally made on clinical and serologic grounds
- Progressive systemic sclerosis diagnosis is generally made from the patient's history and the findings on examination of the skin and other organs
- Positive anticentromere antibody is seen in 70% of patients with CREST syndrome
- Scl-70 is present in approximately 30% of patients with progressive systemic sclerosis and 18% of patients with CREST syndrome
- Elevated antinuclear antibodies are less frequent than in SLE
- Anticentromere antibodies are characteristic of CREST syndrome and may be present in Raynaud phenomenon before systemic sclerosis appears

MANAGEMENT

- Systemic steroids for limited periods early in the disease
- UVA and UVB, aminocaproic acid, D-penicillamine, colchicine, as well as immunosuppressive drugs such as cyclosporine, mycophenolate mofetil, and methotrexate, as well as antimalarials, minocycline, and phenytoin
- Limited benefit from chelation with ethylenediamine tetra-acetic acid (EDTA)
- For Raynaud phenomenon:
  - Warm gloves, thick socks, and slippers
  - It is absolutely essential to discontinue smoking
  - Calcium channel blockers, such as nifedipine
  - Antiadrenergic drugs
  - Statins, pentoxifylline (**Trental**)
  - Sildenafil (**Viagra**), which has been reported to be of benefit
- ✔ **TIP: Raynaud phenomenon: botulinum toxin (Botox) injections have shown some lasting improvement.**

ALSO CONSIDER
- Mixed connective tissue disease
- Graft-versus-host disease
- Overlap syndromes

RARELY
- Nephrogenic systemic fibrosis
- Eosinophilic fasciitis
- Scleromyxedema

Acute Paronychia *vs* Chronic Paronychia

The term *paronychia* refers to inflammation of the nail folds surrounding the nail plate. The condition can be either acute or chronic. Both acute and chronic parony-chias are the result of the breakdown of the protective barrier between the nail plate and the nail fold.

Acute Paronychia

Acute paronychia usually results from an infection caused by *Staphylococcus aureus*; less commonly by *Streptococcus* or *Pseudomonas* species. The condition may occur spontaneously or it may follow trauma or manipulation, such as nail biting, a manicure, or removal of a hangnail.

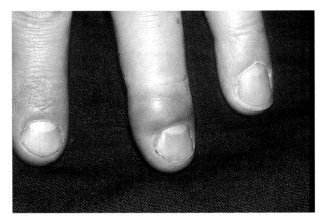

Figure 13-32 Acute paronychia (note preservation of the cuticle).

DISTINGUISHING FEATURES
- Generally, only one nail is involved
- Heralded by the rapid onset of bright red swelling of the proximal or lateral nail fold behind the cuticle, followed by a small, throbbing, tender, and intensely painful pustular lesion (Fig. 13-32)
- Sometimes with purulent exudate

DIAGNOSIS
- Pain and typical clinical appearance
- Bacterial/fungal cultures if the diagnosis is in doubt

MANAGEMENT
- Mild cases may require only warm saline or aluminum acetate (**Burow solution**) soaks for 10 to 15 minutes 2 to 4 times daily
- In more severe cases, simple incision and drainage (with a No. 11 surgical blade) usually affords rapid relief of pain
- Occasionally, systemic therapy with antistaphylococcal antibiotics, such as dicloxacillin, or a cephalosporin, may be needed

Chronic Paronychia

Chronic paronychia results from a combination of chronic moisture, irritation, and trauma to the cuticle and proximal nail fold. It occurs much more often in women than in men, and it is particularly common in persons whose hands are frequently exposed to a wet environment, such as housewives, domestic workers, bartenders, janitors, bakers, dishwashers, dentists, dental hygienists, and children who habitually suck their thumbs. It is also seen more often in patients with diabetes and in persons who manicure their cuticles.

The predisposing factor is usually trauma or maceration that produces a break in the barrier (cuticle) between the nail fold and nail plate. This allows moisture to accumulate and microbial colonization to follow. Clinical evidence suggests that this condition is not primarily a fungal infection at all, but is actually an irritant or eczematous process with secondary yeast colonization.

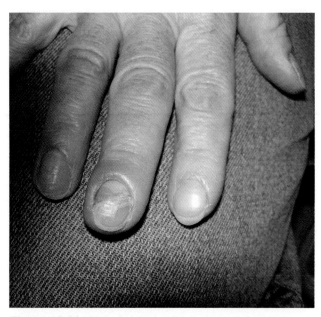

Figure 13-33 Chronic paronychia with nail dystrophy.

DISTINGUISHING FEATURES
- Occasionally, more than one nail is involved
- Usually develops slowly and asymptomatically
- Edema, erythema, of the proximal nail fold, with or without a whitish-yellow discharge (Fig. 13-33)
- Secondary nail plate changes often occur, including onycholysis (see Chapter 14, Fingernails)
- A greenish or brown discoloration along the lateral borders and transverse ridging of the nails may also appear

DIAGNOSIS
- Typical clinical appearance of the fingers and the patient's history
- The presence of a candidal infection can be confirmed with a KOH preparation or fungal culture, if necessary

MANAGEMENT
- Minimize frequent hand washing and manicures
- Wear gloves when performing tasks such as washing dishes
- A superpotent topical steroid such as clobetasol cream or ointment 0.05% applied once or twice daily to the proximal nail fold. Alternatively, **Cordran tape** may be applied nightly to this area (see Appendix A)
- A topical broad-spectrum antifungal agent, such as **clotrimazolE, ketoconazole, econazole,** or **miconazole,** is often combined with a potent topical corticosteroid to provide antifungal as well as anti-inflammatory effects

✔ TIPS:
- **Although *Candida* is frequently isolated from the proximal nail fold of patients with chronic paronychia, a primary pathogenesis for this organism has never been proven. For this reason, topical steroids are often more effective as therapy than topical or even systemic antifungal agents**
- **However, there are instances in which *Candida* may play a primary pathogenic role, such as in patients who are diabetic and in those individuals with primary mucocutaneous candidiasis**

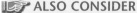

ALSO CONSIDER
- Ingrown finger/toenail
- Contact dermatitis

RARELY
- Mucocutaneous candidiasis

CHAPTER 14

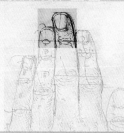

Fingernails

Fingernails are used to help pick up small objects and to scratch itchy areas; they also protect the vulnerable fingertips. Nails also are important contributors to the aesthetic appearance of the hands and feet (see also Chapter 22, Feet). Inflammatory disorders that involve the nail matrix, such as psoriasis and eczema, can result in distinctive deformities of the nails. To the health care provider, nails may represent clinical findings of a skin disorder or be a signal of an underlying systemic disease.

IN THIS CHAPTER

- Onycholysis *vs* onychomycosis *vs* psoriatic nail dystrophy *vs* nail dystrophy secondary to eczematous dermatitis
- Subungual wart *vs* subungual squamous cell carcinoma
- Subungual hematoma *vs* junctional nevus *vs* acral lentiginous melanoma

Onycholysis *vs* Onychomycosis *vs* Psoriatic Nail Dystrophy *vs* Nail Dystrophy Secondary to Eczematous Dermatitis

Onycholysis

Onycholysis represents a separation of the nail plate from its underlying nail bed. Irritants, such as nail polish, nail wraps, nail hardeners, and artificial nails, can cause the problem. Onycholysis may also be seen more frequently in persons who frequently come into contact with water, such as bartenders, hairdressers, manicurists, citrus fruit handlers, and domestic workers. Physiologic onycholysis is seen at the free margin of all healthy nails as they grow. When separation is more proximal, the onycholysis becomes more obvious and may become cosmetically objectionable. Reported causes and associated conditions include:

- Trauma, especially habitual finger sucking, athletic injuries to the toes, preformed artificial nails, and the use of fingernails as a tool
- Certain phototoxic agents (e.g., demethylchlortetracycline)
- Inflammatory skin diseases of the nail matrix (root), such as eczematous dermatitis and lichen planus
- Subungual neoplasms and warts that lift the nail
- Internal causes such as thyroid disease, pregnancy, and anemia
- Psoriasis, fungal infections (e.g., chronic paronychia [see Chapter 13, Hands and Fingers, and Onychomycosis, following])

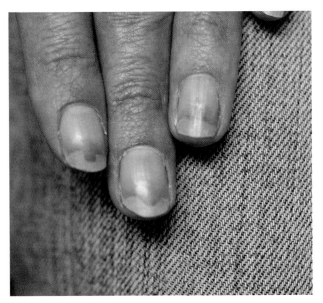

Figure 14-1 Onycholysis.

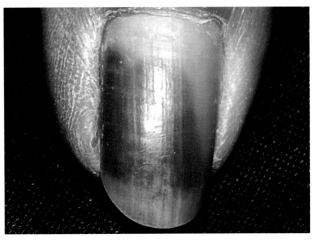

Figure 14-2 Onycholysis and green nail syndrome.

DISTINGUISHING FEATURES

- Most frequently seen in women, particularly in those with long fingernails
- It starts distally and progresses proximally, causing an uplifting of the distal nail plate
- The separated portion is white and opaque, in contrast to the pink translucence of the attached portion of the nail. (Fig. 14-1)
- Green nail syndrome
  - Occurs as a consequence of onycholysis. This asymptomatic discoloration under the nail should not be confused with a subungual fungal infection
  - The "dead space" under the onycholytic nail serves as an excellent breeding ground for microbes.
  - Often, *Pseudomonas* species are present; their presence usually accounts for the green, yellow, or green–black nail color (Fig. 14-2)

DIAGNOSIS

- Clinical

MANAGEMENT

- The goal is to:
  - Keep nails dry and cut closely. Proper trimming (along the contour) on a regular basis can protect the nails from injury and help keep the newly growing nail attached
  - The avoidance of unnecessary manipulation of nails and nail polish
  - Treating or avoiding the underlying cause of the problem, if known
- Green nail syndrome: the affected nails are soaked twice daily in a mixture either of 1 part chlorine bleach and 4 parts water or of equal parts acetic acid (vinegar) and water. This generally eliminates the green discoloration

Onychomycosis

Onychomycosis refers to an infection of the fingernails or toenails (see also Chapter 22, Feet) caused by various fungi, yeasts, and molds. Uncommon in children, the prevalence of onychomycosis increases with advancing age, with rates as high as 30% in those 70 years of age and older. The major causes of onychomycosis are dermatophytes. *Candida* infection of the nail plate generally results from paronychia that becomes established around the proximal the nail fold (see Chapter 13, Hands and Fingers).

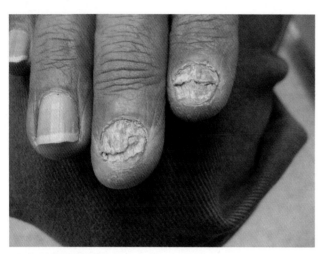

Figure 14-3 Onychomycosis. (Image courtesy of Benjamin Barankin, MD.)

DISTINGUISHING FEATURES

- Nail thickening and subungual hyperkeratosis (scale buildup under the nail) (Fig. 14-3)
- Nail discoloration (yellow, yellow-green, white, or brown)
- Nail dystrophy
- Onycholysis (see previous discussion)
- Generally asymptomatic, aside from footwear causing occasional physical discomfort and the psychosocial liability of unsightly nails

DIAGNOSIS

- Positive potassium hydroxide and/or growth of dermatophyte

MANAGEMENT

- Topical agents are generally ineffective because of poor nail penetration
- Systemic antifungals such as terbinafine (**Lamisil**), itraconazole (**Sporanox**), and griseofulvin (see Appendix A for dosing)
- Pre-existing liver disease is a relative contraindication to the use of systemic antifungal agents for onychomycosis
- Treatment may be required for a prolonged period
- Fingernail infections are usually cured more quickly and effectively than toenail infections

✔ **TIP: Long-term cure with most of these agents is probably no greater than 40% to 50%.**

✔ **TIP: Patients with a family history of onychomycosis are less likely to have a successful treatment outcome than those without such a history.**

- Surgical ablation of nails is rarely indicated and is generally ineffective
- Recently, photodynamic therapy and laser ablation have been used as treatment modalities. The long-term results remain to be determined

Psoriatic Nail Dystrophy

Involvement of nails is very common in patients with psoriasis. **Psoriatic nail dystrophy** is a chronic, primarily cosmetic condition. However, in some instances, thickened psoriatic toenails can become painful, deformed, and may interfere with function.

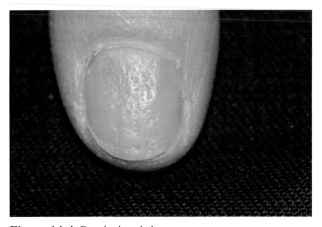

Figure 14-4 Psoriasis: pitting.

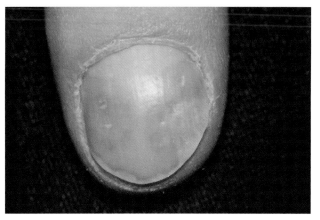

Figure 14-5 Psoriasis: oil spots and onycholysis are evident in this nail.

DISTINGUISHING FEATURES
- **Pitting** is the most characteristic finding. Pits are tiny punctate lesions and appear on the nail plate as it grows (resembling a sewing thimble) (Fig. 14-4)
- **Onycholysis** represents a separation of the nail plate from the underlying pink nail bed (see previous discussion if Onycholysis)
- **"Oil spots"** are orange-brown colorations appearing under the nail plate. They are presumably due to psoriasis of the nail bed (Fig. 14-5)
- **Subungual hyperkeratosis,** similar to onychomycosis (see previous discussion), consists of nail thickening and hyperkeratotic scaling under the nail (Fig. 14-6)

DIAGNOSIS
- Clinical
- Patients usually have psoriasis elsewhere on the body

MANAGEMENT (See Appendix A)
Treatment is generally unrewarding, but some measures can be helpful:
- Careful trimming and paring
- The application of a super-potent (class 1) topical steroid to the proximal nail folds followed by covering with plastic wrap, **Cordran tape,** or a plastic glove

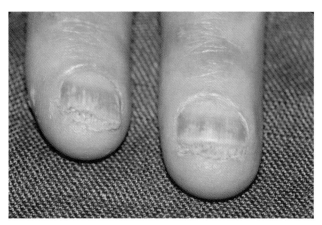

Figure 14-6 Psoriasis: subungual hyperkeratosis and oil spots.

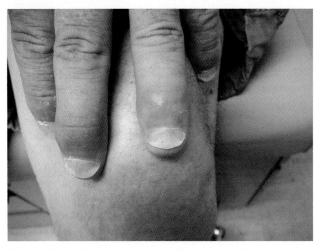

Figure 14-7 Psoriatic arthritis. Note onycholysis.

- Intralesional corticosteroids injected into the nail matrix (see Appendix B)
- Systemic medications are most commonly used to treat severe psoriasis and nail psoriasis: methotrexate, retinoids, and cyclosporine. All have potential serious side effects and toxicities, and, in most cases, the psoriatic nail disease recurs after the systemic therapy is stopped
- Immunologically directed treatment with so-called "biologic" agents such as etanercept (**Enbrel**) and adalimumab (**Humira**) are reserved for intractable cases, particularly when psoriatic arthritis is also present

☑ **TIP: Psoriasis of the nails may be indistinguishable from, or coexist with, onychomycosis.**

⚠ **ALERT: Severe psoriatic nail dystrophy may be an indicator of psoriatic arthritis (Fig. 14-7).**

Nail Dystrophy Secondary To Eczematous Dermatitis

Nail dystrophy secondary to eczematous dermatitis is a problem that is often overlooked in patients with severe atopic dermatitis. It results when eczematous dermatitis involves the distal extensor surface of the fingers. Analogous to the root (matrix) and trunk (nail) of a tree, the associated inflammation also involves the underlying matrix, or "root," of the nail. The inflamed matrix, which underlies the proximal nail fold, consequently gives rise to a dystrophic nail plate.

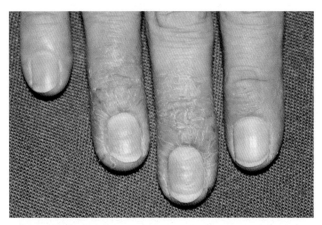

Figure 14-8 Eczematous dermatitis. Eczema of the proximal skin also affects the matrix (root) of the nail, resulting in nail dystrophy.

DISTINGUISHING FEATURES
- Eczematous dermatitis located on the dorsum of the distal part of the finger (proximal nail fold)
- The nails generally have a ripplelike deformity that corresponds to the time of activity of the original inflammation (Fig. 14-8)

DIAGNOSIS
- Clinical (eczematous dermatitis located on dorsal, distal fingers)

MANAGEMENT (see Appendix A)
- Improvement of the appearance of the nail plate follows control of inflammation of the proximal nail fold skin with the use of potent topical steroids

📖 **ALSO CONSIDER**
- Chronic paronychia
- Lichen planus
- Subungual warts (when only 1 or 2 nails are involved)
- Onychogryphosis

RARELY
- Subungual squamous cell carcinoma (when only 1 nail is involved)

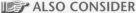

Subungual Wart

A **subungual wart** (Fig. 14-9) can be both a challenging diagnostic as well as therapeutic problem. A solitary wart of the nail bed lifting the nail plate is often mistaken for onychomycosis (see Chapter 13, Hands and Fingers).

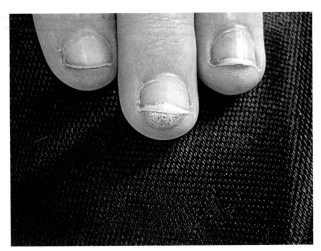

Figure 14-9 Subungual verruca.

Squamous Cell Carcinoma

Although quite rare, the possibility of subungual **squamous cell carcinoma** (Fig. 14-10), basal cell carcinoma, or other neoplasm should always be considered if only one nail or periungual area is involved, particularly in elderly men (see Chapter 1, Hair and Scalp; Chapter 2, Forehead and Temples; Chapter 4, Ears; Chapter 5, Nose and Perinasal Area; Chapter 6, Cheeks).

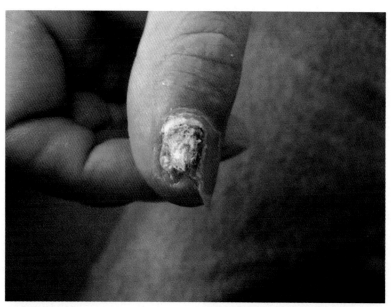

Figure 14-10 Subungual squamous cell carcinoma. (Image courtesy of Haines Ely, MD.)

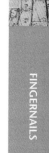

ALSO CONSIDER
• Onychomycosis

Subungual Hematoma *vs* Junctional Nevus *vs* Acral Lentiginous Melanoma

By far, trauma is the most common cause of nail disorders. However, an injury that results in a collection of blood under the nail can be quite unsettling because a neoplasm often is not easy to rule out (see also Chapter 22, Feet).

Subungual Hematoma

Subungual hematoma results from trauma to the nail matrix or nail bed, such as repeated minor injuries (e.g., sports injuries) or substantial impact (as from a hammer). An acute subungual hematoma that results from rapid accumulation of blood under the nail plate can be very painful, whereas small lesions may be painless and may go unnoticed for some time.

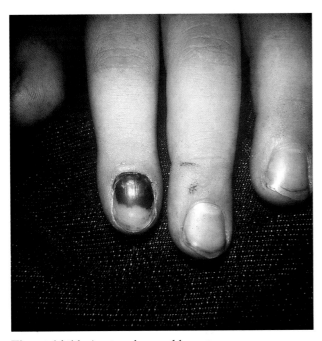

Figure 14-11 Acute subungual hematoma.

DISTINGUISHING FEATURES
- Brown to black subungual pigmentation (Fig. 14-11)
- Painful if acute

DIAGNOSIS
- History and clinical findings
- ✔ **TIP: A rapid method to substantiate the presence of a hematoma is to pare the nail plate gently with a No. 15 scalpel blade or to file it down until the coagulated blood can be visualized (see Chapter 22, Feet; Figures 20-A, 20-B and 20-C).**

MANAGEMENT
- ✔ **TIP: An acute, painful, swollen subungual hematoma may be incised and drained by placing the red-hot end of a heated paper clip on the area elevated by the hematoma. The small hole created with this procedure allows the blood to drain and thus quickly relieves the pain. Twirling a 27-gauge needle to create a similar hole is an alternative method for draining the blood.**
- ⚠ **ALERT: Chronic, painless subungual hematomas that are clearly not the result of trauma may appear similar to a neoplasm, such as an acral lentiginous melanoma (see discussion below). Because the coagulated bloodstains remain until the nail grows out (from 3-4 months for fingernails, 8-12 months for toenails). Consequently, the diagnosis may be in doubt for some time**

Junctional Nevus

Junctional nevus lesions are quite common in dark-skinned people and may be multiple. They are much less common in caucasions.

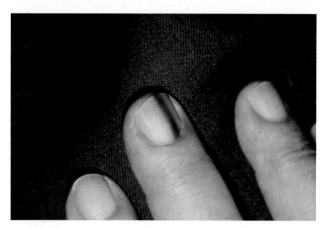

Figure 14-12 Junctional nevus: a brown linear band of longitudinal melanonychia in a child.

DISTINGUISHING FEATURES
- An evenly pigmented linear nevus that emanates from nests of nevus cells in the nail matrix (Fig. 14-12)

DIAGNOSIS
- Clinical
- Dermoscopy (see Appendix B)

MANAGEMENT
⚠ **ALERT: Any smudging or leaching of pigment or variation from the original black band should undergo biopsy immediately to rule out malignant melanoma (see following discussion)**

Acral Lentiginous Melanoma

Acral lentiginous melanoma (ALM) is the least common subtype of melanoma; it is relatively rare. However, it accounts for 29% to 72% of melanoma cases in dark-skinned individuals (i.e., blacks, Asian, and Hispanic persons). Lesions in ALM appear on areas that do not bear hair, such as periungual skin, and beneath the nail plate, especially on the thumb or great toe, as well as on the palms and soles (see Chapter 22, Feet, Plantar Soles).

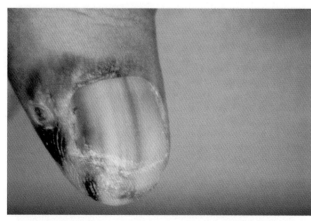

Figure 14-13 Acral lentiginous melanoma (Hutchinson sign). Note spread of pigment to periungual skin.

DISTINGUISHING FEATURES
- A subungual melanoma may manifest as diffuse nail discoloration or a longitudinal pigmented band within the nail plate
- Pigment spread to the proximal or lateral nail folds is termed the *Hutchinson sign*, which is a hallmark for ALM (Fig. 14-13)

DIAGNOSIS
- Dermoscopy (see Appendix B)
- Excisional or punch biopsy is performed on the nail bed
⚠ **ALERT: ALM has a tendency to early metastasis and, because of delays in diagnosis, may be associated with a worse prognosis.**

MANAGEMENT
- Elliptical wide excision should include the entire visible lesion down to the subcutaneous fat
- Sentinel lymph node biopsy (see Chapter 12, Arms), regional lymph node dissection, amputation, and regional chemotherapy perfusion are sometimes necessary for ALM

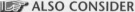 **ALSO CONSIDER**
- Wart
- Onychomycosis
- Pyogenic granuloma
- Fibroma
- Other benign entities

FINGERNAILS

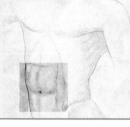

CHAPTER 15

Trunk

The trunk is a large area that incudes a vast assortment of skin disorders that are inflammatory, infectious, or neoplastic. There are many rashes that result from adverse drug reactions, viral, and bacterial infections. As a result of being generally sun-protected by clothing, the trunk is less likely to develop nonmelanoma skin cancers such as solar keratoses, basal cell carcinomas, and squamous cell carcinomas; however, the back and anterior torso are common sites for melanomas to appear, particularly in men.

IN THIS CHAPTER

Upper Back and Chest
- Hypertrophic scars *vs* keloids
- Pruritus and neurotic excoriations *vs* notalgia paresthetica *vs* macular amyloid

Chest, Upper Back, Lower Back, and Abdomen
- Viral exanthems *vs* drug eruptions *vs* erythema multiforme *vs* acute and chronic urticaria
- Tinea corporis *vs* erythema migrans (acute Lyme disease)
- Herpes zoster *vs* herpes simplex
- Pityriasis rosea *vs* generalized plaque psoriasis/acute guttate psoriasis
- Tinea versicolor *vs* vitiligo vulgaris
- Tinea versicolor *vs* confluent and reticulated papillomatosis
- Epidermoid cysts *vs* lipoma
- Cherry angioma *vs* melanocytic nevus
- Halo nevus *vs* atypical nevus *vs* melanoma *vs* seborrheic keratosis
- Superficial basal cell carcinoma *vs* solitary plaque psoriasis

Hypertrophic Scars *vs* Keloids

Hypertrophic Scars

Hypertrophic scars represent an exaggerated formation of scar tissue in response to skin injuries such as lacerations, infections, insect bites, and surgical wounds. These scars are widened, thick, or unsightly scars that *do not* extend beyond the original boundaries of an original injury. Hypertrophic scars may also result from healed inflammatory lesions (e.g., acne, chickenpox). Such exaggerated scars occur less frequently at the extremes of age—the very young and elderly. There is no racial preponderance noted with these scars. In recent years, the popularity of skin-piercing procedures and tattooing has increased the frequency of these undesirable scars and has expanded the sites on the body where they may occur.

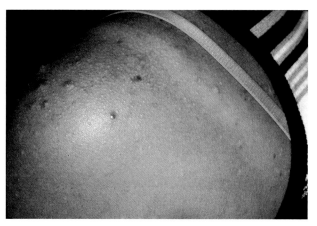

Figure 15-1 Hypertrophic scars. Also note the tiny, white, dome-shaped comedolike acne scars. They are often mistaken for closed comedones.

DISTINGUISHING FEATURES
- Elevated, firm, shiny, hairless, papules, or nodules; they may be flesh-colored, tan, or brown (Fig. 15-1)
- If lesions are inflamed or are of recent onset, they may be red or purple
- Most commonly arise on the sternum, the deltoid region of the upper arm, shoulders, and upper back
- The most common sites on the head and neck are the earlobes, mandibular border, and posterior neck
- Unlike keloids, the hypertrophic scar reaches a certain size and subsequently stabilizes or regresses, whereas keloids (see later discussion) do not regress without treatment and tend to recur after excision

DIAGNOSIS
- Clinical appearance

MANAGEMENT
- Patients who tend to develop hypertrophic scars or keloids should be advised to discontinue or avoid repetitive skin trauma such as tattooing and skin-piercing practices, particularly in areas that are prone to abnormal scarring such as the presternal areas and earlobes
- Conditions such as inflammatory acne and cutaneous infections should be treated promptly to prevent scarring
- Intralesional corticosteroid injections with triamcinolone acetate in varying concentrations (10 to 40 mg/mL) injected directly into the scar are the mainstay of treatment. A 27- to 30-gauge needle at 4- to 6-week intervals often helps flatten the lesions. Additionally, these injections are also useful for diminishing pruritus and tenderness
- Such injections must be administered cautiously to avoid overtreatment, which may result in skin atrophy, telangiectasias, and overdepressed scars
- Topical corticosteroids: clear surgical tape impregnated with flurandrenolide (**Cordran Tape**) has been shown to soften and flatten hypertrophic scars over time
- Pulsed-dye lasers have been used successfully on some persistent hypertrophic scars

Keloids

Keloids are an overgrowth of dense fibrous tissue, a scar whose size far exceeds that which would be expected from the extent and margins of an injury to the skin. "Cheloid," derived from the Greek *chele,* or crab's claw, describes the lateral growth of tissue into unaffected skin. As with hypertrophic scars, keloids are an exaggerated response to a skin injury, inflammatory lesion (e.g., acne), or a surgical wound. However, in contrast to hypertrophic scars, keloids are more likely to occur in individuals of African descent as well as Hispanics and Asians.

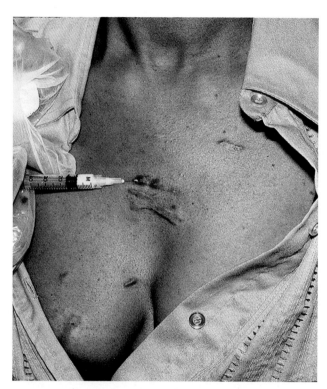

Figure 15-2 Keloids. Injection with triamcinolone.

DISTINGUISHING FEATURES
- Uncontrolled overgrowth of scar tissue with extension beyond the site of the original wound with a tendency to send out clawlike prolongations (Fig. 15-2)
- Usually asymptomatic, although some are pruritic and other may be quite painful and tender
- Keloids, by virtue of their excessive size, are of much greater cosmetic concern to patients than are hypertrophic scars

DIAGNOSIS
- Clinical appearance

MANAGEMENT
- Intralesional corticosteroid injections, often in concentrations as high as 40 mg/mL, can help flatten keloids and diminish itching and erythema (see previous discussion)
- Excision using aseptic operative technique in combination with other postoperative modalities, such as triamcinolone acetate injections, compression dressings, radiotherapy, or injected interferon
- Lasers have been used as alternatives to cold excision for keloids. As with excisional therapy, laser results are best when combined with postoperative injected steroids
- Excision followed by:
  - Topical imiquimod (**Aldara**) cream induces local production of interferon-alpha, which in turn is known to enhance keloidal collagenase activity and reduce the synthesis of collagen
  - Other medications include oral verapamil, intralesional bleomycin, 5-fluorouracil, and botulinum toxin

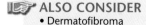 **ALSO CONSIDER**
- Dermatofibroma

RARELY
- Dermatofibrosarcoma protuberans
- Scleredema diabeticorum
- Atrophoderma
- Lichen sclerosis et atrophicus
- Sarcoma

Pruritus and Neurotic Excoriations

Pruritus is the most common symptom of all skin diseases. The pruritus may be due to primary skin disorders such as eczema, or xerosis (dry skin), exogenous causes such as drugs, internal disorders such as chronic renal disease, malignancies (e.g., Hodgkin disease), psychogenic causes such as delusions of parasitosis, or obsessive-compulsive disorder. Itching may sometimes be idiopathic; pruritus of unknown origin is defined as itching lasting for more than 6 weeks with no determined cause.

Neurotic excoriations may be simply defined as skin-picking or scratching episodes that are a conscious response to anxiety or be an unconscious habit. Some individuals with compulsive skin picking often have a coexisting psychiatric disorder, especially obsessive-compulsive disorder. They pick at moles, scabs, sores, acne pimples, or in some cases imagined skin defects that are not actually visible by others.

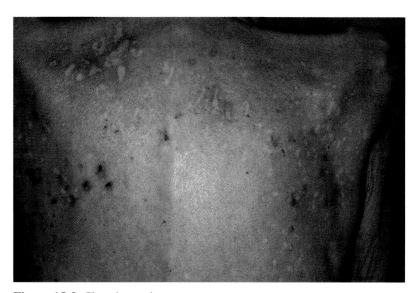

Figure 15-3 Chronic pruritus.

DISTINGUISHING FEATURES
- Linear excoriations, crusts, lichenified plaques, and wheals may be present (Fig. 15-3)
- The lesions may have a bizarre appearance with deep ulcers and scars (factitia or "neurotic excoriations")
- Pruritus with no visible lesions is also quite common

DIAGNOSIS
- A search for the cause of the pruritus is based on:
  - A careful history
  - Physical evidence (linear excoriations, crusts)
- Workup for pruritus of unknown origin includes:
  - Rectal and pelvic examinations, if indicated
  - Complete blood count
  - Stool for parasites and occult blood
  - Chest radiograph
  - Thyroid, renal, liver function tests

MANAGEMENT

- Whenever possible, treatment of underlying systemic disease that is the cause of the pruritus may bring relief
- Antihistamines are of more benefit in the treatment of allergic conditions, urticaria, and drug reactions than they are for the treatment of itching, and may be no more effective than placebo
- Topical therapy that can be soothing and helpful in some patients includes:
  - Menthol, phenol, camphor, calamine lotions (e.g., **Sarna, Prax, PrameGel**)
  - Cold applications of ice packs or packages of frozen vegetables
  - Topical steroids are generally not very helpful when no lesions are apparent
- For pruritus of chronic renal disease:
  - Ultraviolet B (UVB) therapy
  - Oral ingestion of activated charcoal
  - Cholestyramine
- For pruritus due to liver disease:
  - Cholestyramine

- For pruritus due to xerosis:
  - Moisturizers
  - Topical steroids are used only when there are inflammatory skin lesions
  - Antihistamines often exert their antipruritic action by inducing sleep (soporific effect)
  - The dosage of antihistamines should be titrated gradually upward using nonsedating agents during the daytime and sedating agents at bedtime
- For pruritus due to obsessive-compulsive disorder:
  - Often used in conjunction with cognitive behavior therapy, the drugs of choice are the selective serotonin reuptake inhibitors such as fluoxetine, paroxetine, sertraline, and fluvoxamine

☑ **TIP: Angiotensin-converting enzyme (ACE) inhibitors, the "prils," such as benazepril (Lotensin), captopril (Capoten), Enalapril (Vasotec), and lisinopril (Prinivil), and (Zestril), can be a source of pruritus in the elderly.**

⚠ **ALERT: Hodgkin disease may present with a pruritus that precedes the diagnosis by as many as 5 years.**

Notalgia Paresthetica

Notalgia paraesthetica is a relatively common condition of localized itch and/or changed sensation that arises in the areas of skin on or below the shoulder blade on either side of the back. It appears typically in persons over the age of 40. There are two proposed possible causes for its appearance—increased sensory innervation of the affected skin areas and neuropathy from degenerative cervicothoracic disk disease or direct nerve impingement.

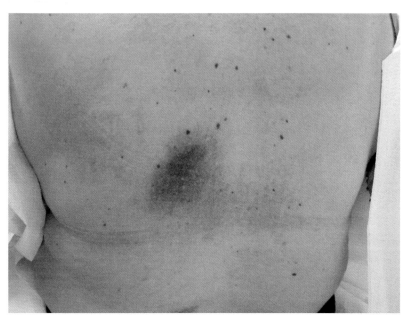

Figure 15-4 Notalgia paresthetica. Note erythema and postinflammatory hyperpigmentation.

DISTINGUISHING FEATURES
- Visible changes arise from rubbing and scratching the affected area. These include erythema, hyperpigmentation, hypopigmentation and possible scarring (Fig. 15-4)

DIAGNOSIS
- Clinical; the postinflammatory hyperpigmentation that often results from the chronic rubbing and scratching reveals the diagnosis

MANAGEMENT
- Treatment is not always successful
- Possible effective measures include the following:
  - Gabapentin (**Neurontin**)
  - Cooling lotions as required (camphor and menthol)
  - Over-the-counter (OTC) capsaicin (**Zostrix**) cream (depletes nerve endings of their chemical transmitters)
  - Local anesthetic creams
  - Amitriptyline tablets at night
  - Transcutaneous electrical nerve stimulation
  - Botulinum toxin

Macular Amyloid

Macular amyloid refers to the deposition of amyloid or amyloidlike proteins in the dermis. It appears to be more common in Asians, South Americans, and individuals from the Middle East. It usually presents in early adult life and appears to affect women more frequently than men. Patients seek medical attention because of intense itching or the hyperpigmentation.

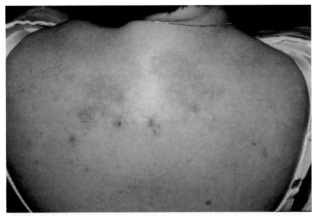

Figure 15-5 Macular amyloid.

DISTINGUISHING FEATURES
- Mild to severe pruritus
- Often a reticulated pattern of small, dusky-brown or grayish pigmented hyperpigmentation (Fig. 15-5)
- Lesions are usually distributed symmetrically over the upper back between the shoulder blades, on the chest, and sometimes on the arms

DIAGNOSIS
- Punch biopsy and special stain (Congo red)

MANAGEMENT
Treatment is focused on relieving itch:
- Sedating antihistamines can be moderately effective
- Topical and intralesional steroids may provide some relief if used with other treatments, which include topical dimethyl sulfoxide and phototherapy (UVB or psoralen plus ultraviolet A), and pulsed-dye laser

ALSO CONSIDER
- Drug abuse (e.g., cocaine, methamphetamine)
- Infestations: scabies, lice
- Foreign body reaction: fiberglass
- Fabric softener dermatitis ("Bounce" dermatitis)
- Pityrosporum folliculitis
- Pregnancy
- Transient acantholytic dermatosis (Grover disease)
- Acne excoriée
- Factitia: self-induced lesions may have a bizarre appearance with deep ulcers and scars
- Internal disorders such as HIV/AIDS, cholestasis, diabetes mellitus, thyroid disease
- Associated malignancies such as leukemia and multiple myeloma
- Psychogenic causes such as delusions of parasitosis

RARELY
- Polycythemia vera
- Carcinoid syndrome
- Primary biliary cirrhosis
- Keratosis follicularis (Darier disease)
- Dermatitis herpetiformis

Viral Exanthems *vs* Drug Eruptions *vs* Erythema Multiforme *vs* Acute and Chronic Urticaria

Viral Exanthems

Viral exanthems are the cutaneous manifestation of an acute viral infection. They are most commonly seen in children and may present as distinct, clinically recognizable illnesses such as measles or chickenpox. More frequently, however, a nonspecific eruption arises, making an exact diagnosis elusive. More than 50 viral agents are known to cause exanthems, and many of these rashes are indistinguishable from each other. Most viral illnesses are benign and self-limited; therefore, a specific diagnosis is often not made. However, there are instances in which the diagnosis of a treatable bacterial infection may be of vital importance (e.g., in rickettsial infection) or eliminating a drug that might be causing a rash accompanied by fever might be life-saving.

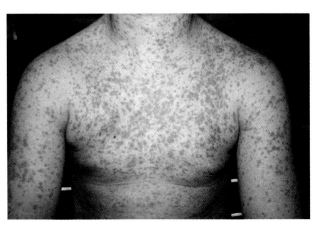

Figure 15-6 Morbilliform eruption (measles). Reprinted with permission from Chung, EK, Atkinson-McEvoy L, Boom JA, Matz PS, eds. *Visual Diagnosis in Pediatrics*. 2nd ed. Philadelphia: Lippincott Williams & Wilkins; 2010.)

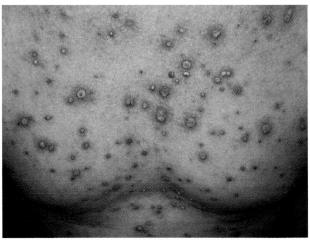

Figure 15-7 Vesicular eruption (varicella). Note pustules.

DISTINGUISHING FEATURES
- Macular and papular (morbilliform) as noted in measles (Figure 15-6)
- Vesicular as seen in varicella (Figure 15-7)

DIAGNOSIS
- It is helpful to be aware of current community infections
- A thorough history and certain laboratory tests may help to exclude bacterial disease as a cause of the rash. These include a throat culture, complete blood count with differential, urine or cerebrospinal fluid testing for bacterial antigens, and a blood culture
- A skin biopsy is rarely valuable in this setting

TIP: Viral or bacterial exanthems generally occur with fever and other symptoms; however, they are often indistinguishable from drug eruptions that may also have similar symptoms (Table 15-1)

MANAGEMENT
- Uncomplicated exanthems in otherwise healthy children are generally treated with supportive care such as antipruritics and antipyretics

Table 15-1 DIFFERENTIAL DIAGNOSIS OF VARIOUS VIRAL EXANTHEMS

	Enterovirus	Rubella	Measles	Roseola	Varicella
Cause	Coxsackievirus, echovirus, or enterovirus	Rubella virus	Measles virus	Herpesvirus 6	Varicella-zoster virus
Incubation period (days)	4–7	12–23	9–11	5–15	11–20
Age	More common in children	Any age	Usually <15 months or >15 years	6 months to 3 years	1–14 years (90%)
Prodrome	Variable fever and malaise	Mild, 1–5 days of fever and malaise	2–4 days of high fever, conjunctivitis, coryza, and cough	Abrupt onset of high fever for 3–5 days, then rash disappears	Rare
Distinguishing features	Variable: macular, papular, urticarial, scarlatiniform, or petechial; may be generalized	Exanthem resolves on the first or second day. Begins on face, spreads centrifugally, and resolution in cephalocaudad direction may be accompanied by fine, branny, desquamation. Lymphadenopathy, with postauricular, suboccipital, and posterior cervical nodes	Pathognomonic Koplik's spots (enanthem). Rash follows cephalocaudad order in its development. Begins as discrete erythematous macules and papules, which soon coalesce into areas of confluent erythema	Discrete rose-pink macules and papules. Begins on face and progresses to trunk and extremities. Mild coryza, and cough	Red macules → papules → vesicles ("dew drops on rose petals") → pustules → crusts. Simultaneous presence of lesions in varying stages of development. Begins on face, scalp, and trunk, and then spreads to centrifugally. Low-grade fever, malaise, pruritus
Duration of illness (days)	3–7	3–5	4–7	5–7	7
Diagnostic techniques	Clinical; viral culture (stool, cerebrospinal fluid, urine)	Clinical; serology (immunoglobulin M or acute and convalescent serology)	Clinical; serology (acute and convalescent serology)	Clinical; (acute and convalescent serology)	Clinical; Tzanck smear; viral culture or direct immunofluorescence; serologic tests

Drug Eruptions

The trunk is a common site for **drug eruptions** to appear. Adverse reactions to drugs are more often seen in the elderly because older people take more drugs than younger people, they frequently take more than one drug at a time, and are more likely to have been previously sensitized. Drug reactions may be allergic (immunologic) or nonallergic (toxic). Certain classes of systemic medications, such as antimicrobial agents, nonsteroidal anti-inflammatory drugs (NSAIDs), chemotherapeutic agents, and psychotropic agents, are associated with a high rate of cutaneous reactions. Nonallergic drug eruptions are more common than allergic-type eruptions. Vertigo due to high-dose oral minocycline and irritant reactions from topical retinoids are examples. Most drug eruptions are exanthematous (red rashes) and usually fade in a few days. More serious reactions include erythema multiforme major (Stevens-Johnson syndrome) and toxic epidermal necrolysis. Other cutaneous reactions to drugs include erythema nodosum, vasculitis, purpura, (see Chapter 21, Legs) and photosensitivity reactions (see Chapter 10, Neck).

DISTINGUISHING FEATURES

Certain drugs are more likely to cause characteristic reactions in the skin:

- *Exanthems and urticarial reactions:* sulfonamides, penicillins, hydantoins, thiazide diuretics, allopurinol, quinidine, ACE inhibitors, barbiturates, carbamazepine, isoniazid, NSAIDs, and phenothiazines
- *Acneiform eruptions:* systemic steroids, topical steroids, lithium, and androgenic hormones
- *Contact dermatitis:* neomycin, preservatives in topical medications
- Pruritus is a common complaint; however, adverse drug reactions also can cause pruritus unaccompanied by a rash (e.g., ACE inhibitors)

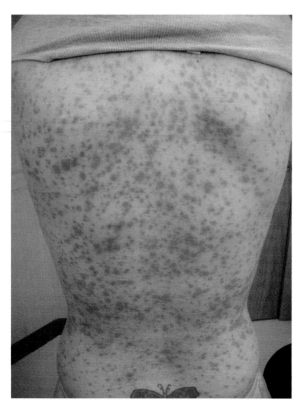

Figure 15-8 Drug eruption: exanthem due to ampicillin.

- Drug eruptions tend to be symmetrical in distribution; however, certain eruptions have specific regional predilections (see fixed drug eruption discussed below)
- Exanthems are noted particularly on the trunk, thighs, upper arms, and face. Lesions are morbilliform (measles-like, macular, and papular); such exanthems are the most common pattern (Figure 15-8)
- There may be areas of confluence
- Lesions are pink, "drug red," or purple in color
- Acute urticarial lesions (see following discussion) usually appear shortly after onset of drug therapy and resolve rapidly when the responsible drug is withdrawn. They usually occur as small wheals that may coalesce or take cyclical or gyrate forms
- A fixed drug eruption may present as a solitary isolated lesion occurring most often on the extremities, glans penis, or trunk; multiple fixed drug lesions may also occur

DIAGNOSIS

- Obtaining a detailed, careful history is paramount
- A drug-induced reaction should be considered in the differential diagnosis of any symmetric cutaneous eruption with sudden onset in a patient who takes medications
- There is occasional eosinophilia
- Skin biopsy of an exanthem showing perivascular lymphocytes and eosinophils may be helpful, but is not diagnostic
- A handy reference to drug eruptions and interactions should be always available

MANAGEMENT

- Often, the decision whether to discontinue a potentially vital drug presents a dilemma
- The presence of urticaria, mucosal involvement, extensive or palpable purpura, or blisters almost always requires discontinuation of the responsible drug
- If a patient is taking multiple medications, it is often impossible to identify the agent responsible for an adverse reaction. In these instances, the drug that is most likely to cause the reaction should be suspected or the number of medications should be reduced to an absolute minimum and the remaining drugs switched to alternative agents when possible
- Oral antihistamines such as diphenhydramine (**Benadryl**), hydroxyzine (**Atarax**), or the nonsedating agents such as cetirizine (**Zyrtec**) or loratadine (**Claritin**) may be helpful
- Systemic steroids are given only in severe cases in which an infectious etiology is ruled out
- If it is necessary to continue the drug (i.e., there is no alternative medication) and the adverse reaction is mild or tolerable, the difficulty may be minimized by decreasing the dosage or treating the adverse drug reaction
- ✔ **TIP: Persons who are immunocompromised have a higher risk of developing a drug eruption than the general population**
- ✔ **TIP: Drug reactions can occur days after a drug has been discontinued.**
- ⚠ **ALERT: A drug eruption may easily be confused as being a feature of the condition that it is intended to treat (e.g., a viral exanthem treated with an antibiotic).**

Erythema Multiforme

Erythema multiforme minor and **major** (Stevens-Johnson syndrome) lesions commonly manifest on mucous membranes and on the palms and soles. They also can be widespread and involve the trunk.

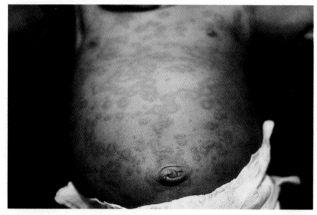

Figure 15-9 Erythema multiforme: target-shaped lesions in an infant. Reprinted with permission from Chung, EK, Atkinson-McEvoy L, Boom JA, Matz PS, eds. *Visual Diagnosis in Pediatrics.* 2nd ed. Philadelphia: Lippincott Williams & Wilkins; 2010.)

DISTINGUISHING FEATURES

Erythema Multiforme Minor

- Lesions begin as round, dull-red macules or urticarial plaques that expand over 24 to 48 hours
- Some lesions evolve to form targetoid plaques (iris lesions) (Figure 15-9) with a dark center that may become vesicobullous
- Lesions persist (are "fixed") for at least 1 week; thereafter, erosions and crusts form
- Bilateral and symmetric

- The palms and soles, dorsa of hands (see Fig. 13-16) and feet, extensor forearms, face, and legs may be affected
- Most commonly seen in late adolescence and in young adulthood
- Patients are generally well with, at most, mild systemic symptoms
- When present, mucous membrane lesions are limited to the mouth and lips
- The eruption is acute, relatively mild, self-limited, and often recurrent
- An active vesicle or a crusted lesion of recurrent herpes simplex virus (HSV) may be present on the vermillion border of the lip during an outbreak or the patient may have a history of recurrent HSV (see Fig. 8-7)

Erythema Multiforme Major

- Severe, extensive, painful mucous membrane involvement; may be located in multiple sites, including the mouth, pharynx, eyes, and genitalia
- As in erythema multiforme minor, target lesions may also be present
- Often accompanied by symptoms of fever, malaise, and myalgias
- At least 2 mucosal surfaces are affected in erythema multiforme major and are characterized by hemorrhagic crusting of the lips and ulceration of the mucosa (see Fig. 8-8)

DIAGNOSIS/MANAGEMENT

- See Chapter 8, Oral Cavity and Tongue; Chapter 13, Hands and Fingers

Acute and Chronic Urticaria

Acute urticaria, also known as *hives* (see Chapter 13, Hands and Fingers), may be caused by an obvious precipitant such as an acute upper respiratory infection, a drug reaction (see previous discussion), parasitic infection, or bee sting. The most common drugs that may cause acute urticaria are antibiotics (especially penicillin and sulfonamides), pain medications such as aspirin, NSAIDs, narcotics, radiocontrast dyes, diuretics, and opiates such as codeine. The most common foods associated with acute urticaria are milk, wheat, eggs, chocolate, shellfish, nuts, fish, and strawberries. Food additives and preservatives such as salicylates and benzoates may also be responsible. Systemic diseases such as lymphomas and collagen vascular diseases may have an associated urticaria. **Chronic urticaria,** often referred to as chronic idiopathic urticaria, is defined as urticaria that lasts for more than 6 weeks.

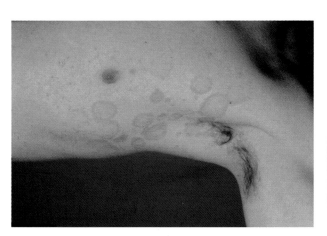

Figure 15-10 Urticaria, annular, gyrate erythema.

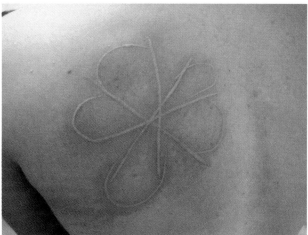

Figure 15-11 Dermatographism.

DISTINGUISHING FEATURES
- Annular or gyrate shapes (Figure 15-10)
- Pruritus without excoriations
- Individual lesions, by definition, last less than 24 hours

Physical urticarias: physical factors are the most commonly identified causes of chronic urticaria. Physical urticarias are diagnosed by challenge testing. The following is a list of some of the physical urticarias and their causes:
- *Dermatographism* ("skin writing"), which results from firm stroking or scratching or from tight garments (e.g., bras). Linear erythematous wheals occur 3 to 4 minutes after firmly stroking the skin with the wooden handle of cotton swab; they fade within 30 minutes (Figure 15-11)
- *Cold urticaria,* which results from cold exposure. Itchy hives occur at sites of cold exposure, such as areas exposed to cold winds or immersion in cold water
- *Aquagenic urticaria,* which results from contact with water
- *Cholinergic urticaria,* which results from heat or exercise
- *Solar urticaria,* which results from sun exposure

DIAGNOSIS

- The diagnosis of acute and chronic urticaria (see also Chapter 13, Hands and Fingers, Palmar Surface) is usually made on clinical observation and history. If a complete review of systems is normal and a physical urticaria is ruled out, it is often futile to perform multiple laboratory tests to determine a cause of chronic urticaria
- Nonetheless, a positive symptom-directed search for underlying illness (e.g., systemic lupus erythematosus, thyroid disease, lymphoma, and necrotizing vasculitis) may warrant evaluations such as:
  - Complete blood count
  - Erythrocyte sedimentation rate
  - Fluorescent antinuclear antibody test
  - Thyroid function studies
  - Hepatitis-associated antigen test
  - Assessment of the complement system
  - Radioallergosorbent test for immunoglobulin E antibodies
  - In the presence of eosinophilia, stool examination for ova and parasites
  - A CD203c assay, used to detect autoimmune urticaria, is now available

MANAGEMENT (see Appendix A)

- Cool soaks/ice packs
- First-generation antihistamines H_1 blockers such as diphenhydramine and hydroxyzine
- Nonsedating fexofenadine (**Allegra**), cetirizine (**Zyrtec**), or loratadine (**Claritin**)
- Doxepin can be given at a much lower dosages than when it is used as an antidepressant

🛈 **ALERTS:**
- **Epinephrine, which is often administered by intramuscular or subcutaneous injection for acute urticaria, should not be used for routine cases of hives. It should be reserved for cases of acute anaphylaxis**
- **Patients with severe reactions should consider wearing a Medic Alert bracelet that describes their problem**

🐾 ALSO CONSIDER
- Bacterial exanthem (e.g., scarlet fever, Kawasaki syndrome)
- Atypical measles in those vaccinated with the killed virus vaccine
- Erythema infectiosum
- Pityriasis rosea

RARELY
- Reticulated erythematous mucinosis
- Disseminated granuloma annulare
- Erythema annulare centrifugum
- Hansen disease (leprosy)
- Tuberculosis

Tinea Corporis

Tinea corporis ("ringworm") is most often acquired by contact with an infected animal, usually kittens and occasionally dogs (see also Chapter 6, Cheeks). It may also spread from person-to-person contact (e.g., transmission from wrestling [tinea gladiatorum]).

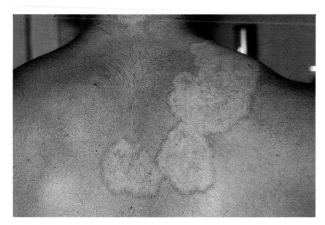

Figure 15-12 Tinea corporis.

DISTINGUISHING FEATURES
- Lesions often annular with peripheral enlargement and central clearing (Fig. 15-12)
- Single or multiple lesions
- May be pruritic or asymptomatic

DIAGNOSIS
- A history of a newly adopted kitten, or of another infected contact, is helpful
- Diagnosis is confirmed by a positive potassium hydroxide (KOH) examination or fungal culture best taken from the border (see Appendix B) or from periodic acid–Schiff stain on biopsy specimens

MANAGEMENT (see Appendix A)
- Topical antifungal agents such as ketoconazole 2% twice daily
- Systemic antifungal agents such as terbinafine (**Lamisil**), itraconazole (**Sporanox**), ketoconazole, or griseofulvin are sometimes necessary
- If pets appear to be the source of infection, they may also need antifungal treatment after evaluation by a veterinarian

Erythema Migrans (Acute Lyme Disease)

Lyme disease, or Lyme borreliosis (LB), is a systemic infection caused by the spirochete, *Borrelia burgdorferi.* The bacteria are introduced into the skin by a bite from an infected *Ixodes* tick. Transmission of the spirochete requires 48 to 72 hours, thus affording the tick (usually the larva or nymph) enough time to embed in the skin. Once in the skin, the spirochete may stay localized at the site of inoculation, or it may disseminate via the blood and lymphatic glands. Hematogenous dissemination can occur within days or weeks of the initial infection. The organism can travel to other parts of the skin, the heart, the joints, the central nervous system, and other parts of the body.

The tick vector of LB, *Ixodes dammini,* is found in the northeastern and midwestern United States, where most cases are reported. *Ixodes scapularis* in the southeastern United States, *Ixodes pacificus* on the Pacific coast, and *Ixodes ricinus,* the sheep tick in Europe, are also vectors. Lyme borreliosis can occur in any season, although it is most prevalent during the nymphal stage of the tick (the warmer months from May through September). The ticks cling to vegetation (not trees) in grassland, marshland, and woodland habitats. They transfer to animals and humans brushing against the vegetation.

DISTINGUISHING FEATURES
Initial Phases
- Initially, the LB lesion is a red macule or papule at the site of a tick bite. The bite itself usually goes unnoticed. Approximately 2 to 30 days after infection, the rash appears
- Common sites are the trunk (Fig. 15-13), groin, and thigh
- Usually asymptomatic, the initial lesion expands to form an annular erythematous lesion, erythema migrans, which is the classic lesion of LB
- It measures from 4 to 70 cm in diameter, generally with central clearing
- The center of the lesion, which corresponds to the putative site of the tick bite, may become darker, vesicular, hemorrhagic, or necrotic

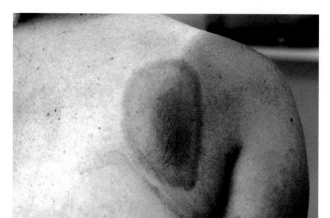

Figure 15-13 Erythema migrans (acute Lyme disease).

- Lesions may be confluent (not annular), and concentric rings may form
- Multiple lesions sometimes occur, likely the result of bacteremia
- At the early stage of disease, flulike symptoms, such as malaise, arthralgias, headaches, and a low-grade fever and chills, may occur. Other symptoms include stiffness of the neck and difficulty in concentrating

Intermediate, Chronic, and Late Phases
- Some of the signs and symptoms of LB may not appear for weeks, months, or even years after the initial tick bite and are believed to be caused by immunopathogenic mechanisms. They include:
  - Arthritis, nervous system problems, Bell's palsy, headaches, memory loss, and cardiac dysrhythmias
  - Rarely, a lesion of lymphocytoma cutis
  - Acrodermatitis chronica atrophicans
- Late Lyme disease refers to symptoms, primarily rheumatologic and neurologic, that occur months to years after initial infection

DIAGNOSIS
Early Diagnosis
To diagnose early LB, the following are important:
  - There is a history of tick exposure or bite in an area endemic for LB
  - The specific tick is identified as a potential vector of LB

Laboratory Testing
- Serologic testing, using enzyme-linked immunosorbent assay (ELISA) and Western blot analyses for *B. burgdorferi*, are notoriously unreliable. Furthermore, most patients at the erythema migrans stage are seronegative
- After 4 to 6 weeks, approximately 75% of these patients test positive, even after antibiotic therapy
- Enzyme-linked immunosorbent assay or immunofluorescent assay followed by a confirmatory Western immunoblot test on any samples with positive or equivocal results on ELISA

MANAGEMENT
Tick Recognition
- *Ixodes* ticks are much smaller than dog ticks. In their larval and nymphal stages, they are no bigger than a pinhead; unengorged adult ticks are the size of the head of a match

Tick Removal
- An attached tick should be removed carefully by using a pair of tweezers. The tick should be grasped by the head (not the body) as close as possible to the skin, to avoid force that may crush it

Treatment
- Oral antibiotics are effective. The duration of recommended therapy ranges from 10 to 30 days. Use one of the following:
  - Doxycycline (100 mg twice per day for 21 days [do not use in children younger than 10 years or in pregnant women]) *or*
  - Amoxicillin (500 mg 3 times per day for 21 days) *or*
  - Ceftriaxone or cefuroxime (500 mg twice per day for 21 days [expensive; use if patient is unable to tolerate the other antibiotics])
- Azithromycin (**Zithromax**) and erythromycin: second-line drugs that should be considered in pregnant patients who are allergic to beta-lactam antibiotics

Prevention
- People who are outdoors in endemic areas in the summer should wear long pants and socks, use insect repellents, and frequently examine themselves and their clothing for ticks

☑ **TIP: Doxycycline: a single dose of 200 mg given in less than 72 hours of tick removal is reported to prevent the disease.**

ALSO CONSIDER
- Granuloma annulare
- Annular urticaria
- Insect bites
- Cutaneous sarcoidosis
- Subacute cutaneous lupus erythematosus
- Syphilis
- Erythema multiforme
- Viral infections, such as influenza and mononucleosis, also may manifest with rash, aches, fever, and fatigue.
- Drug eruptions and insect bite reactions other than those caused by the *Ixodes* tick

RARELY
- Hansen disease (leprosy)
- Actinic granuloma

Herpes Zoster *vs* Herpes Simplex

Herpes Zoster

Herpes zoster (HZ) (shingles) is caused by the same herpesvirus that causes varicella, or chickenpox. In childhood, the virus first manifests as varicella, the primary infection. Subsequently, when the same latent virus is reactivated, its second episode manifests as HZ. After the primary varicella infection resolves, the virus retreats to the dorsal root ganglion where it remains in a dormant state. Reactivation—into dermatomal shingles—may be caused by severe illness, infection with HIV, or after organ transplantation, but most often it occurs spontaneously without an obvious precipitating cause. The likelihood and degree of pain (acute and chronic), disease severity, complications such as postherpetic neuralgia (PHN), and dissemination are significantly increased in the elderly and immunocompromised patients. Second episodes of HZ in immunocompetent people are rare, probably because of the immunologic "boosting" effect of the first episode.

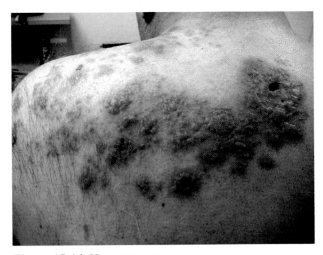

Figure 15-14 Herpes zoster.

DISTINGUISHING FEATURES
- Pain is often the first symptom
- Lesions initially arise as nonbullous erythematous papules (urticaria-like) that rapidly mature into clustered vesicles or bullae nesting on top of an erythematous base (Fig. 15-14)
  - Successive crops continue to appear for 6 to 8 days
  - The blisters sometimes umbilicate (sag in the middle); occasionally, they become pustular and hemorrhagic
- Although HZ can affect any dermatome, it most commonly is noted on the thoracic, trigeminal, lumbosacral, and cervical areas
- Lesions occur in a characteristic unilateral dermatomal ("zosteriform") distribution

- Occasionally, lesions involve contiguous dermatomes or extend beyond the midline
- In time, lesions dry into crusts or erosions that may heal and disappear completely or resolve with postinflammatory hyperpigmentation or hypopigmentation and, possibly, scarring (particularly in HIV-infected patients)
- Some individuals experience pain without a rash ("zoster sine herpete"), which makes diagnosing HZ more difficult.
- Immunocompromised patients have a greater risk of multidermatomal zoster and recurrent zoster
- In children, HZ may be asymptomatic
- PHN is defined as pain persisting for more than 1 month after the eruption of the initial HZ lesions. The frequency of PHN increases with age

✔ **TIP: Gabapentin (Neurontin) with valacyclovir taken within 72 hours of HZ may significantly reduce pain.**

⚠ **ALERT: Infection in pregnant women with primary varicella (chickenpox) may result in severe fetal abnormalities; however, the development of HZ during pregnancy does not appear to harm the developing fetus.**

DIAGNOSIS
- HZ can most often be diagnosed on the basis of clinical appearance and the presence of pain in a dermatomal distribution
- Lesions tend to vary more in size than do the lesions of HSV
- If necessary, a Tzanck smear should be obtained from the base of a fresh lesion (see Appendix B). A positive result suggests either HSV *or* varicella-zoster virus infection

MANAGEMENT (see Appendix A)
- Topical therapy
  - Wet dressings with **Burow solution** are soothing and drying

- Topical anesthetic "caines" such as benzocaine, which may be helpful for pain relief
- Capsaicin **(Zostrix)** available OTC and is applied 3 to 5 times daily
- Systemic therapy
  - Oral analgesics, such as acetaminophen, aspirin, and other NSAIDs, well as mild narcotics, are helpful in mild, self-limited cases
  - Oral antiviral medications are used to reduce the duration and severity of symptoms. They include acyclovir **(Zovirax),** valacyclovir **(Valtrex),** or famciclovir **(Famvir).** Ideally, they should be taken within 72 hours of the first sign of the rash
  - Prednisone is occasionally used to reduce inflammation and lower the risk of PHN
- Postherpetic neuralgia
  - Lidocaine patches
  - Low-dose tricyclic antidepressants (e.g., amitriptyline)
  - Gabapentin **(Neurontin),** an antiseizure drug, has been helpful in some patients

- Neurosurgical procedures include nerve blocks with local anesthetics
- Intralesional corticosteroids may be given as subcutaneous injections
- Transcutaneous electrical stimulation
- Vaccination
  - The recent introduction of the vaccine **Zostavax,** a live attenuated virus, promises to reduce both the risk of developing HZ zoster as well as resulting in less frequent, less painful, and shorter courses of PHN
  - Vaccination is recommended for everyone older than 60 years of age
- **ALERT: Herpes zoster, particularly if it is recurrent or disseminated, may be an early indicator of an immunosuppressive disorder or a lymphoproliferative disease. Also, patients with HZ can transmit the virus as chickenpox to persons who have not already been infected with this virus (e.g., newborns, immunocompromised, and pregnant women)**

Herpes Simplex

When HSV presents in a site usually occupied by HZ, or when it occurs in a semidermatomal distribution, it may be clinically indistinguishable from HZ.

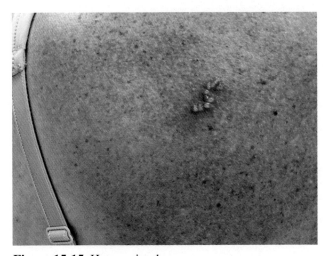

Figure 15-15 Herpes simplex.

DISTINGUISHING FEATURES
- The vesicles of herpes simplex tend to be more uniform in size and are much less painful than those seen in HZ (Fig. 15-15)
- Recurrence strongly suggests HSV infection

DIAGNOSIS/MANAGEMENT
- See Chapter 7, Lips and Perioral Area

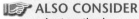

ALSO CONSIDER
- Acute urticaria
- Folliculitis
- Insect bite reaction
- Acute Lyme (erythema migrans)

RARELY
- Bullous pemphigoid

Pityriasis Rosea *vs* Generalized Plaque Psoriasis/Acute Guttate Psoriasis

Pityriasis Rosea

Pityriasis rosea (**PR**) is a common, acute, self-limiting eruption that has a characteristic clinical course. It tends to occur in the spring and fall, and although it may occur at any age, it is seen mostly in young adults and older children. The cause is unknown; however, the occasional clustering of cases and seasonal appearances suggest an infectious, transmissible etiology. Reports have suggested a role for human herpesvirus 7; however, PR does not appear to be contagious because household contacts and schoolmates generally do not develop the rash.

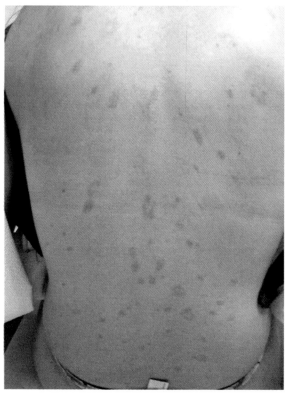

Figure 15-16 Pityriasis rosea. Note Christmas tree pattern.

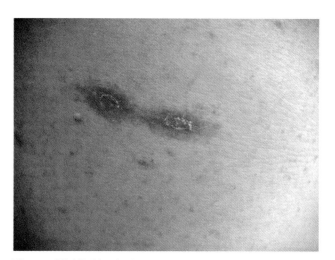

Figure 15-17 Pityriasis rosea: close-up view. Note elliptical shape and fine central scale.

DISTINGUISHING FEATURES
- Usually asymptomatic but may itch
- Often begins with the larger herald patch, a scaly lesion that may exhibit central clearing and therefore mimics tinea corporis (Fig. 15-16)
- A few days later, smaller similar scaly erythematous patches appear, scattered mainly on the trunk but may spread to the thighs, upper arms, and neck in an *old-fashioned bathing suit* distribution
- Lesions are oval or elliptical with fine, thin scale on their surface (Fig. 15-17)
- The long axis of individual lesions run parallel to skin tension lines. This yields a *Christmas tree* pattern on the trunk

- A self-limiting benign disorder; it usually lasts for 6 to 8 weeks
- On resolution, postinflammatory pigment changes (hyperpigmentation) can occur, particularly in dark-skinned people
- Recurrences are rare
- Clinical variants
  - In dark-skinned patients, lesions may be vesicular and uncharacteristically pruritic
  - PR may be limited in its distribution or it may present in an inverse fashion involving the groin, axillae, or distal extremities (inverse pityriasis rosea)

DIAGNOSIS

- The diagnosis is made clinically in most cases
- In general, laboratory tests are not necessary or helpful, with the following exceptions:
  - A KOH examination may be helpful when only the herald patch is present, to help rule in or rule out tinea corporis
- A skin biopsy may be performed when the eruption is atypical, the diagnosis is uncertain, or the disease has not resolved after 3 to 4 months

⚠ **ALERT: Secondary syphilis should be considered in the differential diagnosis, especially when lesions are also present on the palms and soles.**

MANAGEMENT

- Treatment is often unnecessary in most cases because PR is usually self-limiting and asymptomatic
- Pruritus, when it occurs, is always mild and tolerable
- Exposure to sunlight may speed resolution of the eruption
- Extensive or persistent cases can be treated by phototherapy (UVB)

Generalized Plaque Psoriasis/Acute Guttate Psoriasis

Generalized plaque psoriasis and the **acute guttate psoriasis** variant often present on the trunk. Psoriasis is essentially an inflammatory skin condition with abnormal epidermal differentiation and hyperproliferation. It is suggested that the inflammatory process is immunologically based and most likely set off, and maintained by, T cells in the dermis. Psoriasis affects 1% to 2% of the world's population. Much less common in West Africans, African-Americans, Native Americans, and Asian than in Caucasians; it is seen equally in men and women. Patients may also develop psoriatic arthritis, which may precede or follow the onset of skin lesions.

Psoriasis most frequently begins in the second or third decade of life, but it can first present in infants or in the elderly. About 30% of patients with psoriasis have a positive family history. It can flare very quickly and unexpectedly to cover 20% to 80% of the body. Therapy for widespread psoriasis differs from that used for more localized disease (see Chapter 12, Arms, Elbows).

Acute guttate psoriasis is characterized by multiple small areas of psoriasis that tend to affect most of the body. The rash comes on very quickly, usually within a couple of days, and may follow a streptococcal infection of the throat. It tends to affect children and young adults.

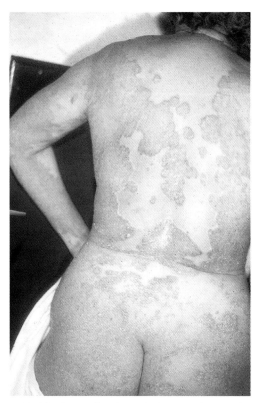

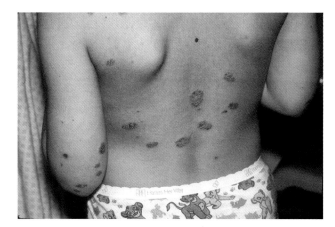

Figure 15-18 Generalized psoriasis. (Reprinted with permission from Goodheart HP. *Goodheart's Photoguide to Common Skin Disorders: Diagnosis and Management.* 3rd ed. Philadelphia: Lippincott Williams & Wilkins, 2009.)

Figure 15-19 Acute guttate psoriasis.

DISTINGUISHING FEATURES
- Well-demarcated erythematous plaques with characteristic overlying white or silvery (micaceous) scale (Fig. 15-18)

DIAGNOSIS
- Clinical
- Biopsy if diagnosis is in doubt
- Acute guttate psoriasis
  - The diagnosis of guttate psoriasis (Fig. 15-19) is made by the combination of history, clinical appearance of the rash, and evidence for preceding streptococcal infection

- Psoriatic papules and plaques are usually concentrated around the trunk and upper arms and thighs

MANAGEMENT (see Appendix A)

Generalized Plaque Psoriasis

- Topical therapy
  - Soak and smear with class 1 superpotent topical steroid (see Appendix B), followed by less-potent topical steroids
  - Besides topical steroids, coal tar, anthralin, calcipotriene (**Dovonex**), calcitriol (**Vectical ointment**), calcipotriene, and betamethasone dipropionate (**Taclonex ointment**) may be prescribed. No single topical agent is ideal, and many are often used concurrently in a combined approach. Auxiliary agents such as scale-removing keratolytics (e.g., **Salex cream and Keralyt gel**) can often be used
- Phototherapy
  - UVB and narrowband UVB are used only in the presence of extensive and widespread moderate-to-severe plaque psoriasis that is not responding to topical treatment
  - Broadband UVB, excimer laser UVB

- Systemic therapy
- Methotrexate in a low-dose weekly regimen, cyclosporine, acitretin (**Soriatane**), azathioprine, and mycophenolate mofetil (**CellCept**)
- Biologics such as:
  - Adalimumab (**Humira**): tumor necrosis factor (TNF)-alpha inhibitor
  - Alefacept (**Amevive**): CD4 inhibitor
  - Infliximab (**Remicade**): TNF-alpha inhibitor
  - Etanercept (**Enbrel**): TNF-alpha inhibitor
  - Ustekinumab (**Stelara**): targets interleukins 12 and 23
- ☑ **TIP: Rotational therapy—by using a rotational approach with the various topical and systemic agents, the toxic effects of long-term treatment with any of the agents can be minimized.**

Acute Guttate Psoriasis

- Spontaneous clearing may occur
- Anti-streptococcal antibiotic therapy

ALSO CONSIDER
- Tinea versicolor
- Tinea corporis
- Pityriasis rosea–like drug eruption (lesions are redder, less scaly, and tend to be itchier than seen in pityriasis rosea)
- Nummular eczema
- Atopic dermatitis/eczema
- Contact dermatitis
- Lichen planus
- Secondary syphilis
- Erythema migrans
- Grover disease

RARELY
- Pityriasis rubra pilaris
- Pemphigus foliaceus
- Erythema annulare centrifugum
- Small plaque parapsoriasis or digitate dermatosis
- Subacute cutaneous lupus erythematosus
- Darier disease
- Hansen disease

Tinea Versicolor vs Vitiligo Vulgaris

Tinea Versicolor

Tinea versicolor (TV), also known as pityriasis versicolor, is a very common superficial yeast infection caused by the hyphal form of *Pityrosporum ovale* (also known as *Malassezia furfur*). Seen mostly in young adults, TV is unusual in very young and elderly persons. TV is primarily of cosmetic concern and is generally asymptomatic. It is a chronic relapsing condition because the causative fungus is part of the skin's normal flora. TV is ubiquitous in tropical and subtropical countries and recurs during the summer in more temperate zones. The term *versicolor* refers to the varied coloration that tinea versicolor can display.

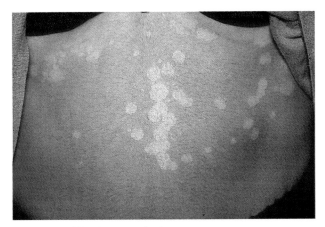

Figure 15-20 Tinea versicolor.

DISTINGUISHING FEATURES
- The primary lesions are well-defined round or oval macules with an overlay of fine scales; the lesions often coalesce to form larger patches
- The color of the lesions may vary from a whitish to pink to tan or dark brown (see following discussion) (Fig. 15-20)
- Lesions are most often distributed on the trunk, upper arms, and neck

DIAGNOSIS
- If scale is present, KOH examination is positive, and the typical "spaghetti and meatball" hyphae are abundant and easily found
- Wood lamp examination is used to demonstrate the extent of the infection and may help to confirm the diagnosis because lesions often fluoresce an orange mustard color when the light is held close to lesions in a dark room

MANAGEMENT (see Appendix A)
Topical Agents
- For mild, limited tinea versicolor, topical therapy is applied. Daily applications of selenium sulfide (**Selsun Blue**) shampoo, pyrithione zinc (**Head & Shoulders**) shampoo, and ketoconazole 1% (**Nizoral**) cream or shampoo are inexpensive OTC methods that often clear the eruption
- Also, application of topical OTC antifungals such as clotrimazole (**Lotrimin**) or terbinafine (**Lamisil**). These topical agents are used once or twice daily. Alternatively, prescription strength ketoconazole 2% (**Nizoral**) cream and shampoo may be applied
- This treatment regimen may be repeated for 3 or 4 weeks

Systemic Therapy
- For stubborn, widespread, or recurrent disease, short-term (4 to 5 days) systemic therapy with ketoconazole or fluconazole (**Diflucan**) may be prescribed
- Patients should be advised that the uneven coloration of the skin may take several months to disappear after the fungus has been successfully eliminated
- Recurrences are very common, especially in warm weather

✔ **TIP: Topical therapy with anti-fungal cream or shampoo should be repeated 1 week before the next exposure to warm weather.**

Vitiligo Vulgaris

Vitiligo vulgaris is characterized by depigmentation of the epidermis due to a partial or complete loss of melanocytes. The cause is unknown, but it is thought to result from an autoimmune process resulting in the loss of melanocytes.

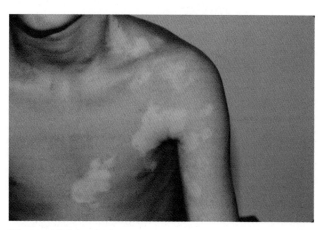

Figure 15-21 Vitiligo.

DISTINGUISHING FEATURES
- Hypopigmented or depigmented, chalk-white macules (Fig. 15-21)
- In dark-skinned people, pigmentary loss may be observed at any time of year, whereas in light-skinned people, the lesions may be most obvious in the summer because the tanning effects of the summer sun can accentuate the contrast between the light and dark skin

- Lesions tend to have a bilateral, symmetric distribution
- Occur on the hands and feet, body folds, bony prominences, and external genitals
- Lesions characteristically appear around orifices (e.g., the mouth, eyes, nose, and anus), but they may also involve the eyebrows, eyelashes, and scalp hair, resulting in white hairs (leukotrichia)

DIAGNOSIS
- Clinical
- Aided by Wood lamp examination; this should reveal a "milk-white" fluorescence

MANAGEMENT
- See Chapter 6, Cheeks, as well as Appendices A and B

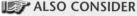**ALSO CONSIDER**
- Postinflammatory hypopigmentation

RARELY
- Small plaque parapsoriasis or digitate dermatosis
- Hypopigmented cutaneous T-cell lymphoma (mycosis fungoides)

Tinea Versicolor

Tinea versicolor (TV) can present as a tan, brown, or even black coloration (Figs. 15-22, 15-23). See previous discussion.

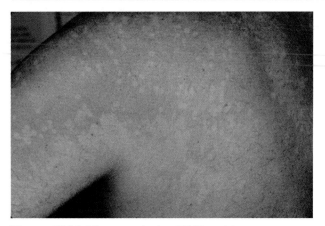

Figure 15-22 Tinea versicolor KOH positive.

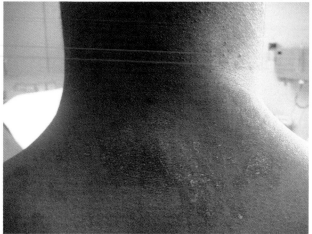

Figure 15-23 Tinea versicolor. Darkly pigmented patches that are KOH positive. Note similarity to Fig. 15-24A and 15-24B.

Confluent and Reticulated Papillomatosis

Confluent and reticulated papillomatosis (CRP), also known as confluent and reticulated papillomatosis of Gougerot and Carteaud, is a relatively uncommon skin disorder that typically affects young persons. It closely resembles darkly pigmented tinea versicolor. Confluent and reticulated papillomatosis is typically located on the trunk. The etiology is unknown. Various theories about its cause include an endocrine disturbance, a disorder of keratinization, or an abnormal host reaction to fungi or bacteria. The successful use of antibiotics in the treatment of CRP has led to the concept that bacteria are the etiologic agents. It is not unusual for it to coexist with acanthosis nigricans, which it both resembles clinically and histopathologically. The eruption is chronic with exacerbations and remissions.

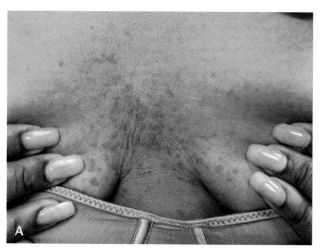 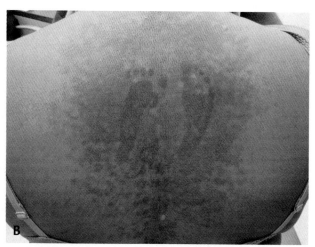

Figure 15-24 A: Confluent and reticulated hyperkeratosis. **B:** Confluent and reticulated hyperkeratosis (same patient as in Fig. 15.24A).

DISTINGUISHING FEATURES
- The onset usually occurs shortly after puberty
- Tan-brown, often grayish, hyperkeratotic papules and plaques in a confluent pattern centrally and lesions coalesce to form a reticular pattern peripherally (Fig. 15-24)
- Distribution most often is on the intermammary, interscapular, and abdominal areas
- Often asymptomatic, but may experience mild pruritus

DIAGNOSIS
- Clinical
- KOH examination is negative
- Shave biopsy if diagnosis is in doubt

MANAGEMENT
- Many different topical and systemic modalities have been used in the treatment of CRP, with variable results. The most consistent results may be seen with minocycline or other oral tetracycline derivatives
- It is responsive to treatment with antibiotics but may recur after discontinuation of therapy

ALSO CONSIDER
- Acanthosis nigricans
- Pityriasis rosea
- Erythema dyschromicum perstans

RARELY
- Dermatopathia pigmentosa reticularis
- Small plaque parapsoriasis or digitate dermatosis
- Erythrokeratodermia variabilis
- Keratosis follicularis (Darier disease)
- Macular amyloidosis
- Pityriasis rubra pilaris

Epidermoid Cysts

Epidermoid cysts are the most common type of cyst. As with other "true" cysts, they have an epithelial lining within which there is semisolid or liquid material composed of keratin and lipid-rich debris. They occur most often on the face, behind the ears, neck, trunk, scrotum, and vaginal labia. Cysts are derived from the epithelium of the hair follicle and connect to the surface of the skin with a keratin-filled central pore that looks like a blackhead. Such cysts tend to be hereditary, arise in adulthood, and may occur as multiple lesions. **Pilar cysts,** the second most common type, occur on the scalp.

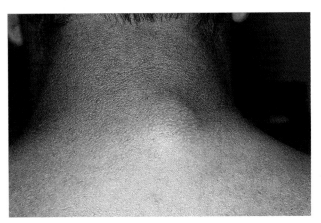

Figure 15-25 Epidermoid cyst.

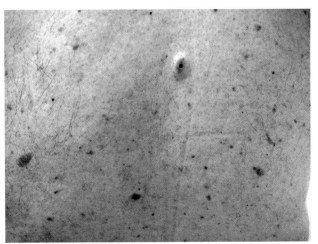

Figure 15-26 Giant comedones.

DISTINGUISHING FEATURES

- Lesions arise as smooth, discrete, freely moveable, dome-shaped nodules (Fig. 15-25)
- Usually asymptomatic, unless inflamed or infected
- Cysts that have previously been infected, ruptured, drained, or scarred may be firmer and less freely movable
- Lesions range from 0.5 to 5.0 cm in diameter
- Often, there is a central pore from which cheesy-white, malodorous keratin material can be expressed
- Giant comedones (Fig. 15-26) are superficial cysts
  - Exceptionally large blackhead (can be up to 1 cm)
  - Usually single, but occasionally several can be found
  - Frequently occur in the absence of previous acne
  - Occur more in the middle-aged and elderly population
  - Usually on the back and chest
  - The diagnosis is usually straightforward as it is normally very easy to press gently to squeeze out the contents. However, it will refill over a period of 2 to 3 months

DIAGNOSIS

- Most often, cysts can be diagnosed clinically because on palpation, an intact epidermoid feels smooth; when compressed, it feels like an eyeball or a fully expanded balloon
- If necessary, a biopsy or an incision and drainage can be performed to confirm the diagnosis

MANAGEMENT

- Complete excision. The entire cyst wall does not have to be completely removed to prevent recurrence
- Alternatively, a large epidermoid can be removed through a small hole created by a punch biopsy tool
- A fluctuant, inflamed, or infected cyst may be incised with a No. 11 blade, drained, and then packed with iodoform gauze
- ✔ **TIP: The contents of inflamed or so-called infected cysts are most often sterile or contain normal skin flora; thus, the necessity of pre- or postoperative antibiotics treatment is generally unnecessary.**

Lipoma

A **lipoma** is a benign, subcutaneous tumor composed of fat cells. **Dercum disease** is a syndrome of multiple tender lipomas that develops in middle-aged women. Angiolipomas may be tender or painful.

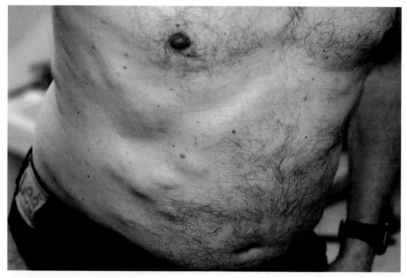

Figure 15-27 Multiple lipomas.

DISTINGUISHING FEATURES

- Rubbery consistency, generally asymptomatic masses; ranging in size from small nodules to large tumors (Fig. 15-27)
- Usually irregular in shape and may be greater than 7 cm in length
- Occur most commonly on the trunk, back of neck, upper arms, and forearms

DIAGNOSIS

- The diagnosis is made on clinical grounds
- A biopsy should be performed if the diagnosis is uncertain
- As noted previously, a lipoma may be confused with an epidermoid cyst. However, the latter feels "like an eyeball" and has a regular dome shape

MANAGEMENT

- Lesions may be excised or removed using liposuction

ALSO CONSIDER

- Neurofibroma
- Angiolipoma

RARELY

- Multiple angiolipomas (Dercum disease)
- Liposarcoma
- Dermatofibrosarcoma protuberans
- Metastasis

Cherry Angioma *vs* Melanocytic Nevus

Cherry Angioma

Cherry angiomas, which are also known as *Campbell De Morgan spots, ruby spots,* and *senile angiomas,* are extremely common benign vascular neoplasms. The angiomas are found in fair-skinned adults older than 40 years.

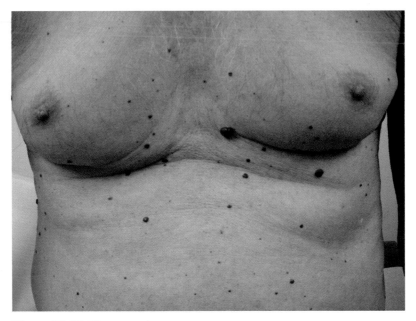

Figure 15-28 Cherry angioma.

DISTINGUISHING FEATURES
- Asymptomatic, cherry- to plum-colored papules that develop primarily on the trunk (Fig. 15-28)

DIAGNOSIS
- Easily diagnosed
- Dermoscopy (see Appendix B)

MANAGEMENT
- Lesions are benign and usually do not undergo spontaneous involution
- For those patients who have concern regarding the cosmetic appearance of the lesions:
  - Shave excision or performing electrocautery
  - Pulsed dye laser ablation
  - Cryotherapy with liquid nitrogen

Melanocytic Nevus

Melanocytic nevi (MN) are extremely common on the trunk. Congenital and acquired nevi are much more often seen in patients with fair skin than in blacks or Asians. Large congenital nevi (see Chapter 2, Forehead and Temples; Chapter 12, Arms) have a low, but real risk, for malignant transformation and the development of melanoma.

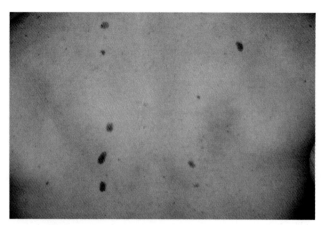

Figure 15-29 Multiple melanocytic nevi.

DISTINGUISHING FEATURES

- Compound MN:
  - Elevated, dome-shaped papules or papillomatous nodules that are uniformly brown to dark brown
  - May contain hairs
  - Seen most often on the face, arms, legs, and trunk
- Junctional MN:
  - Small, macular (flat), frecklelike; uniform in color; vary from brown to dark brown to black (Fig. 15-29)
  - Acquired or congenital, junctional nevi are most prevalent on the face, arms, legs, trunk, genitalia, palms, and soles

DIAGNOSIS

- Based on clinical appearance or, if necessary, a histopathologic evaluation

MANAGEMENT

- All MN should be carefully examined and considered for biopsy, particularly if there is any suggestion of clinical atypia
- Removed for cosmetic purposes or because of repeated irritation by clothing, such as a bra strap
- Shave removal/shave biopsy (see Appendix B)

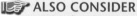

ALSO CONSIDER
- Seborrheic keratosis
- Pigmented basal cell carcinoma
- Melanoma
- Angiokeratoma

RARELY
- Blue rubber bleb nevus syndrome

TRUNK

Halo Nevus *vs* Atypical Nevus *vs* Melanoma *vs* Seborrheic Keratosis

Halo Nevus

A **halo nevus (Sutton's nevus)** is a melanocytic nevus that is encircled by a white halo of depigmentation. The halo represents a regression of a pre-existing nevus caused by a lymphocytic infiltrate. Frequently, the entire nevus disappears and the area ultimately regains normal pigmentation.

Most often, halo nevi are seen on preadolescents; they usually appear on the trunk. The pigmented nevus in the center of a halo is rarely malignant. Antibodies and T cells attack the pigment cells. This causes the central mole to fade from dark brown to light brown to pink, eventually disappearing completely, causing the white halo.

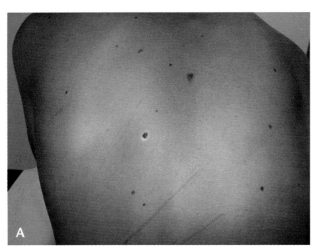 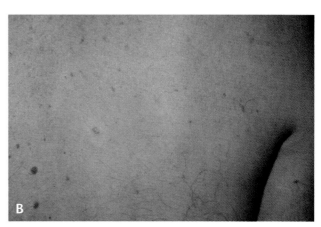

Figure 15-30 A: Halo nevus. **B:** Halo nevus: Note lesion is becoming pink and fading away.

DISTINGUISHING FEATURES
- Stage 1: A rim of hypopigmented skin surrounds a nevus (Fig. 15-30A)
- Stage 2: The nevus may become pinker and fades away (Fig. 15-30B)
- Stage 3: A circular area of depigmentation persists
- Stage 4: The affected skin returns to its normal color

DIAGNOSIS
- Clinical

MANAGEMENT
- No treatment is normally required
- ⚠ **ALERT: If a halo nevus appears on an adult, 2 very rare possibilities should be considered: the lesion may be malignant, or a melanoma may be present elsewhere on the body. Biopsy and removal are indicated.**

Atypical Nevus

Atypical nevus (dysplastic nevus, Clark's nevus) is a controversial and confusing lesion. Even among dermatopathologists, there is no consensus regarding the histopathologic criteria for its diagnosis. Furthermore, differentiating these nevi clinically from melanoma is often difficult. There are basically 2 types of atypical nevi: sporadically occurring atypical nevi and familial (inherited) atypical nevi. It is commonly agreed that when a patient has numerous atypical nevi and there is a positive family history of melanoma, the potential for melanoma in that patient and in his or her family is extremely high. Such dysplastic nevi may be inherited as an autosomal dominant trait (see following discussion of familial atypical mole syndrome). Atypical nevi are rarely seen in African-American, Asian, or Middle Eastern populations.

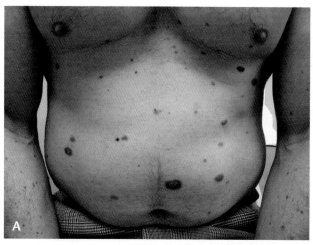
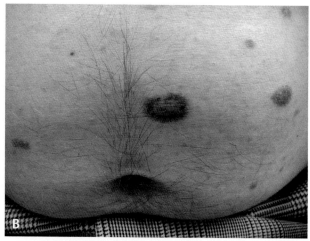

Figure 15-31 A: Atypical nevus. **B:** Atypical nevus: close-up view of Figure 15.31A.

DISTINGUISHING FEATURES
- Unlike other nevi, these lesions often continue to appear into adulthood
- Atypical nevi have some or all of the following features:
  - They are usually larger than common moles and frequently measure 5 to 15 mm in diameter
  - Their borders are usually irregular, notched, and ill-defined
  - Coloration (tan, brown, black, pink, or red) is irregular
  - They have a macular appearance, but the centers may be raised (for this reason, they are sometimes called "sunny-side-up egg lesions") (Fig. 15-31B)
  - Most often found on the trunk, less often on the legs, and arms; generally, the face is spared
- Sporadic atypical nevi
  - A patient with an isolated atypical nevus and no family history of multiple atypical nevi or melanoma probably carries little risk of developing melanoma. Some individuals have only a few atypical nevi, and their risk of melanoma may not be much higher than the general population
- Multiple atypical nevi
  - The exact risk of an individual nevus developing into a melanoma is uncertain
  - In certain situations, atypical nevi are considered possible precursors to, as well as potential markers for, the development of melanoma

- Familial atypical mole syndrome also known as the dysplastic nevus syndrome
  - Those persons who meet the following criteria are considered to have an extremely high potential fo developing malignant melanoma:
    - A first-degree (e.g., parent, sibling, or child) or second-degree (e.g., grandparent, grandchild, aunt, uncle) relative who has a history of malignant melanoma
    - Many nevi—often more than 50—are present, and some of them are atypical moles

DIAGNOSIS (see Appendix B)
- It is not always easy even for an experienced dermatologist to tell whether a lesion is an atypical nevus or a melanoma. Dermoscopy in trained hands may be helpful. A suspicious or changing atypical nevus should be biopsied
- If melanoma is suspected, complete excision should be performed

MANAGEMENT
- ⚠ **ALERT: The risk of melanoma is greatly increased in patients with multiple atypical nevi and a personal or family history of melanoma.**
- Once a diagnosis of multiple atypical nevi is established, other family members should be examined
- Patients with many atypical nevi should avoid excessive sun exposure and should routinely use a sunscreen with a sun protective factor of 15 or greater

Melanoma

Melanoma is more likely to occur on the backs and anterior torso of men and the arms and legs of women (see Chapter 12, Arms; Chapter 21, Legs). Melanoma is very rare in dark-skinned persons and Asians; however, when it does occur, it tends to be present on acral, non-sun-exposed areas such as the palms of the hands, soles of the feet, or in the nail bed (see Chapter 14, Hands and Fingers; Chapter 22, Feet).

The main risk factors for developing melanoma include:

- Sun exposure, particularly during childhood
- Fair skin that burns easily; an inability to tan
- Blistering sunburn, especially when young
- Previous melanoma
- Previous nonmelanoma skin cancer (basal cell carcinoma, squamous cell carcinoma)
- Family history of melanoma (first-degree relatives), especially if 2 or more members are affected
- Large numbers of nevi (especially if there are more than 100)
- Abnormal nevi (atypical or dysplastic nevi)

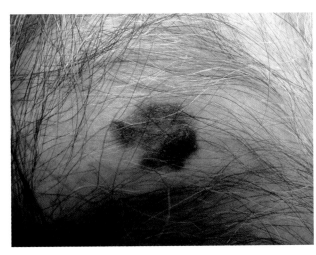

Figure 15-32 Melanoma.

DISTINGUISHING FEATURES
- New, changing (evolving), or unusual appearing nevi that arise de novo or in a pre-existing nevus
- Symptomatic nevi (e.g., those that itch, burn, or are painful)

- Superficial spreading melanoma, by far the most common type, may arise de novo or in a pre-existing nevus. An initial in situ slow horizontal growth phase, if left untreated, is followed in months or years by a vertical growth phase, which indicates invasive disease and potential metastasis
- White coloration may indicate regression or scarring
- May conform to some or all of the "ABCDE" criteria for melanoma (Figure 15-32):
  A: Asymmetry
  B: Border irregularity
  C: Color variation
  D: Diameter over 6 mm
  E: Evolving (size, color, shape)

DIAGNOSIS (see Appendix B)
- Clinical diagnosis is based on ABCDE criteria (see Chapter 12, Arms)
- Dermoscopy
- Elliptic excisional biopsy should include the entire visible lesion down to the subcutaneous fat

MANAGEMENT/SURGICAL TREATMENT/PROGNOSIS/ WORKUP/LONG-TERM MANAGEMENT
- See Chapter 12, Arms

Seborrheic Keratosis

A **seborrheic keratosis** (see Chapter 2, Forehead and Temples) is an extremely common benign skin growth seen in people over age 40. Lesions are most often located on the back, chest, arms (see Chapter 12, Arms; Chapter 21, Legs), and face, particularly along the frontal hairline and scalp (see Chapter 1, Hair and Scalp). Seborrheic keratoses are mainly a cosmetic concern, except when they are inflamed or irritated.

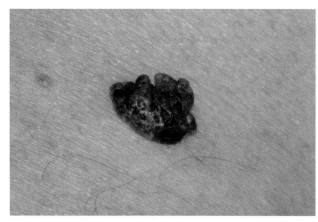

Figure 15-33 Seborrheic keratosis.

DISTINGUISHING FEATURES
- Typically, a warty, "stuck-on" appearance (Fig. 15-33)
- Color ranges from tan to dark brown to black
- "Dry," crumbly, keratotic surface
- Appearance of individual lesions tends to vary considerably, even on the same patient: warty, tortoise shell-like, scaly, flat or almost flat

DIAGNOSIS
- With experience, seborrheic keratoses are easily recognized
- A biopsy (generally a shave biopsy) is performed if necessary to confirm the diagnosis
- ⚠ **ALERT: To the untrained eye, however, these lesions may resemble melanomas. An excisional biopsy is unnecessary unless a melanoma is suspected.**

MANAGEMENT (see Appendix B)
- No treatment at all or:
  - Cryosurgery performed with liquid nitrogen spray or cotton swab
  - Electrocautery and curettage

👉 ALSO CONSIDER
- Other benign melanocytic nevi
- Pigmented basal cell carcinoma
- Warts

Superficial Basal Cell Carcinoma

Superficial basal cell carcinomas (BCCs) most often appear on the trunk and have little tendency to become invasive. There is no clear association between superficial BCC and sun exposure. Lesions may mimic psoriasis (see following discussion), squamous cell carcinoma in situ, or eczema.

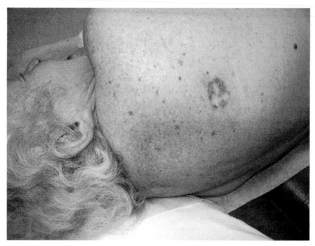

Figure 15-34 Superficial basal cell carcinoma.

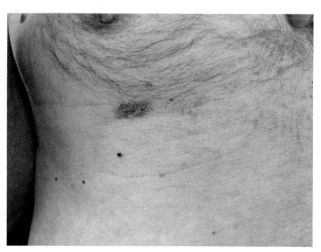

Figure 15-35 Superficial basal cell carcinoma. Note resemblance to a plaque of psoriasis.

DISTINGUISHING FEATURES

- Arises as a scaly pink to red-brown patch with a threadlike border (Figs. 15-34, 15-35)
- Lesions tend to be indolent, asymptomatic, and the least aggressive of BCCs
- Often multiple, occurring primarily on the trunk and proximal extremities

DIAGNOSIS (see Appendix B)

- A shave biopsy is all that is necessary

MANAGEMENT (Appendix A)

- Electrodesiccation and curettage
- Cryosurgery with liquid nitrogen
- The application of the topical immunomodulator 5% imiquimod cream (**Aldara**) is used for the treatment of multiple superficial BCCs

Solitary Plaque Psoriasis

Psoriasis may arise as a solitary plaque with no other signs or evidence of psoriasis elsewhere.

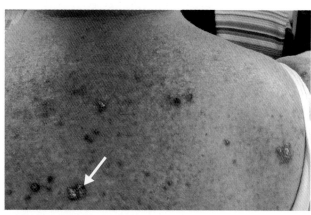

Figure 15-36 Psoriasis. This patient has typical psoriatic papules and plaques. The lower left lesion is a superficial basal cell carcinoma.

DISTINGUISHING FEATURES
- A well-demarcated erythematous plaque with or without an overlying white or silvery (micaceous) scale (Fig. 15-36)

DIAGNOSIS
- Clinical
- Biopsy if diagnosis is in doubt

MANAGEMENT
- Responsive to topical psoriatic therapy
- See Appendix A as well as Chapter 12, Arms, Elbows

☞ **ALSO CONSIDER**
- Squamous cell carcinoma in situ (Bowen disease)
- Seborrheic keratosis

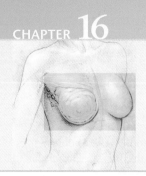

CHAPTER 16

Breasts and Inframammary Area

The breasts are subject to the same dermatoses as the rest of the cutaneous surface of the trunk; however, the occasional appearance of eczema and the relatively rare Paget disease of the nipples and areola require special attention.

The intertriginous inframammary area, where opposing skin surfaces rub against each other, have similar problems and dermatoses as the axillary, inguinal, intragluteal, and abdominal folds.

IN THIS CHAPTER

Nipples and Areolae
- Paget disease of the breast *vs* atopic dermatitis (eczema) of areolae
- Seborrheic keratoses *vs* superficial basal cell carcinoma

Inframammary Area
- Intertrigo *vs* inverse psoriasis *vs* candidiasis

Paget Disease of the Breast *vs* Atopic Dermatitis (Eczema) of Areolae

Paget Disease of the Breast

Paget disease of the breast is an intraepidermal skin cancer that is often indicative of a more severe underlying malignancy. It is a relatively uncommon clinical presentation of intraductal carcinoma of the breast. The disease occurs almost exclusively in postmenopausal women; men are rarely affected. Paget disease of the breast has a subtle, insidious course and tends to be ignored, misdiagnosed, or unrecognized by patients and clinicians alike. A high index of suspicion and prompt identification and treatment can be lifesaving. Furthermore, Paget disease of the breast is often mistakenly diagnosed as a chronic eczematous condition (see following discussion). A similar condition that involves the skin of female and male genitalia is known as extramammary Paget disease (see Fig. 20-7).

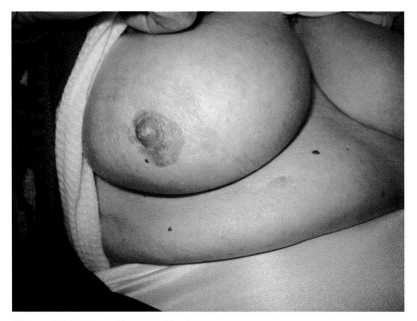

Figure 16-1 Paget disease of the breast.

DISTINGUISHING FEATURES
- Often presents with a chronic *unilateral* "rash" on the nipple, areola, or surrounding skin (Fig. 16-1); less commonly, the lesion originates and remains on the nipple
- Typically, the lesion appears as a sharply marginated red plaque with an irregular border and eczemalike appearance
- When the nipple is involved, it may become scaly, crusted, have a bloody discharge, become deformed, or retracted

DIAGNOSIS (see Appendix B)
- Punch, wedge, or excisional biopsy of the lesional skin of the nipple-areola complex, including the dermal and subcutaneous tissue for microscopic examination

MANAGEMENT
- As in other types of confirmed breast carcinoma, treatment can include surgery, radiation therapy, chemotherapy, and hormonal treatment as indicated

Atopic Dermatitis (Eczema) of Areolae

Atopic dermatitis of the nipples and areolae often presents bilaterally but may present unilaterally. It occurs in association with a personal or family history of atopy.

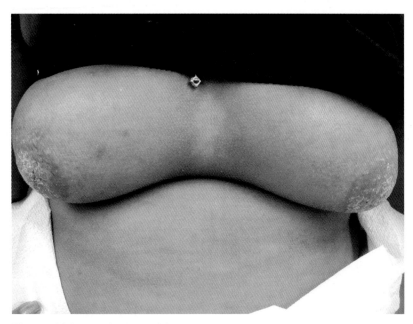

Figure 16-2 Atopic dermatitis.

DISTINGUISHING FEATURES
- Usually *bilateral* pruritic eczematous eruption (Fig. 16-2)

DIAGNOSIS
- Clinical

MANAGEMENT (see Appendix A)
- Atopic dermatitis should respond rapidly to topical corticosteroid therapy

👉 **ALSO CONSIDER**
- Psoriasis
- Irritant contact dermatitis
- Mastitis, commonly affects women who are breast-feeding
- Nipple duct adenoma
- Erosive adenomatosis of the nipple
- Bowen disease (squamous cell carcinoma in situ)
- Superficial basal cell carcinoma

RARELY
- Melanoma

Seborrheic Keratoses

Seborrheic keratoses (see Chapter 2, Forehead and Temples) is an extremely common benign skin growth seen in people over age 40 (see Chapter 1, Hair and Scalp; Chapter 12, Arms; Chapter 21, Legs). These lesions are mainly a cosmetic concern, except when they are inflamed or irritated.

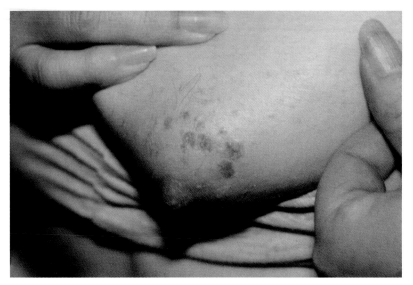

Figure 16-3 Seborrheic keratoses.

DISTINGUISHING FEATURES
- Typically, a warty, "stuck-on" appearance (Fig. 16-3)
- On the breast, lesions may appear similar to pigmented skin tags
- Color ranges from tan to dark brown to black
- "Dry," crumbly, keratotic surface

DIAGNOSIS
- Clinical
- A biopsy (generally a shave biopsy) is performed if the diagnosis is in doubt

MANAGEMENT (see Appendix B)
- Cryosurgery performed with liquid nitrogen (LN_2) spray or cotton swab
- Light electrocautery and curettage

Superficial Basal Cell Carcinoma

Superficial basal cell carcinomas (see Chapter 15, Trunk) have no clear association with sun exposure. Most often, they appear on the trunk, particularly on the back.

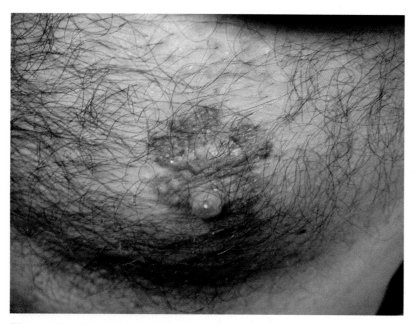

Figure 16-4 Superficial basal cell carcinoma.

DISTINGUISHING FEATURES

- Arises as a scaly pink to red-brown patch with a threadlike border (Fig. 16-4)
- Lesions tend to be indolent, asymptomatic, and the least aggressive of basal cell carcinomas

DIAGNOSIS

- A superficial shave biopsy is all that is necessary for these thin lesions

MANAGEMENT (see Appendix A)

- Electrodesiccation and curettage
- Cryosurgery with LN_2 for rapid treatment
- Application of the topical immunomodulator 5% imiquimod cream (**Aldara**)

ALSO CONSIDER

- Atopic dermatitis
- Psoriasis
- Melanocytic nevi
- Skin tag (acrochordon)
- Warts
- Bowen disease (squamous cell carcinoma in situ)
- Paget disease of the breast

RARELY

- Melanoma

Intertrigo *vs* Inverse Psoriasis *vs* Candidiasis

Intertrigo

Intertrigo is a very common superficial inflammatory process that occurs in places where opposing skin surfaces rub against each other: the axillae, creases of the lips (see Chapter 7, Lips and Perioral Area) inguinal, intragluteal creases (see Chapter 19, Buttocks and Perineal Area, Gluteal Cleft; Chapter 20, Inguinal Area), under the breasts (see Chapter 11, Axillae), and the abdominal folds. Complicating factors may include atopy, hyperhidrosis, diabetes, and obesity as well as colonization by secondary infections such as *Candida albicans* (see later discussion).

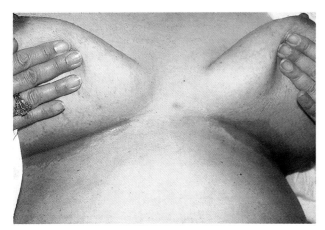

Figure 16-5 Intertrigo.

DISTINGUISHING FEATURES
- Begins as a mild erythema followed by erythematous, well-demarcated patches or plaques that oppose each other on either side of the skin folds (mirror image) (Fig. 16-5)
- Often pruritic; may progress to erosions, oozing, exudation, and painful fissures
- Particularly common in those who are obese or in those who have pendulous breasts

DIAGNOSIS
- Clinical

- Exclusion of other diagnoses (e.g., contact dermatitis, psoriasis, seborrheic dermatitis, as well as bacterial or fungal infection (negative potassium hydroxide [KOH] and/or fungal culture), although such infections may be may be secondary phenomena

MANAGEMENT
- Treatment (see Appendix A)
  - **Burow solution** compresses to exudative, oozing areas
  - Lowest-potency nonfluorinated topical steroids are used to avoid atrophy and striae. To achieve rapid improvement, treatment may be initiated with a higher-potency (class 5) steroid that is used for several days before it is changed to a lower-potency (class 6 or 7) agent
- ⚠ **ALERT: Intertriginous areas are inherently moist and occluded; therefore, the penetration and potency of topical agents are increased in these regions**
  - For longer-term use:
    - Tacrolimus **(Protopic)** ointment 0.1% once or twice daily
    - Pimecrolimus **(Elidel)** cream 1% once or twice daily
- Prevention
  - Promote air drying or use of hair dryer with heat off
- Nonrestrictive clothing
- Weight loss, if necessary
- Zeasorb powder

Inverse Psoriasis

Psoriasis that is localized in the intertriginous areas such as the axillae (see Chapter 11, Axillae), inframammary, perineal, and inguinal creases is referred to as **inverse psoriasis** (see also Chapter 19, Buttocks and Perineal Area, Gluteal Cleft; Chapter 20, Inguinal Area). Inverse psoriasis is often difficult to distinguish from atopic dermatitis, seborrheic dermatitis, intertrigo, and candidiasis.

DISTINGUISHING FEATURES
- Deep pink to red color and well-defined borders characteristic of psoriasis may be obvious; however, lesions generally lack scale (constant rubbing of two apposing surfaces does not allow scale to build up) (Fig. 16-6)

- May be pruritic
- Fissures may occur

DIAGNOSIS
- Clinical
- Psoriasis may be present elsewhere on the body
- Negative KOH and/or fungal culture

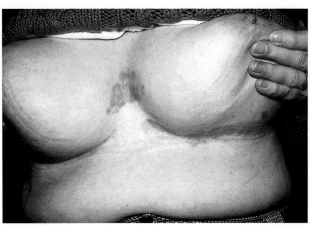

Figure 16-6 Inverse psoriasis.

MANAGEMENT (see Appendix A)
- Low-potency, nonfluorinated topical steroids (class 6 or 7) or, if necessary, a higher-potency (class 5) steroid that is used for several days before it is changed to a lower-potency agent
- Tacrolimus (**Protopic**) ointment 1% or pimecrolimus (**Elidel**) cream 1% is applied once or twice daily for longer-term use

☑ **TIP: Inverse psoriasis is commonly misdiagnosed by nondermatologists as tinea or candidiasis. Accordingly, it is often incorrectly treated with topical antifungal agents.**

Candidiasis

Cutaneous candidiasis (see also Chapter 17, Umbilicus; Chapter 19, Buttocks and Perineal Area, Gluteal Cleft; Chapter 20, Inguinal Area) is characterized by infection with *Candida* species. This genus is a common secondary and sometimes primary cause of intertrigo in both elderly, diabetic, and immunocompromised patients. Most cases of cutaneous candidosis occur in skin folds, where occlusion by clothing produces warm, moist conditions. Candidal infection of the skin under the breasts occurs when such areas become macerated under pendulous breasts.

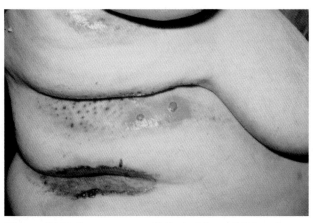

Figure 16-7 Cutaneous candidiasis. Note additional involvement in axilla and abdominal folds.

DISTINGUISHING FEATURES
- "Beefy red" color to the lesions (Fig. 16-7)
- Satellite pustules may be seen beyond the border of the plaques (see Figs. 11-5 and 18-13A)
- Maceration and fissures may be present
- Discomfort and/or pruritus

DIAGNOSIS
- Positive KOH examination for budding yeast or positive culture for *Candida* species

MANAGEMENT (see Appendix A)
- The skin should be patted dry or dried with a hair dryer (no heat)
- Topical nystatin powder, ketoconazole, clotrimazole, or miconazole twice daily
- Patients with extensive infection may require the addition of oral fluconazole (**Diflucan**), itraconazole (**Sporanox**) or ketoconazole
- For acute candidal intertrigo, **Burow solution** compresses to exudative, oozing areas

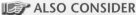 **ALSO CONSIDER**
- Tinea corporis
- Atopic dermatitis
- Contact dermatitis
- Intertriginous seborrheic dermatitis

RARELY
- Paget disease

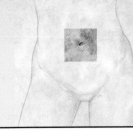

CHAPTER 17

Umbilicus

Aside from psoriasis, seborrheic dermatitis, or the nondescript excoriated lesions of scabies, there are few dermatoses that present in the umbilical and periumbilical area. Rarely, the occurrence of a malignant umbilical tumor associated with metastasizing intra-abdominal cancer or the granulomatous skin lesions of Crohn disease may appear in the umbilicus.

IN THIS CHAPTER
- Psoriasis vs seborrheic dermatitis
- Umbilical pyogenic granuloma vs umbilical hernia

Psoriasis and **seborrheic dermatitis** of the umbilicus both present as scaly red eruptions.

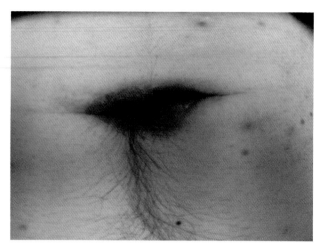

Figure 17-1A Psoriasis of the umbilicus

DISTINGUISHING FEATURES
- Well-demarcated erythematous plaque (Fig. 17-1A)
- With or without pruritus

DIAGNOSIS
- Clinical
- Psoriasis elsewhere on the body (Fig. 17-1B)

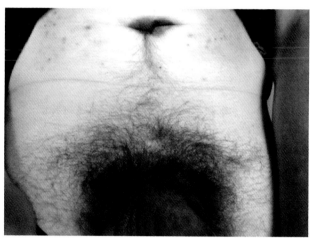

Figure 17-1B Psoriasis. Note the characteristic, well demarcated psoriatic plaque on the pubic area as well as the papules on the shaft of the penis

MANAGEMENT (see Appendix A)
- Low-potency, nonfluorinated topical steroids (class 6 or 7) or, if necessary, a higher-potency (class 5) steroid that is used for several days before it is changed to a lower-potency agent
- Tacrolimus **(Protopic)** ointment 1% or pimecrolimus **(Elidel)** cream 1% is applied once or twice daily for longer term use

Seborrheic Dermatitis

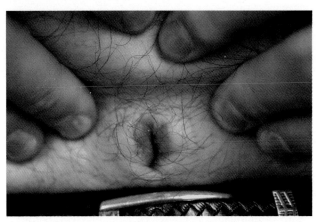

Figure 17-2 Seborrheic dermatitis of the umbilicus. This patient also has involvement of his face and scalp. Note similarity to Figure 17-1A.

DISTINGUISHING FEATURES
- Similar to psoriasis above with well-demarcated erythematous plaque (Fig. 17-2)

DIAGNOSIS
- Clinical
- Seborrheic dermatitis usually present elsewhere on the body

MANAGEMENT (Similar to psoriasis)

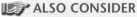 **ALSO CONSIDER**
- Impetigo
- Atopic dermatitis
- Scabies
- Cutaneous candidiasis

Umbilical Pyogenic Granuloma

Umbilical pyogenic granulomas are common, benign abnormalities in neonates that appear within the first few weeks of life. They form from excess granulation tissue persisting at the base of the umbilicus after cord separation.

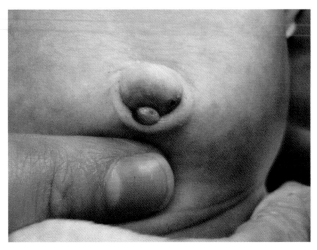

Figure 17-3 Umbilical pyogenic granuloma

DISTINGUISHING FEATURES
- Red, moist, velvety nodule with a soft, velvety appearance without a fistulous tract (Fig. 17-3)

DIAGNOSIS
- Clinical
- Biopsy if no response to therapy or if the lesion is persistent

MANAGEMENT
- Air drying with alcohol wipes should be tried before cauterizing with silver nitrate
- Conventional management has been to dry the umbilical stump and carefully cauterize the granuloma with a 75% silver nitrate stick
- Cryosurgery, electrocautery, salt, and ligature are other treatment options

Umbilical Hernia

Umbilical hernias are very commonly seen at birth.

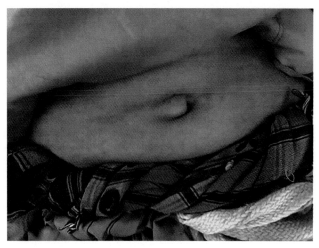

Figure 17-4 Umbilical hernia. Note that lesion is covered with skin.

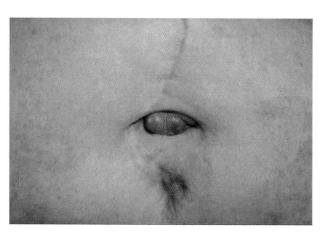

Figure 17-5 Sister Mary Joseph's nodule.

UMBILICUS

DISTINGUISHING FEATURES
- Covered with skin, which helps distinguish them from granulomas (Fig. 17-4)

DIAGNOSIS
- Clinical

MANAGEMENT
- Spontaneously close in most children by approximately 3 years of age and rarely become incarcerated
- Surgical repair, if necessary

ALSO CONSIDER
In Infants
- Umbilical polyp
- Patent urachus
- Omphalomesenteric duct remnant
- Bilious or fecal discharge from umbilicus
- Omphalocele

In Older Children and Adults
- Fibroepithelial papilloma
- Nevus
- Seborrheic keratosis
- Crohn disease

- Cysts
- Foreign body of talc granuloma
- Hypertrophic scar/keloid

RARELY
- Umbilical endometriosis
- Melanoma
- Basal cell carcinoma, squamous cell carcinoma, myosarcoma, and adenosarcoma
- Sister Mary Joseph nodule, a malignant umbilical tumor that is usually associated with metastasizing intra-abdominal cancer (Fig. 17- 5)

CHAPTER 18

Genital Area

A large number of conditions involve the skin and mucous membranes of the pubic and genital regions, including sexually transmitted diseases such as syphilis, venereal warts, herpes virus infections, molluscum contagiosum, and pediculosis pubis ("crabs"). However, the vast number of cutaneous disorders that are found elsewhere on the body, such as psoriasis, seborrheic dermatitis, and lichen planus, should also be considered here.

IN THIS CHAPTER

Pubic Area
- Molluscum contagiosum *vs* folliculitis *vs* pediculosis pubis
- Diaper rash *vs* atopic dermatitis

Scrotum/Vulva
- Lichen simplex chronicus/atopic dermatitis *vs* allergic or irritant contact dermatitis
- Cysts *vs* angiokeratomas of Fordyce

Male and Female External Genitalia
- Candidiasis *vs* lichen sclerosis *vs* lichen planus
- Psoriatic balanitis *vs* nonspecific balanitis
- Condyloma acuminata *vs* vestibular papillae and pearly penile papules *vs* molluscum contagiosum
- Herpes simplex genitalis *vs* primary syphilis *vs* chancroid

Molluscum Contagiosum

Molluscum contagiosum is spread by skin-to-skin contact and caused by a large DNA-containing poxvirus. It is seen most often in young, healthy children (see Chapter 3, Eyelids and Periorbital Area), in the genital region in sexually active young adults, and in patients with HIV/AIDS.

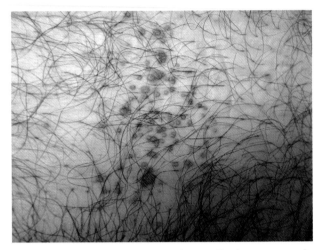

Figure 18-1 Molluscum contagiosum. Lesions are inflamed in this patient.

DISTINGUISHING FEATURES
- Dome-shaped waxy or pearly papules with a central white core (umbilication)
- Lesions generally 1 to 3 mm in diameter but may coalesce into double or triple lesions and become "giant" mollusca
- Generally asymptomatic; may itch and become inflamed (Fig. 18-1)

DIAGNOSIS
- Clinical
- A handheld magnifier often reveals the central core
- A short application of cryotherapy with liquid nitrogen accentuates the central core (see Figs. 2-2A and 2-2B)
- Shave or curettage biopsy if diagnosis is in doubt ("molluscum bodies")

MANAGEMENT (see Appendices A and B)
- Cryotherapy with liquid nitrogen
- Electrocautery
- Imiquimod 5% cream (**Aldara**) applied at bedtime

Folliculitis

Folliculitis (see also Chapter 9, Chin and Mandibular Area; Chapter 10, Neck) of the pubic area has become more common because of the increase in the practice of shaving this area in young adults. Besides shaving, irritants such as waxing, depilatories, electrolysis, and hair plucking can result in folliculitis.

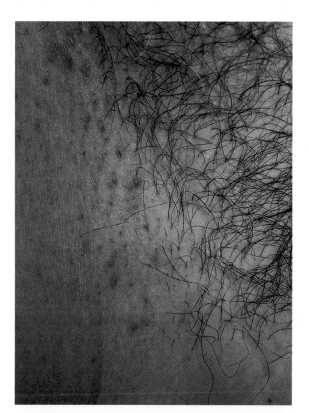

Figure 18-2 Folliculitis from shaving. Note the small erythematous papules in a grid-like pattern. (Reproduced with permission from Edwards L. *Genital Dermatology Atlas.* Philadelphia: Lippincott Williams & Wilkins; 2004.)

DISTINGUISHING FEATURES
- Superficial, small red papules and/or pustules (Fig. 18-2)

DIAGNOSIS
- Clinical
- Bacterial culture, if necessary

MANAGEMENT (see Appendix A)
Nonbacterial
- Discontinuance or removal of external causes and irritants (e.g., waxing, shaving)

Bacterial
- Mild cases of bacterial folliculitis can sometimes be prevented or controlled with antibacterial soaps (e.g., **Hibiclens**)
- Topical antibiotics, such as clindamycin (**Cleocin**) 1% solution, foam or gel, may be applied twice daily
- If staphylococcal colonization is present, mupirocin 2% (**Bactroban**) ointment should be applied
- If necessary, a systemic antibiotic for coverage of *Staphylococcus aureus*. Dicloxacillin or a cephalosporin is generally the first choice

Pediculosis Pubis

Pubic lice (crab lice, pediculosis pubis) are insects that infest the pubic hair and survive by feeding on human blood. They are most often spread by sexual contact. The pubic louse gets the nickname of "crab" from its large front claws. The claws enable the lice to grasp the coarser pubic hairs in the groin, perianal, and axillary areas. Heavy infestation with *Pediculus pubis* can also involve the eyelashes, eyebrows, and facial hair. The lice cannot survive off the human host for more than one day.

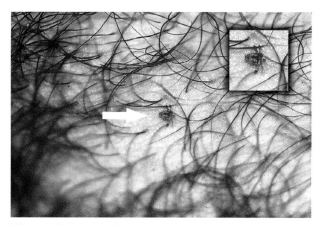

Figure 18-3 Pubic lice. (Reproduced with permission from Goodheart HG. *Photoguide to Common Skin Disorders: Diagnosis and Management.* 3rd ed. Philadelphia: Lippincott Williams & Wilkins; 2009.)

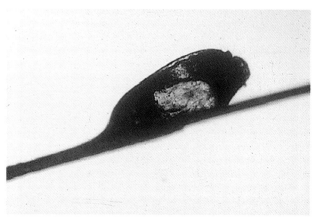

Figure 18-4 Pubic lice: nits. (Reproduced with permission from Goodheart HG. *Photoguide to Common Skin Disorders: Diagnosis and Management.* 3rd ed. Philadelphia: Lippincott Williams & Wilkins; 2009.)

DISTINGUISHING FEATURES
- The primary symptom of infestation is pubic itching
- Often, a sexual partner has "crabs"

DIAGNOSIS
- Pubic lice are diagnosed easily because they are visible to the naked eye at the base of hairs (Fig. 18-3). They are pinhead size, oval in shape, and grayish, but they appear reddish-brown when full of blood from their host
- Nits (ova), the tiny white eggs, also are visible and usually are observed clinging to the base of pubic hair (Fig. 18-4)

- Blue macules (maculae caeruleae) may occur on nearby skin

MANAGEMENT (see Appendix A)
- Lotions and shampoos that will kill pubic lice are available both over the counter (OTC) and by prescription
- Permethrin agents are usually the first line of treatment, although resistance to permethrin has become an increasingly important problem
- Permethrin 1% is available OTC as **Nix** and **Rid**
- A 5% permethrin (**Elimite**) is available only by prescription

- Benzyl alcohol lotion 5% **(Ulesfia),** an OTC product effective against head lice, may be tried
- Malathion **(Ovide),** approved only for use against head lice, may be effective against *P. pubis*
- Mercuric oxide ointment and petrolatum (twice daily for 7 to 10 days) is often used, with good results, for eyelash infestation

- Treatment should include contacts of infested patients, especially sexual partners
- Shaving of pubic or body hair is not necessary to treat lice
- ☑ **TIP: In resistant cases, particularly after repeated treatment failures, "delusions of parasitosis" should be considered in the differential diagnosis in adult patients.**

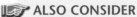

ALSO CONSIDER
- Scabies
- Atopic dermatitis
- Delusions of parasitosis

RARELY
- Fox-Fordyce disease in females

Diaper Rash

Diaper rash, diaper dermatitis, referred to as *napkin dermatitis* in the United Kingdom, is a type of irritant contact dermatitis. Diaper dermatitis is by far the most common rash in infancy, and it can also affect persons of any age group who wear diapers, such as incontinent patients. It is essentially the result of overhydration of the skin that is irritated by chafing, by soaps and detergents, and by prolonged contact with urine and feces. It may also be caused or exacerbated by the presence of atopic dermatitis, seborrheic dermatitis, or by a primary or secondary infection by *Candida albicans*.

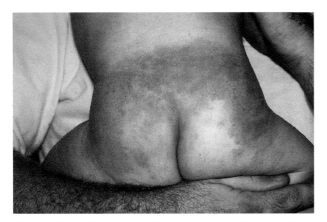

Figure 18-5 Diaper rash. Note the rash conforms to the shape of the diaper. (Reproduced with permission from Goodheart HG. *Photoguide to Common Skin Disorders: Diagnosis and Management.* 3rd ed. Philadelphia: Lippincott Williams & Wilkins; 2009.)

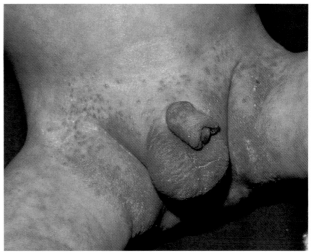

Figure 18-6 Diaper rash (candidal). Note involvement of inguinal creases and "satellite" pustules. (Reproduced with permission from Edwards L. *Genital Dermatology Atlas.* Philadelphia: Lippincott Williams & Wilkins; 2004.)

DISTINGUISHING FEATURES

- Erythema, scale, and possibly papules and plaques; infrequently, vesicles and bullae occur
- Lesions typically spare the creases (genitocrural folds) because such areas do not come in direct contact with a diaper
- "Beefy" redness and satellite papules and pustules suggest a primary or secondary infection with *C. albicans*
- The eruption may conform to, and be limited to, the diaper area (Fig. 18-5), or it may also involve the lower abdomen, genitalia, and perineum

DIAGNOSIS

- Clinical
- Potassium hydroxide (KOH)/fungal culture if patient is not responding to treatment
- ✔ **TIP: Primary candidal diaper dermatitis should be considered in an immunocompromised patient, particularly if the creases are involved (Fig. 18-6).**

MANAGEMENT (see Appendix A)

General Preventive Measures

- Use of disposable or superabsorbent diapers
- The diaper area should be gently dried and aired out after changing
- Frequent diaper changes
- Soap-free cleansers such as **Cetaphil Lotion**
- Absorbent baby powders such as **Desitin** cornstarch powder, **Zeasorb** powder, and **Johnson's Baby Powder**
- **Aquaphor** ointment and pure white petrolatum ointment **(Vaseline Petroleum Jelly)** act by trapping water beneath the epidermis

Specific Treatment Measures

- Many inexpensive OTC products contain zinc oxide such as **Balmex, Desitin, and A and D Ointment**
- Low-potency (class 7) OTC hydrocortisone 1% or 0.05% cream or ointment is often all that is necessary for uncomplicated diaper dermatitis

- Stronger topical steroids (class 6) such as desonide 0.05% or hydrocortisone valerate 0.02% cream (class 5) or ointment (class 4) may be used for very short periods, if necessary
- If the presence of *C. albicans* is suspected, particularly if there is no improvement after several days, a topical antifungal preparation such as the OTC miconazole 2% cream (**Micatin**) or miconazole combined with 15% zinc oxide (**Vusion ointment**) is another option that is available only with a prescription
- Consider adding nonabsorbable oral nystatin in recalcitrant cases

⚠ **ALERT: Potent topical steroids, particularly fluorinated preparations such as contained in Lotrisone, are to be avoided in the diaper area.**

Atopic Dermatitis

Atopic dermatitis (AD) and diaper dermatitis, seborrheic dermatitis, and psoriasis may be indistinguishable from one another in the diaper area. Atopic dermatitis occurs in association with a personal or family history of atopy.

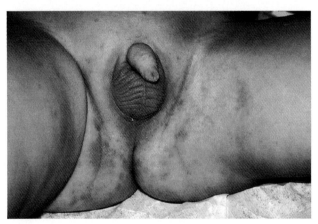

Figure 18-7 Atopic dermatitis. Note involvement of inguinal creases. (Reproduced with permission from Goodheart HG. *Photoguide to Common Skin Disorders: Diagnosis and Management.* 3rd ed. Philadelphia: Lippincott Williams & Wilkins; 2009.)

DISTINGUISHING FEATURES
- Often in patients with AD, the diaper area is remarkably spared (Fig. 18-7)

DIAGNOSIS
- Clinical
- There may be AD elsewhere on the body

MANAGEMENT (see Appendix A)
General Preventive Measures
- See previous discussion (as for Diaper Rash)

Specific Treatment Measures
- Low-potency OTC hydrocortisone 1% or 0.05% cream or ointment is often all that is necessary for uncomplicated AD
- Stronger topical steroids (class 6) such as desonide 0.05% or hydrocortisone valerate 0.02% cream (class 5) or ointment (class 4) may be used for very short periods, if necessary

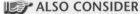 **ALSO CONSIDER**
- Seborrheic dermatitis: creases usually involved; the patient may have seborrheic dermatitis elsewhere such as in the axillae or on the scalp ("cradle cap")
- Psoriasis
- Candidiasis
- Tinea cruris
- Impetigo
- Child abuse (severe or repeated ulcerations)

RARELY
- Kawasaki disease
- Langerhans cell histiocytosis
- Acrodermatitis enteropathica (from zinc deficiency)
- Leiner disease is associated with diarrhea and a failure to thrive

GENITAL AREA

Lichen Simplex Chronicus/atopic Dermatitis

Lichen simplex chronicus (LSC) is a localized form of eczema. Scrotal and vulvar eczema is the most common cause of chronic genital itching. Most patients who have LSC also have atopic dermatitis, which generally implies that they have signs of eczema elsewhere on their body or have a positive atopic diathesis. Lichen simplex chronicus refers to localized areas of lichenification. It is seen most often on the nape of the neck (see Chapter 10, Neck), scalp, wrists, extensor forearms, ankles, pretibial areas, and inner thighs and vulva. It is most often noted in adults (see Chapter 12, Arms, Antecubital Fossae, Flexor Forearms, and Wrists; Chapter 21, Legs), who are more apt to develop genital LSC than children.

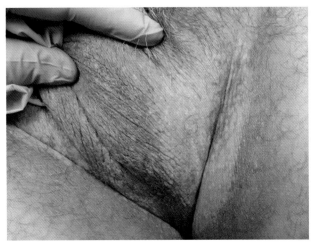

Figure 18-8 Note lichenification. Chronic scratching and rubbing has destroyed melanocytes resulting in areas of hypo and depigmentation.

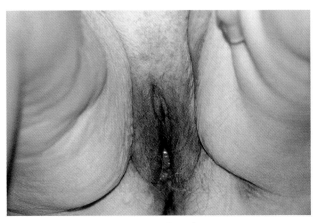

Figure 18-9 Lichen simplex chronicus.

DISTINGUISHING FEATURES

- Chronic or paroxysmal pruritus is the primary symptom
- Thick, leathery skin due to constant scratching and rubbing results in thickening of the skin and exaggeration of the normal skin markings (lichenification) with little or no scale
- Men: occurs particularly in the posterior portion of the scrotum and the crural crease (Fig. 18-8); the penis is spared
- Women: the labia majora is most often affected (Fig. 18-9)
- The perianal skin is often involved in both sexes

DIAGNOSIS

- The diagnosis is readily apparent and is made on clinical grounds
- Atopic history often obtained
- The exclusion of candidiasis
- The diagnosis is confirmed by the rapid response to topical anti-inflammatory therapy with topical steroids

☑ **TIP: A chronic itchy scrotal or vulvar rash is rarely the result of a fungal infection.**

☑ **TIP: Tinea infections tend to involve the inguinal areas and spare the scrotum.**

MANAGEMENT (see Appendix A)

- Avoid scratching and rubbing. This can be very difficult if the condition is chronic
- Eliminate harsh soaps, scrubbing, irritants, and over-washing
- Unfortunately, many patients scratch themselves in their sleep; consequently, a soporific antihistamine such as doxepin (10 to 20 mg at bedtime) can help reduce nocturnal pruritus
- The application of a potent class two such as fluocinonide or a superpotent class 1 topical steroid such as clobetasol, even for a week or two, if necessary, followed by lower-potency, intermediate-strength (class 3 or 4) topical steroids, helps break the chronic itch-scratch cycle

- Patients should be advised that recurrences are to be expected; therefore, the long-term use of the lowest-potency topical steroids and less frequent applications should be encouraged
- Alternatively, for longer-term use:
  - Tacrolimus (**Protopic**) ointment 0.1% once or twice daily
- Pimecrolimus (**Elidel**) cream 1% once or twice daily

☑ **TIP: Many physicians prescribe low-potency topical steroids, thus undertreating eczema, and the condition persists. The use of potent or superpotent topical steroids for several weeks is often the most effective means to interrupt the itch-scratch cycle. This promotes patient confidence and sets a goal for ongoing therapy.**

Allergic or Irritant Contact Dermatitis

Allergic or **irritant contact dermatis** on the scrotum or vulva is an eczematous eruption in response to an irritant or an allergen. Causes include overwashing, feminine hygiene products, spermicides, and various topical medications such as benzocaine agents, neomycin, fragrances, and latex (condoms and diaphragms).

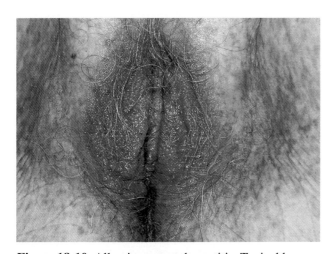

Figure 18-10 Allergic contact dermatitis. Topical benzocaine has resulted in this ill-defined erythematous eruption. (Reproduced with permission from Edwards L. *Genital Dermatology Atlas.* Philadelphia: Lippincott Williams & Wilkins; 2004.)

DISTINGUISHING FEATURES

- Poorly demarcated erythematous plaques with or without mild scaling (Fig. 18-10); or excoriations and lichenification similar to LSC and atopic dermatitis (see previous discussion)
- Soreness, pruritus, and irritation

DIAGNOSIS

- Clinical grounds
- Patient may have an atopic history
- The diagnosis is primarily confirmed by the response to the elimination of all irritants and/or allergens

☑ **TIP: Soaps, toilet paper, and laundry detergents can be irritants, but they are rarely causes of allergic contact dermatitis.**

MANAGEMENT (see Appendix A)

- Identification and elimination of all irritants and/or allergens
- Topical anti-inflammatory therapy with topical steroids (see Lichen Simplex Chronicus)

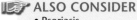 **ALSO CONSIDER**
- Psoriasis
- Seborrheic dermatitis
- Candidiasis

RARELY
- Vulvodynia
- Red scrotum syndrome
- Tinea (due to *Epidermophyton floccosum*)
- Bowen disease (squamous cell carcinoma in situ)
- Extramammary Paget disease

Cysts

Epidermoid **cysts** are sacs that contain semisolid or liquid material (keratin and lipid-rich debris). They are derived from the epithelium of the hair follicle are most often seen on the scalp (see Chapter 1, Hair and Scalp), ears, back (Chapter 15, Trunk), face, and upper arm. Another common place for them to develop is on the scrotum, they appear less often on the vulva.

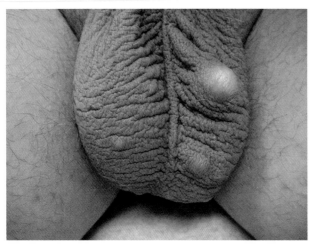

Figure 18-11 Scrotal cysts.

DISTINGUISHING FEATURES
- Solitary or multiple white milialike lesions (Fig. 18-11)
- When incised, a cheesy-white, rancid, malodorous keratin material can be expressed
- Scrotal cysts may calcify

DIAGNOSIS
- Clinical grounds

MANAGEMENT (see Appendix B)
- Reassurance of benign nature of these lesions
- If the patient wishes, destructive measures such as incision and drainage may be performed
- Excision for large lesions

Angiokeratomas of Fordyce

Angiokeratomas of Fordyce are typically blue-to-red papules located on the scrotum, shaft of the penis, labia majora, and inner thigh. Histologically, they are composed of ectatic thin-walled vessels in the superficial dermis with overlying epidermal hyperplasia. Patients usually give a history of many years of a progressive appearance of asymptomatic papules. The patient is often not aware of these lesions.

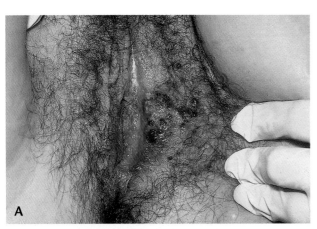 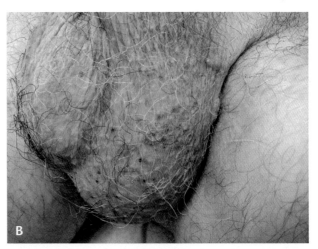

Figure 18-12 A: Angiokeratomas of Fordyce of vulva. **B:** Angiokeratomas of Fordyce of scrotum.

DISTINGUISHING FEATURES
- Asymptomatic 2 to 3 mm red-to-blue papules; solitary or multiple
- They occur on the medial labia minora in women and the scrotum in men (Fig. 18-12A and 18-12B)
- The overlying surface may show slight scales (hyperkeratosis)
- Bleeding from vulvar lesions may occur during pregnancy or after intercourse

DIAGNOSIS
- Clinical
- Shave biopsy only if diagnosis is in doubt

MANAGEMENT (see Appendix A)
- Reassurance of benign nature of these lesions
- If the patient desires: destructive measures such as cryotherapy, electrodesiccation, or laser ablation

☞ ALSO CONSIDER
- Genital wart
- Pyogenic granuloma
- Lymphangioma
- Seborrheic keratosis
- Vestibular cysts
- Bartholin's gland duct cyst

RARELY
- Angiokeratoma corporis diffusum (Fabry disease)
- Blue rubber bleb nevus syndrome

GENITAL AREA

Candidiasis

Candidiasis is a very common cause of vaginal irritation or vaginitis. It can also occur on the uncircumcised male genitals as *candidal balanitis*, particularly in immunocompromised patients. Although uncommon, penile candidiasis may be due to sexual intercourse with an infected individual. Broad spectrum antibiotics and diabetes mellitus are also predisposing factors.

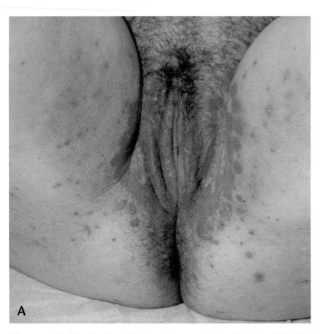
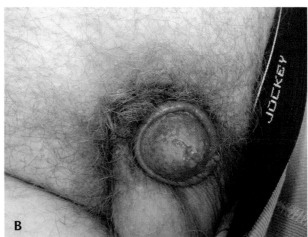

Figure 18-13 A: Candidal vulvovaginitis. **B:** Candidal balanitis.

DISTINGUISHING FEATURES
- Infection of the vagina or vulva may cause severe itching, burning, soreness, irritation, and a whitish or whitish-gray cottage cheese–like discharge, often with a curdlike appearance (Fig. 18-13A)
- On the glans penis, an erythematous, erosive, plaque with or without whitish scale (Fig. 18-13B)

DIAGNOSIS
- KOH or fungal culture demonstrates pseudohyphae and budding yeast

MANAGEMENT (see Appendix A)
- The antifungal drugs commonly used to treat candidiasis are topical clotrimazole, topical nystatin, fluconazole, and topical ketoconazole
- A one-time dose of fluconazole (**Diflucan** 150-mg tablet taken orally) is very effective in treating a vaginal yeast infection
- Local treatment may include vaginal antifungal suppositories or medicated douches

Lichen Sclerosis

Lichen sclerosis (LS), formerly referred to as *lichen sclerosis et atrophicus*, is a chronic inflammatory condition of unknown etiology that most commonly affects perimenopausal and postmenopausal women. Genital skin and mucosa are affected most frequently, but extragenital lesions of LS also occur. *Kraurosis vulvae* is an older term that was used to describe LS that was limited to the vulvar area. Lichen sclerosis that involves the glans penis, *balanitis xerotica obliterans*, is seen almost exclusively in uncircumcised men and boys.

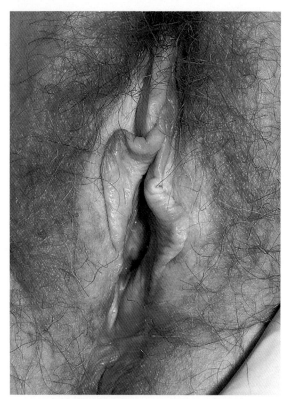

Figure 18-14 Lichen sclerosus. Vulvar plaques with atrophy and scarring. (Reproduced with permission from Edwards L, Lynch PJ. *Genital Dermatology Atlas.* 2nd ed. Philadelphia: Lippincott Williams & Wilkins; 2010.)

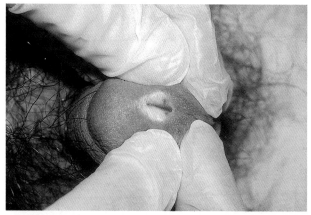

Figure 18-15 Penile lichen sclerosus (balanitis xerotica obliterans).

DISTINGUISHING FEATURES
Females
- When patients complain of itching, which is the most common presenting symptom, LS may cause diagnostic problems and may be considered to be a manifestation of eczematous dermatitis, candidiasis, or nonspecific vaginal pruritus
- Lesions consist of white plaques with epidermal atrophy. The vaginal mucosa may also become involved and display a whitish color with hemorrhages, telangiectasias, or bullae
- Lichen sclerosis can be quite pruritic and result in self-induced excoriations and erosions
- Dyspareunia may come about as the vaginal mucosa becomes increasingly sclerotic and atrophic
- Lesions may be confined to the labia majora but usually involve, and may eventually obliterate, the labia minora and stenose the introitus
- In chronic LS, the labia majora, labia minora, clitoris, perineum, and perianal skin may all be affected (Fig. 18-14)

Males
- Single or multiple discrete erythematous papules or macules progress and coalesce into atrophic ivory, white, or purple-white patches or plaques

- Itching, burning
- Lesions most commonly affect the glans and prepuce, frenulum, and urethral meatus (Fig. 18-15)
- Progression may lead to symptoms such as hypoesthesia, dysuria, painful erections, phimosis, urine retention, and significant scarring

DIAGNOSIS
- For genital biopsies, a snip excision or shave biopsy may suffice, but a punch biopsy is the preferable method to obtain tissue for histopathologic examination

MANAGEMENT (see Appendix A)
Both Males and Females
- Potent topical corticosteroids especially in the superpotent class 1 such as clobetasol cream or ointment 0.05%, applied twice daily, aides in reducing inflammation and pruritus and, in some cases, helps resolve the lesions. Pulse dosing (two consecutive days per week) may be used long term. On off days, a milder steroid such as triamcinolone cream or ointment 0.1% or topical (**Protopic**) ointment 1% tacrolimus may be applied
- In those patients who are refractory to topical therapy, intralesional injections of (**Kenalog**) 5 mg/mL once per month may be effective (see Appendix B)

- Oral retinoids: combining a retinoid with a potent topical corticosteroid as previously described may be beneficial in refractory cases

Females

- Topical testosterone may not be more effective than placebo and can be associated with virilization

- Vulvar surgery is not recommended unless an associated malignancy is present

- ⚠ **ALERT: The relation of LS to vulvar or penile malignancy has been the source of ongoing debate; however, ulcerative or vegetative genital lesions may need to be biopsied to screen for squamous cell carcinoma.**

Lichen Planus

Lichen planus is noted for oral mucosal and cutaneous involvement (see Chapter 8, Oral Cavity and Tongue; Chapter 12, Arms); however, vulvar and penile lesions do occur. Adhesions and sclerosis may be clinically indistinguishable from LS; therefore a biopsy may be necessary to differentiate one from another. Vulvar involvement is sometimes noted in adult women. A common place for genital lichen planus in adult men is on the glans penis.

DISTINGUISHING FEATURES
Females

- Vulvar lesions present as whitish, slightly elevated reticulated (Wickham striae) or papules and plaques (Fig. 18-16)
- Pruritus can be intense

- Vulvar involvement can range from reticulate papules to severe vulvar and vaginal erosions with resultant dyspareunia and postcoital bleeding (Fig. 18-17)

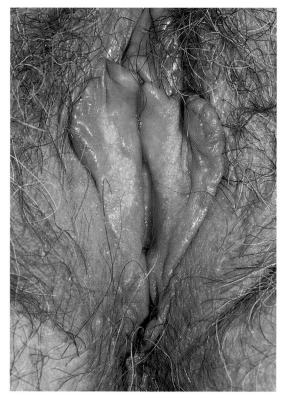

Figure 18-16 Vulvar lichen planus. Note white reticulated pattern of Wickham's striae on labia minorum. (Reproduced with permission from Edwards L. *Genital Dermatology Atlas.* Philadelphia: Lippincott Williams & Wilkins; 2004.)

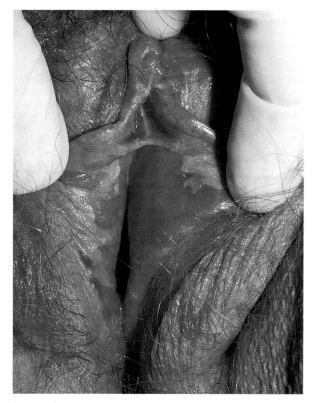

Figure 18-17 Vulvar lichen planus. Note erosive vaginitis. (Reproduced with permission from Edwards L. *Genital Dermatology Atlas.* Philadelphia: Lippincott Williams & Wilkins; 2004.)

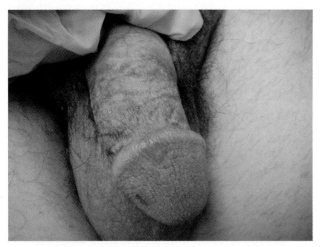

Figure 18-18 Penile lichen planus. Note characteristic violaceous flat-topped papules.

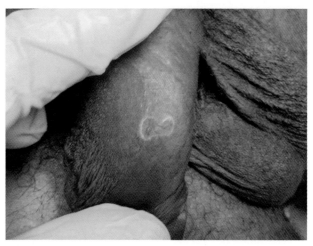

Figure 18-19 Penile lichen planus: typical annular lesion on shaft of penis.

Males

- Lesions on the glans penis are usually well demarcated, red, flat-topped, and shiny (Fig. 18-18)
- Often asymptomatic
- Frequently, a characteristic annular configuration is seen (Fig. 18-19)

DIAGNOSIS (see Appendix B)

- Shave biopsy or snip excision (especially for lesions on the shaft of the penis)

MANAGEMENT

- Topical steroids (class 6) such as desonide 0.05% or hydrocortisone valerate 0.02% cream (class 5) or ointment (class 4) may be used for very short periods, if necessary
- Alternatively, for longer-term use:
  - Tacrolimus **(Protopic)** ointment 0.1% once or twice daily
- Pimecrolimus **(Elidel)** cream 1% once or twice daily

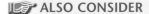 **ALSO CONSIDER**

Females
- Nonspecific vaginal pruritus
- Candidiasis
- Trichomonal vaginitis

Males
- Reiter disease
- Lichen nitidus

Males and Females
- Sexually transmitted disease
- Atopic dermatitis and lichen simplex chronicus
- Allergic or irritant contact dermatitis
- Squamous cell carcinoma
- Bowen disease (squamous cell carcinoma in situ, also referred to as *erythroplasia of Queyrat*)
- Vitiligo

RARELY
- Extramammary Paget disease
- Hailey-Hailey disease
- Chronic cutaneous lupus erythematosus (discoid)
- Plasma cell mucositis (vulvitis, balanitis), Zoon's (vulvitis, balanitis)

Psoriatic Balanitis

Balanitis refers to inflammatory conditions that affect the glans penis. Specific diagnostic causes include: contact dermatitis (e.g. to rubber condoms) or topical medications, psoriasis, eczematous dermatitis, and lichen planus

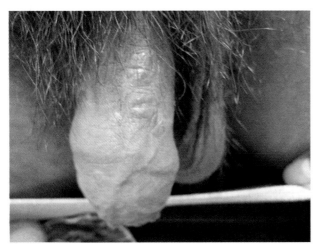

Figure 18-20 Psoriasis on shaft of penis.

DISTINGUISHING FEATURES
- Psoriatic balanitis; lesions may be typically well-demarcated erythematous plaques (Fig. 18-20)
- Lichen planus; may demonstrate characteristic flat-topped violaceous papules (Fig. 18-18)
- Reiter syndrome; psoriasislike plaques (Fig. 18-21)

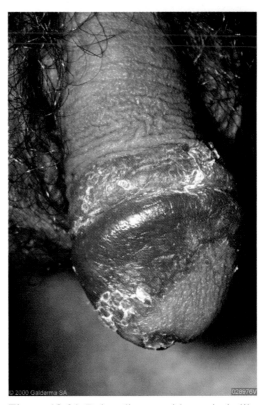

Figure 18-21 Reiter disease with psoriasis-like plaques.

DIAGNOSIS
- Clinical; history
- Shave biopsies may be necessary to make a definitive diagnosis (see Appendix B)

MANAGEMENT (see Appendix A)
- Potent topical steroids should only be used for a short time; less potent topical steroids are for longer-term application

Nonspecific Balanitis

When the conditions previously described are ruled out, the origin of the balanitis is best considered to be a type of irritant intertrigo or **nonspecific balanitis.** It nearly always affects uncircumcised men, as the tissue under the foreskin may fail to dry out adequately. Predisposing factors include:
- Excessive moisture and sweating and/or failure to dry the glans after washing
- Infrequent washing; conversely, overwashing
- Obesity
- Diabetes mellitus, which especially increases the likelihood of *C. albicans* infection (Fig. 18-13B)
- A sexual partner who has vaginal candidiasis
- Trauma, which may include friction during sexual intercourse

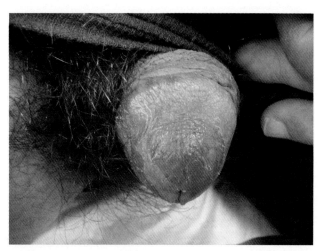

Figure 18-22 Nonspecific balanitis.

DISTINGUISHING FEATURES
- An ill-defined, erythematous, sometimes scaly eruption with or without itching and discomfort (Fig. 18-22)
- In severe cases, it may be difficult to retract the foreskin (phimosis)

DIAGNOSIS (see Appendix B)
- Clinical
- Other diagnostic procedures such as a negative KOH scrapings or shave biopsies may be necessary to rule out a specific diagnosis as previously described

MANAGEMENT
- The main aim of treatment is to keep the head of the penis and foreskin clean and dry
- Astringent compresses using dilute vinegar (acetic acid 1%), **Burow solution,** or potassium permanganate
- Topical antifungal medication
- Mild topical steroid; potent topical steroids should only be used for a short time (see Appendix A)

✔ **TIP: For phimosis or in refractory cases, circumcision may be necessary to prevent recurrence.**

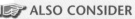
ALSO CONSIDER
- Fixed drug eruption
- Syphilis
- Scabies

RARELY
- Lichen sclerosus
- Plasma cell balanitis
- Bowen disease

Condyloma Acuminata

Condyloma acuminata (anogenital warts) for the most part are sexually transmitted viral warts caused by infection with specific types of human papillomavirus (HPV) (see also Chapter 19, Buttocks and Perineal Area; Chapter 20, Inguinal Area). Despite the generally benign nature of the proliferations, certain types of HPV can place patients at a high risk for anogenital cancer. Treatment can be difficult and lengthy. The incubation period is variable, ranging from 3 weeks to 8 months. Human papillomavirus has been identified in the skin of infected persons at a distance of up to 1 cm from the actual lesion; this feature may explain the high recurrence rate. The HPV types 16, 18, 31 to 35, 39, 42, 48, and 51 to 54 have been identified in cervical and anogenital cancers. Lesions tend to be more extensive and recalcitrant to treatment in immunocompromised persons. In addition, they tend to grow larger and more numerous during pregnancy.

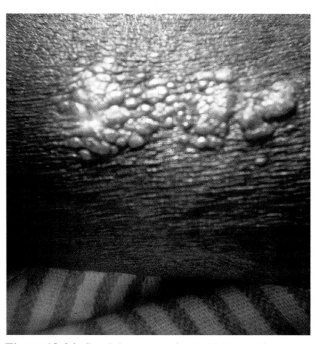

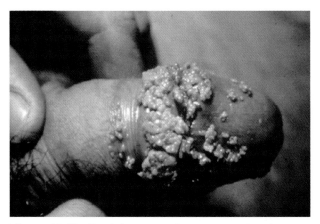

Figure 18-23 Condyloma acuminata. (Reproduced with permission from Goodheart HG. *Photoguide to Common Skin Disorders: Diagnosis and Management.* 3rd ed. Philadelphia: Lippincott Williams & Wilkins; 2009.)

Figure 18-24 Condyloma acuminata. Note papular lesions. (Reproduced with permission from Goodheart HG. *Photoguide to Common Skin Disorders: Diagnosis and Management.* 3rd ed. Philadelphia: Lippincott Williams & Wilkins, 2009.)

DISTINGUISHING FEATURES
- May resemble small cauliflowers (condyloma acuminatum) (Fig. 18-23)
- Warts may appear as smooth, dome-shaped, or relatively flat, papular lesions (Fig. 18-24)
- They can look like typical verrucous papules or plaques that resemble common warts
- In men, lesions occur on the penis, scrotum, mons pubis, inguinal crease, and perianal area
- In women, the vagina, labia, mons pubis, perianal area, and uterine cervix are the most common locations (Figure 18-25)
- Usually asymptomatic but may become pruritic, painful, or bleed, particularly perianal and inguinal lesions

- Bowenoid papulosis
  - Clinically similar to, and often indistinguishable from, flat or dome-shaped genital warts; associated with HPV type 16 or 18
  - Histologically, bowenoid papulosis demonstrates squamous cell carcinoma in situ; however, it follows a largely benign clinical course

DIAGNOSIS (see Appendix B)
- Generally straightforward when the patient presents with the typical cauliflowerlike lesions; however, when lesions are papular (flat-topped), pigmented, moist, or erosive, the diagnosis may not be as clinically obvious
- Snip excisional biopsy from the labia minora or perianal area or a shave biopsy, if necessary

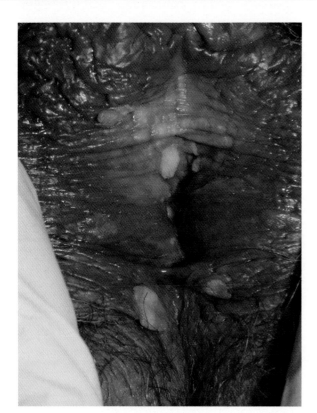

Figure 18-25 Condyloma acuminata.

- A biopsy is used to rule out bowenoid papulosis or frank squamous cell carcinoma in atypical or recalcitrant lesions

MANAGEMENT
Counseling
- Patients should be advised about the long latency period of HPV; thus, a patient may not have contracted condyloma from his or her current partner
- Male patients should use condoms at least 1 year after clinical infection is treated; however, condoms are not perfect protection because warts can occur on genital areas other than the penis or vagina

⚠ **ALERT: In affected women, there is a risk of malignant degeneration to cervical intraepithelial neoplasia or squamous cell carcinoma**
- It is recommended that anogenital warts be treated in pregnant women during the second and third trimesters and that vaginal delivery be performed if possible

Surgical Therapy
- Cryosurgery with liquid nitrogen: effective for treating multiple, small, warts (e.g., lesions on the shaft of the penis and vulva). Cryotherapy is also safe for pregnant women
- Electrodesiccation and curettage: effective for a limited number of lesions on the shaft of the penis
- Surgical excision (useful for debulking large "cauliflower" lesions) followed by electrocautery

Intralesional Therapy
- Interferon alpha-2b (not recommended by the Centers for Disease Control and Prevention because of high expense and no increased efficacy over other treatments)

Topical Therapy (Table 18-1)

Vaccines
- The HPV vaccine works by preventing the most common types of HPV that cause cervical cancer and genital warts. It is given as a three-dose vaccine. Vaccines can protect males and females against some of the most common types of HPV. The vaccines are most effective when given before a person's first sexual contact, when he or she could be exposed to HPV
- Girls and women
  - Two vaccines (**Cervarix** and **Gardasil**) are available to protect females against the types of HPV that cause most cervical cancers. One of these vaccines (**Gardasil**) also protects against HPV subtypes 6, 11, 16, and 18
- Both vaccines are recommended for 11- and 12-year-old girls, as well as for females age 13 through 26 years who did not get any or all of the shots when they were younger. These vaccines can also be given to girls as young as 9 years of age

⚠ **ALERT: Pregnant women *should not* be vaccinated.**
- Boys and men
  - **Gardasil** protects males against most genital warts.
- The vaccine is available for boys and men, 9 through 26 years of age

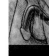

Table 18-1   TOPICAL THERAPY

	Treatment	Application
Patient-applied therapies	Imiquimod (**Aldara**) 5% cream	Three times weekly for up to 16 weeks. Works by increasing local production of interferon. Safety for use in pregnancy is not known.
	Sinecatechins (**Veregen**) 15% ointment	Recommended in adults (≥18 years old) 3 times per day until all warts clear completely. Therapy should not exceed 16 weeks.
Provider-applied therapies	Podophyllin resin 10% to 25% in tincture of benzoin	Carefully applied to the wart surface. The patient is instructed to wash the area in 4 to 6 hours, and this interval is increased in subsequent treatments. Most effective on mucosal warts
	Trichloroacetic or bichloroacetic acid 80% to 90%.	Most effective on small warts and on nonmucosal surfaces.

Vestibular Papillae and Pearly Penile Papules

Vestibular papillae (vulvar papillomatosis) and **pearly penile papules** are normal anatomic structures. Unlike warts, vestibular papillae (vulvar papillomatosis) occur near the vaginal vestibule in symmetric clusters or in a linear pattern.

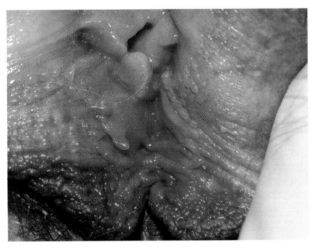

Figure 18-26 Vestibular papillae. Note grouped soft, fleshy, papules with rounded tips. (Reproduced with permission from Goodheart HG. *Photoguide to Common Skin Disorders: Diagnosis and Management.* 3rd ed. Philadelphia: Lippincott Williams & Wilkins; 2009.)

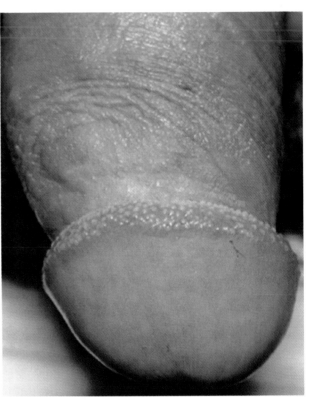

Figure 18-27 Pearly penile papules. (Reproduced with permission from Goodheart HG. *Photoguide to Common Skin Disorders: Diagnosis and Management.* 3rd ed. Philadelphia: Lippincott Williams & Wilkins; 2009.)

DISTINGUISHING FEATURES
Females
- Grouped, soft papules with rounded tips located in the vaginal vestibule (Fig. 18-26)

Males
- Uniform, small, smooth projections that resemble cobblestones
- Commonly occur around the corona and are sometimes seen on the shaft near the frenulum (Fig. 18-27)

DIAGNOSIS
- Clinical
- Shave biopsy only if diagnosis is in doubt
- ✔ **TIP: Pearly penile papules, vestibular papillae, and other normal anatomic structures are often mistaken for condyloma acuminata.**

MANAGEMENT
- Reassurance regarding the benign nature of these lesions

Molluscum Contagiosum

Molluscum contagiosum (see Pubic Area in this chapter and Chapter 3, Eyelids and Periorbital Area) commonly arise on the penis, vulva, and pubic area in sexually active young adults and in patients with HIV/AIDS.

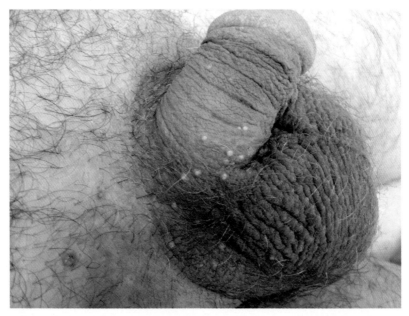

Figure 18-28 Molluscum contagiosum.

DISTINGUISHING FEATURES
- Dome-shaped, waxy, or pearly papules with a central white core (Fig. 18-28)

DIAGNOSIS
- Clinical
- Shave biopsy only if diagnosis is in doubt

MANAGEMENT
- See Pubic Area and Appendices A and B

ALSO CONSIDER
- Skin tags
- Seborrheic keratoses
- Melanocytic nevi

RARELY
- Malignant neoplasms:
  - Bowenoid papulosis
  - Giant condyloma acuminatum (Buschke-Löwenstein tumor)
  - Squamous cell carcinoma

Herpes Simplex Genitalis

Herpes simplex genitalis is caused most commonly by herpes simplex virus-2 (HSV-2), although HSV-1 can also infect genital skin. Herpes simplex virus, which is most often but not invariably sexually transmitted, is the most common cause of ulcerative genital lesions. The disease is highly contagious during the prodrome and while the lesions are active, becoming noncontagious when all lesions are crusted over. The HSV establishes latency in the dorsal root ganglia and reappears following different triggers in individual patients. Triggers include psychological or physiologic stress, physical trauma (e.g., intercourse), menses, and immunosuppression. Recurrences may be infrequent or a once-monthly phenomenon. As with HSV-1, primary herpes simplex (HSV-2) may be more severe than recurrent infections (see Chapter 7, Lips and Perioral Area). Alternatively, the initial outbreak may be mild or asymptomatic, so that the patient sheds the virus intermittently without realizing that he or she is infected. Up to 30% of U.S. adults have antibodies against HSV-2. A mother who is infected with the herpesvirus may transmit it to her newborn during vaginal delivery, especially if she has an active infection at the time of delivery, even if there are no symptoms or visible lesions.

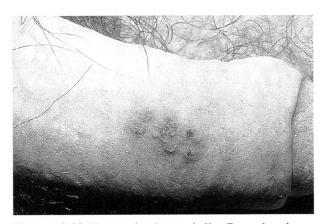

Figure 18-29 Herpes simplex genitalis. (Reproduced with permission from Goodheart HG. *Photoguide to Common Skin Disorders: Diagnosis and Management.* 3rd ed. Philadelphia: Lippincott Williams & Wilkins; 2009.)

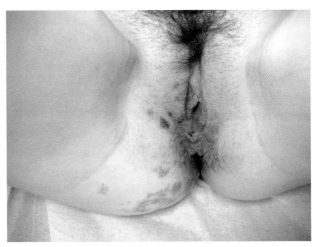

Figure 18-30 Herpes simplex genitalis.

DISTINGUISHING FEATURES

- Lesions initially appear as grouped vesicles on an erythematous base (Fig. 18-29)
- Lesions may then become pustular, crusted, and eroded (Fig. 18-30)
- Crusting of the lesions occurs over 15 to 20 days before reepithelialization begins
- Chronic ulcerations or crusted or verrucous papules may develop in immunocompromised patients
- In women, the vulva, perineum, inner thighs, buttocks, and sacral area are the most common sites
- In men, the penis, scrotum, thigh, and buttocks are the typical locations

Primary Herpes Simplex Virus
- May be more severe than recurrent infections
- Duration is generally from 10 to 14 days
- Regional adenopathy may be present
- Fever, dysuria, and constipation may also occur

- Alternatively, the patient may be asymptomatic so that initial outbreak looks like recurrent HSV
- ⚠ **ALERT: Risk of neonatal infection is greatest in patients with primary HSV at the time of delivery. If maternal HSV is acquired near the time of delivery, caesarian section is usually advised.**

Recurrent Herpes Simplex Virus
- There is often a prodrome of itching, burning, numbness, tingling, or pain 1 to 2 days before clinical outbreak
- Lesions are localized and recur at the same site or in close proximity each time
- Regional adenopathy may be present
- Vulvar and periurethral involvement may cause dysuria
- Duration is generally from 3 to 5 days
- Chronic ulcerative lesions are indicative of immunosuppression
- Risk of neonatal transmission is less than 3%

DIAGNOSIS

- Most often, diagnosis is based on the clinical appearance
- Tzanck preparation may be helpful (see Appendix B)
- Viral culture is the gold standard of diagnosis, but the sensitivity declines rapidly as the lesions begin to heal
- Diagnosis in tissue culture using monoclonal antibodies or polymerase chain reaction is sensitive but expensive
- Serologic testing is of little value

MANAGEMENT

Patient Education

- The patient should be given written educational materials and clear instructions regarding safe sexual practices
- The use of condoms should be encouraged
- The patient should be advised about asymptomatic viral shedding

Topical Therapy

- Topical antivirals are of limited effectiveness and are not recommended
- Symptomatic relief may be achieved with cold compresses, viscous lidocaine (**Xylocaine**), lidocaine and prilocaine (**EMLA**), or oral analgesics

Systemic Antiviral Therapy

- **Primary herpes simplex**
  - Acyclovir (200 mg 5 times per day daily or 400 mg 3 times daily for 10 days) *or*
  - Famciclovir (**Famvir**) (250 mg 3 times daily for 10 days) *or*
  - Valacyclovir (**Valtrex**) (1 g twice daily for 10 days)
- **Recurrent herpes simplex: episodic therapy**
  - Treat at the first sign of the prodrome.
    - Acyclovir (400 mg 3 times daily for 5 days) or (800 mg twice daily for 5 days, or 800 mg 3 times daily for 3 days) *or*
    - Famciclovir (125 mg twice daily for 5 days) or (1000 mg twice daily for 1 day) *or*
    - Valacyclovir (500 mg twice daily for 3 days) or (1000 mg daily for 5 days)
- **Daily suppressive therapy (more than 6 recurrences per year)**
  - Acyclovir 400 mg twice daily) *or*
  - Famciclovir (250 mg twice daily) *or*
  - Valacyclovir (500 mg once daily)
- **Acyclovir-resistant herpes simplex**
  - This is seen in patients with AIDS. Intravenous **Foscarnet** can be given
- ✔ TIP: Oral antiviral treatment should be initiated, if possible, during the prodromal phase.

Primary Syphilis

Syphilis is a sexually transmitted systemic disease caused by the spirochetal bacterium *Treponema pallidum*. It is divided into primary, secondary, early latent, late latent, and tertiary stages. Our discussion is limited to the primary lesions of this disease.

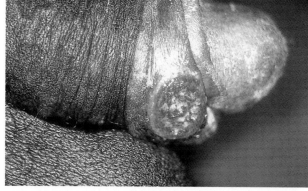

Figure 18-31 Primary syphilis.

DISTINGUISHING FEATURES

- Usually asymptomatic; an ulceration (chancre) with a rolled, indurated border (Fig. 18-31)
- Lesions are usually single, but they may be multiple
- The base of the ulcer is "clean" unless it is superinfected
- There are no vesicles
- The primary chancre most often presents on or near the glans penis in men; it appears less commonly on shaft of the penis
- A visible chancre is less common in women
- In women, lesions may occur on the labia majora or minora, the clitoris, or the posterior commissure
- Anal lesions may occur after receptive anal intercourse
- Less frequently, extragenital chancres can occur
- Regional adenopathy may be present
- An untreated chancre heals within 3 months

DIAGNOSIS

- The following diagnostic methods are used:
  - Darkfield examination of the ulceration
  - Skin biopsy
  - Nontreponemal serologic tests such as Venereal Disease Research Laboratory (VDRL), rapid plasma reagin (RPR), and the automated reagin test. These become positive at a rate of 25% of patients per week of infection

MANAGEMENT

- Test for HIV infection and retest 3 months later if negative

Non–Penicillin-Allergic Patients

- Benzathine penicillin G (2.4 million units intramuscularly in a single dose)

Penicillin-Allergic Nonpregnant Patients

- Doxycycline (100 mg orally twice daily for 2 weeks)

  or

- Tetracycline (500 mg 4 times daily for 2 weeks)

Penicillin-Allergic Pregnant Patients

- Desensitization to penicillin
- Subsequent treatment with benzathine penicillin G (2.4 million units intramuscularly, with a second dose 1 week later)

HIV-Infected Patients

- Benzathine penicillin G (2.4 million units intramuscularly in 1 dose)
- Some experts recommend repeated treatment

Chancroid

Chancroid is an ulcerative sexually transmitted disease that is most common in developing countries and is rare in the United States and western Europe. In the United States, it is associated with the use of crack cocaine. The causative organism, *Haemophilus ducreyi*, a Gram-negative rod, is fastidious and requires specific conditions for culture. Chancroid occurs as a mixed infection with syphilis or herpes simplex in 10% of cases. Clinical infection is more common in men than in women.

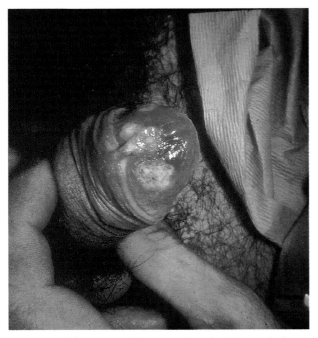

Figure 18-32 Chancroid. (Reproduced with permission from Goodheart HG. *Photoguide to Common Skin Disorders: Diagnosis and Management.* 3rd ed. Philadelphia: Lippincott Williams & Wilkins; 2009.)

DISTINGUISHING FEATURES

- The earliest manifestation is a papule, which becomes a pustule and ulcerates
- Fully developed lesions are painful, with undermined borders and peripheral erythema (Fig. 18-32)
- Unilateral or bilateral inguinal adenopathy (buboes) may be present
- Borders are not indurated
- There may be satellite ulcers
- The location of lesions depends on the site(s) of inoculation
- In men, the prepuce, balanopreputial fold, and the shaft of the penis are the typical sites
- In women, lesions are noted on the labia majora, posterior commissure, or perianal area.
- The incubation period is 25 days
- Tenderness and pain are common

DIAGNOSIS

- Often made based on the clinical appearance
- A negative darkfield examination, syphilis serologic testing, and HSV cultures help exclude other diagnoses
- Obtaining a culture is difficult
- A Gram stain shows characteristic "schools of fish" or "Chinese characters"
- Polymerase chain reaction may help in making a diagnosis

MANAGEMENT

- Azithromycin (1 g orally in a single dose) *or*
- Ceftriaxone (250 mg intramuscularly in a single dose) *or*
- Erythromycin (500 mg orally 4 times daily for 7 days) *or*
- Ciprofloxacin (500 mg orally twice daily for 3 days)
- ⚠ **ALERT: Always test for coinfection with HIV, syphilis, and HSV.**

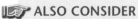 **ALSO CONSIDER**
- Erythema multiforme
- Trauma (e.g., human bite)
- Fixed drug eruption

RARELY
- Lymphogranuloma venereum
- Granuloma inguinale
- Behçet syndrome

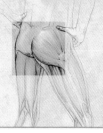

CHAPTER 19

Buttocks and Perineal Area

Many lesions and dermatoses that occur on the buttocks, gluteal cleft, and perianal areas are often associated with lesions on other parts of the body. Examples include acne, folliculitis, furunculosis, psoriasis, and tinea corporis. There are also findings that are characteristically seen in the perineal and perianal areas such as condyloma lata of secondary syphilis and external hemorrhoids. For practical purposes, most eruptions are inflammatory rather than neoplastic in nature; the relatively rare, but increasing incidence, of cutaneous T-cell lymphoma (mycosis fungoides) is an exception.

IN THIS CHAPTER

Buttocks
- Tinea corporis *vs* psoriasis *vs* cutaneous T-cell lymphoma (mycosis fungoides)
- Hot tub folliculitis *vs* folliculitis *vs* herpes simplex

Gluteal Cleft
- Intertrigo *vs* inverse psoriasis

Perianal Area
- Condyloma acuminata *vs* condyloma lata *vs* anal hemorrhoids
- Pruritus ani *vs* eczema/lichen simplex chronicus

Tinea Corporis *vs* Psoriasis *vs* Cutaneous T-cell Lymphoma (Mycosis Fungoides)

Tinea Corporis

Tinea corporis ("ringworm") on the buttocks is most often acquired by spread from other parts of the body via autoinoculation, most often from tinea cruris or tinea pedis (see also Chapter 15, Trunk; Chapter 20, Inguinal Area; Chapter 22, Feet). It is most often seen in adult and elderly men.

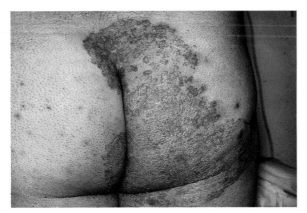

Figure 19-1 Tinea corporis.

DISTINGUISHING FEATURES
- Distribution of lesions is usually asymmetrical
- Lesions of tinea corporis are generally annular, with peripheral enlargement and central clearing; however, lesions on the buttocks have a propensity to be more blended into one or more confluent scaly patches, and therefore the entire lesion tends to be scaly (Fig. 19-1)
- Often asymptomatic

DIAGNOSIS
- Confirmed by a positive potassium hydroxide (KOH) examination or fungal culture (it is especially easy to find hyphae in patients who have been previously treated unsuccessfully with topical steroids)

MANAGEMENT (see Appendix A)
- Topical antifungal agents such as ketoconazole 2% twice daily
- Systemic antifungal agents such as terbinafine (**Lamisil**), itraconazole (**Sporanox**), ketoconazole, or griseofulvin are most often necessary to cure this condition

Psoriasis

Plaques of **psoriasis** often appear on the buttocks (see also Chapter 15, Trunk).

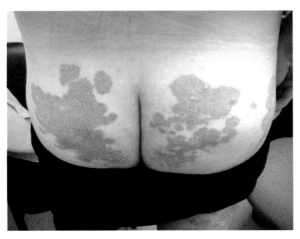

Figure 19-2 Psoriasis.

DISTINGUISHING FEATURES
- Well-demarcated, symmetric erythematous plaques with characteristic overlying white or silvery (micaceous) scale (Fig. 19-2)

DIAGNOSIS
- Clinical
- Biopsy if diagnosis is in doubt

MANAGEMENT
- See Appendix A

Cutaneous T-cell Lymphoma

Cutaneous T-cell lymphoma (CTCL), also known as *mycosis fungoides*, is a malignancy of helper T cells (CD4+); it accounts for almost 50% of all primary cutaneous lymphomas. In advanced stages, the disease may progress to extracutaneous manifestations, such as involvement of internal organs. Most often, CTCL has an indolent clinical course with slow progression over years or decades. However, patches may develop into more infiltrated plaques and, eventually, tumors. Cutaneous T-cell lymphoma is more common in men; the male-female ratio is approximately 2:1.

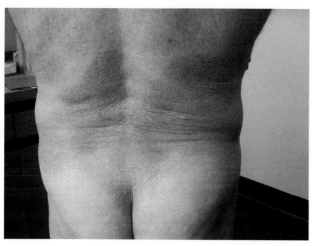

Figure 19-3 Patch stage cutaneous T-cell lymphoma.

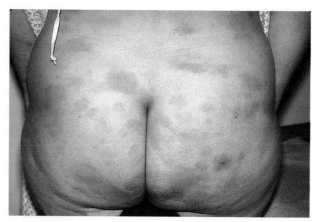

Figure 19-4 Cutaneous T-cell lymphoma. Note "smudgy patches". (Reproduced with permission from Goodheart HG. *Photoguide to Common Skin Disorders: Diagnosis and Management.* 3rd ed. Philadelphia: Lippincott Williams & Wilkins; 2009.)

DISTINGUISHING FEATURES
- Classic CTCL is divided into 3 stages: patch (atrophic or nonatrophic), plaque, and tumor
- Often, the first stage goes on for many years and is characterized by a subtle nonspecific dermatitis usually consisting of patches on the lower trunk and buttocks (Fig. 19-3) and other "double-clothed" areas of the body: axillae, breasts, and groin
- Patches are initially poorly defined, thin, red, scaly, "smudgy" lesions (Fig. 19-4)
- At times, patches may have a wrinkled quality, often with reticulated pigmentation
- May progress over years to decades to plaque stage and later to tumor stage

DIAGNOSIS
- CTCL may be difficult to diagnose; in fact, eczema and psoriasis are the two most commonly diagnosed conditions before a definitive diagnosis of CTCL is made (a latent period between onset and diagnosis may take many years)
- Well-developed plaques that are clinically diagnostic for CTCL are usually intensely pruritic
- A skin biopsy (sometimes several shave biopsies) is usually necessary to demonstrate the disease

- Rarely, CTCL appears from the beginning as tumors (tumour d'emblee)
- An erythrodermic variant of CTCL, Sézary syndrome, has been defined historically by the triad of erythroderma, generalized lymphadenopathy, and the presence of neoplastic T cells (Sézary cells) in skin, lymph nodes, and peripheral blood

MANAGEMENT
Treatment
- Treatments for CTCL confined to the skin consist of topical corticosteroids, heliotherapy, photochemotherapy, topical application of nitrogen mustard (mechlorethamine) or carmustine (BCNU), or radiotherapy, including total skin electron-beam irradiation, and chemotherapy with bexarotene (**Targretin**) or vorinostat (**Zolinza**)
- A detailed explanation of the various modalities is beyond the scope of this discussion
Prognosis
- The prognosis for patients with mycosis fungoides depends on stage and, in particular, the type and extent of skin lesions and the presence of extracutaneous disease
- In many cases, the disease never progresses beyond the patch/plaque stage, and the prognosis is quite good

 ALSO CONSIDER
- Atopic dermatitis/eczema
- Nonspecific dermatitis
- Contact dermatitis
- Small-plaque parapsoriasis
- Large-plaque parapsoriasis

RARELY
- Pityriasis rubra pilaris
- Erythema annulare centrifugum

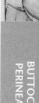

BUTTOCKS AND PERINEAL AREA

Hot Tub Folliculitis *vs* Folliculitis *vs* Herpes Simplex

Hot Tub Folliculitis

Hot tub folliculitis (*Pseudomonas* folliculitis) often appears on the buttocks ("hot tub buns"). It is most often acquired from communal hot tubs and caused by infection by *Pseudomonas aeruginosa*. Jacuzzis, therapeutic whirlpools ("whirlpool folliculitis"), public swimming pools, and the use of loofah sponges may also be a source of this infection.

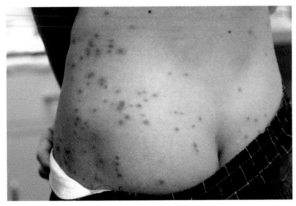

Figure 19-5 Hot tub folliculitis. (Reproduced with permission from Goodheart HG. *Photoguide to Common Skin Disorders: Diagnosis and Management.* 3rd ed. Philadelphia: Lippincott Williams & Wilkins; 2009.)

DISTINGUISHING FEATURES
- Lesions consist of intensely pruritic or tender follicular papules, and less commonly, pustules that are most often found on the trunk and buttocks (areas generally covered by a bathing suit)
- Pruritic lesions occur 1 to 3 days after bathing in a hot tub, whirlpool, or public swimming pool (Fig. 19-5)

DIAGNOSIS
- Clinical, and based on a history of exposure
- *Pseudomonas* organisms can sometimes be isolated if intact pustules are present

MANAGEMENT
- Hot tub folliculitis usually resolves spontaneously, but it may not if it is very extensive or symptomatic
- Symptomatic treatment with class 1–2 topical steroids
- If necessary, it may be treated with oral ciprofloxacin (500 mg twice a day for 5 days)

Folliculitis

Folliculitis often appears on the buttocks. It can occur from occlusion, heat, and sweat retention. It can be sterile or bacterial (*Staphylococcus aureus*) (see also Chapter 9, Chin and Mandibular Area).

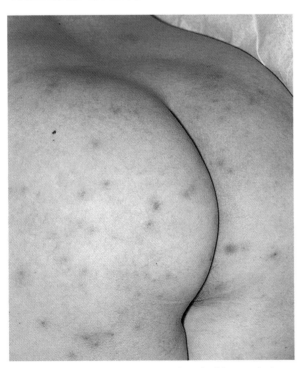

Figure 19-6 Folliculitis. (Reproduced with permission from Edwards L, Lynch PJ. *Genital Dermatology Atlas.* 2nd ed. Philadelphia: Lippincott Williams & Wilkins; 2010.)

DISTINGUISHING FEATURES
- Red papules and occasional pustules, many with crusts, are characteristic of folliculitis in this area (Fig. 19-6)

DIAGNOSIS
- Clinical diagnosis
- Culture for bacteria can aid in selecting an appropriate treatment

MANAGEMENT
- Depends on the cause:
  - Staphylococcal folliculitis is treated with cephalexin or dicloxacillin
  - Sterile folliculitis can be effectively treated with topical clindamycin or an oral tetracycline derivative

Herpes Simplex

Herpes simplex of the sacral and buttock area is caused most commonly by herpes simplex virus type 2 (HSV-2), although HSV-1 can also infect these areas (see also Chapter 18, Genital Area). The disease is most commonly, but not invariably, sexually transmitted.

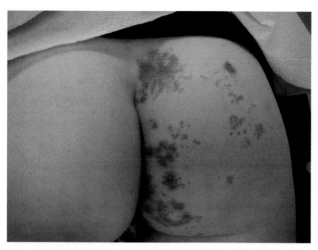

Figure 19-7 Herpes simplex virus type 2.

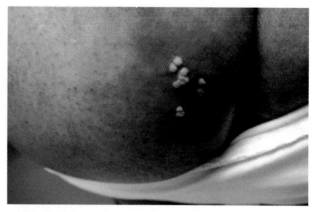

Figure 19-8 Herpes simplex virus type 2 grouped pustules on an erythematous base.

DISTINGUISHING FEATURES
- In women, the buttocks and sacral area are the most common sites
- Initially lesions appear as grouped vesicles on an erythematous base (Fig. 19-7)
- Lesions may then become pustular (Fig. 19-8), crusted, and eroded
- Symptoms: burning and/or itching
- Affected patients may have recurrences that are infrequent or as common as once monthly

DIAGNOSIS
- See Appendix A and Chapter 18, Genital Area

MANAGEMENT
- See Appendix A and Chapter 18, Genital Area

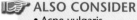

ALSO CONSIDER
- Acne vulgaris
- Scabies
- Arthropod bite reaction

RARELY
- Dermatitis herpetiformis

Intertrigo *vs* Inverse Psoriasis

Intertrigo

Intertrigo occurs in places where opposing skin surfaces rub against each other: the axillae (see Chapter 11, Axillae), under the breasts (see Chapter 16, Breasts and Inframammary Area), the inguinal creases (see Chapter 20, Inguinal Area), and the intragluteal creases. *Candida albicans* is a common secondary, and sometimes primary, cause of intertrigo in both elderly, diabetic, and immunocompromised patients.

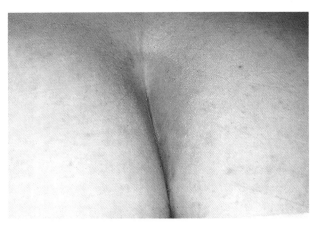

Figure 19-9 Intertrigo. Note fissure. (Reproduced with permission from Goodheart HG. *Photoguide to Common Skin Disorders: Diagnosis and Management.* 3rd ed. Philadelphia: Lippincott Williams & Wilkins; 2009.)

DISTINGUISHING FEATURES
- Intertrigo begins as a mild erythema followed by erythematous, well-demarcated patches or plaques that oppose each other on either side of the skin folds (mirror image)
- Often pruritic, painful fissures may occur (Fig. 19-9)

DIAGNOSIS
- Clinical
- Exclusion of other diagnoses (e.g., contact dermatitis, psoriasis, seborrheic dermatitis, as well as bacterial or fungal infection [negative KOH and/or fungal culture])

MANAGEMENT
Treatment (see Appendix A)
- Application of **Burow solution** compresses to exudative, oozing areas
- To achieve rapid improvement, treatment may be initiated with a high-potency (class 5) topical steroid that is used for several days before it is changed to a lower-potency (class 6 or 7) agent

Prevention
- Promote air drying or use of hair dryer with heat off
- **Zeasorb powder**
- For longer-term use:
  - Tacrolimus (**Protopic**) ointment 0.1% once or twice daily
  - Pimecrolimus (**Elidel**) cream 1% once or twice daily

Inverse Psoriasis

Psoriasis localized in the intertriginous areas such as the axillae (see Chapter 11, Axillae), inframammary, perineal, and inguinal creases is referred to as *inverse psoriasis* (see also Chapter 16, Breasts and Inframammary Area; Chapter 20, Inguinal Area). This condition is often difficult to distinguish from atopic dermatitis, seborrheic dermatitis, intertrigo, and candidiasis.

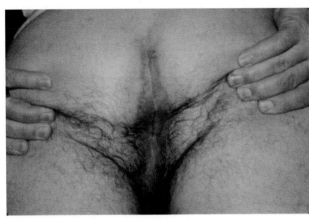

Figure 19-10 Inverse psoriasis.

DISTINGUISHING FEATURES
- The deep pink to red color and well-defined borders characteristic of psoriasis may be obvious (Fig. 19-10)
- May be pruritic
- Fissures may occur

DIAGNOSIS
- Clinical
- Psoriasis may be present elsewhere on the body
- Negative KOH and/or fungal culture

MANAGEMENT (see Appendix A)
- A higher-potency (class 5) steroid used for several days before it is changed to a lower-potency agent
- Tacrolimus (**Protopic**) ointment 1%, or pimecrolimus (**Elidel**) cream 1% applied once or twice daily for longer-term use

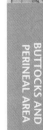

ALSO CONSIDER
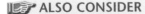
- Tinea corporis
- Atopic dermatitis
- Contact dermatitis
- Intertriginous seborrheic dermatitis

Condyloma Acuminata

Intra-anal and perianal **condyloma acuminata (anogenital warts)** warts are seen in patients who have engaged in receptive anal intercourse as well as in infants whose mothers have transmitted the virus during childbirth (see also Chapter 18, Genital Area; Chapter 20, Inguinal Area).

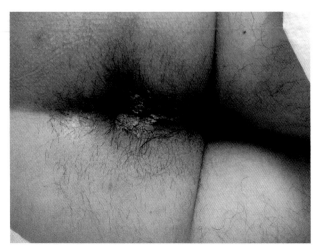

Figure 19-11 Condyloma acuminata.

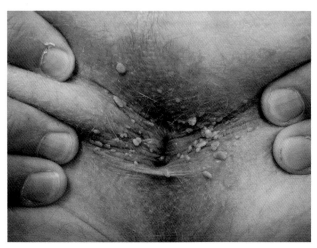

Figure 19-12 Condyloma acuminata.

DISTINGUISHING FEATURES
- May resemble small cauliflowers (Fig. 19-11)
- May appear as smooth, dome-shaped, or relatively flat, papular lesions (Fig. 19-12)
- Usually asymptomatic but may become pruritic or painful; they may bleed

DIAGNOSIS (see Appendix B)
- Clinical
- If necessary, snip excisional biopsy from the perianal area or a shave biopsy. A biopsy is used to rule out anogenital bowenoid papulosis or frank squamous cell carcinoma in atypical or recalcitrant lesions

MANAGEMENT (see Appendices A and B)
Surgical Therapy
- Cryosurgery with liquid nitrogen: effective for treating multiple, small, warts. Cryotherapy is also safe for pregnant women
- Electrodesiccation and curettage: effective for a limited number of lesions
- Surgical excision (useful for debulking large "cauliflower" lesions) followed by electrocautery of the remaining tissue down to the skin surface
- ⚠ **ALERT: In affected men with perianal warts, there is a risk of malignant degeneration to anal intraepithelial neoplasia or anal carcinoma. Atypical lesions should be biopsied.**
- ✔ **TIP: Patients who have internal anal or rectal warts tend to have continual recurrences of external warts and should be referred to a rectal surgeon.**

Topical Therapy
- See Table 18-1

Condyloma Lata

Condyloma latum, wartlike lesions of secondary syphilis, appear in moist areas of the body (usually vulva, scrotum, and perianal areas).

DISTINGUISHING FEATURES
- Lesions are "moist," smooth-surfaced, and usually whitish and flat-topped (Fig. 19-13)
- These lesions are highly contagious ("teeming with spirochetes")

DIAGNOSIS
- Serologic tests for syphilis are positive (see Chapter 18, Genital Area)

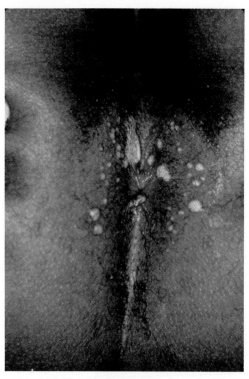

Figure 19-13 Condyloma lata.

External Anal Hemorrhoids

Not infrequently, **anal hemorrhoids** are mistaken for anogenital warts. External hemorrhoids develop as a result of distention and swelling of the external hemorrhoidal venous system. Engorgement of a hemorrhoidal vessel with acute swelling may allow blood to pool and, subsequently, clot. This leads to the acutely thrombosed external hemorrhoid, a bluish-purplish discoloration often accompanied by severe incapacitating pain. The prevalence of this condition peaks between 45 to 65 years of age.

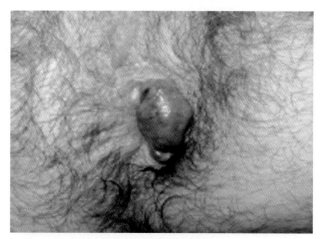

Figure 19-14 External anal hemorrhoid.

MANAGEMENT
- Penicillin remains the treatment of choice for treating syphilis; a single intramuscular injection (**Bicillin L-A**) of 2.4 million units
- Alternatively, erythromycin, tetracycline, or intramuscular ceftriaxone (**Rocephin**) are useful

DISTINGUISHING FEATURES
- Smooth and compressible, flesh-colored or bluish nodules (Fig. 19-14)
- Possible history of bleeding, tenderness, and pruritus

DIAGNOSIS
- Clinical (physical examination)

MANAGEMENT
- Most hemorrhoids can be treated with simple changes to diet and bowel habits; most do not require surgery or other treatment unless the hemorrhoids are very large and painful
- Fixative procedures include tying off the hemorrhoids with a rubber band (rubber band ligation) or using heat, lasers, or electric current to create scar tissue (coagulation therapy)
- Surgical removal of hemorrhoids (hemorrhoidectomy)

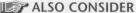
ALSO CONSIDER
- Tinea corporis
- Atopic dermatitis
- Contact dermatitis
- Intertriginous seborrheic dermatitis

Pruritus Ani *vs* Eczema/Lichen Simplex Chronicus

Pruritus Ani

Pruritus ani, itching of the skin around the anus, a common complaint, is usually an isolated skin complaint in otherwise healthy persons. However, it may be part of a disorder involving other areas of the skin, especially the vulva in women and children. Common factors that may underlie pruritus ani include psoriasis, eczema, and *C. albicans.* Exacerbating factors include diarrhea, straining at stool, scratching, vigorous use of toilet tissue, scrubbing with soap and water, and eating spicy foods.

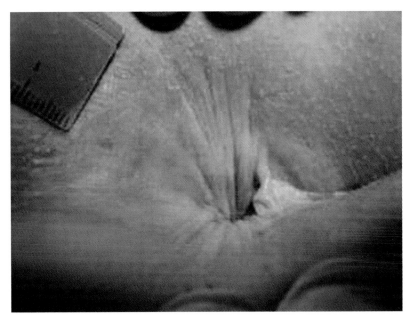

Figure 19-15 Pruritus ani. Note erythema and lichenification from chronic scratching and rubbing.

DISTINGUISHING FEATURES
- Pruritus, often unremitting

DIAGNOSIS
- Clinical
- Lichenification when chronic (Fig. 19-15)

MANAGEMENT
Prevention
- Reduce irritation of the anal skin
- **Tucks Pads;** careful cleansing and thorough and gentle washing after bowel movements
- Wash the anus using lukewarm water
- Moistened tissues or soft toilet paper are next best
- Use aqueous cream, mineral oil, or other soap-free cleanser. Avoid soap and rough toilet paper
- High-fiber foods (cereals, fruit, and vegetables)

Treatment
- The application of a potent class 2 topical steroid such as fluocinonide or a superpotent class 1 topical steroid such as clobetasol, even for a week or two, if neces-

sary, followed by lower-potency intermediate-strength (class 3 or 4) topical steroids, helps break the chronic itch-scratch cycle
- Patients should be advised that recurrences are to be expected; therefore, the long-term use of lower-potency topical steroids (class 1) and less frequent applications should be encouraged
- Alternatively, for longer-term use:
  - Tacrolimus **(Protopic)** ointment 0.1% once or twice daily
  - Pimecrolimus **(Elidel)** cream 1% once or twice daily
- ✔ **TIP: The use of potent or superpotent topical steroids for several weeks is often the most effective means to interrupt the itch-scratch cycle. This promotes patient confidence and sets a goal for ongoing therapy.**

Eczema/Lichen Simplex Chronicus

Eczema/lichen simplex chronicus (see also Chapter 18, Genital Area) is a common problem in the anal and perianal area, and a frequent cause of pruritus.

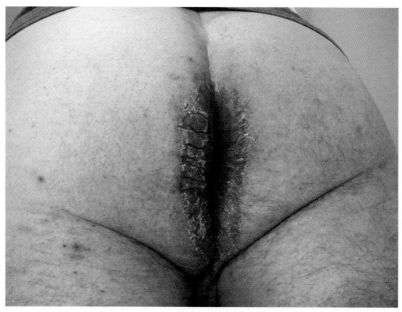

Figure 19-16 Chronic pruritus ani with fissuring and lichenification.

DISTINGUISHING FEATURES
- Pruritus, often unremitting (Fig. 19-16)
- Lichenification and fissuring

DIAGNOSIS
- Atopic history often obtained
- Exclusion of candidiasis
- The diagnosis is confirmed by the rapid response to topical anti-inflammatory therapy with topical steroids

MANAGEMENT (see Appendix A)
- Treatment and preventive measures are similar to those described previously for pruritus ani
- ☑ **TIP: A chronic itchy anal rash is rarely the result of a fungal infection.**

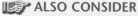 **ALSO CONSIDER**
- Contact dermatitis
- Intertriginous seborrheic dermatitis
- Perianal streptococcal disease
- Inverse psoriasis
- Candidiasis
- Pinworm (*Enterobius vermicularis*): in school-age children
- Anodynia

BUTTOCKS AND
PERINEAL AREA

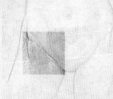

CHAPTER 20

Inguinal Area

Similar to the axillary and inframammary regions, the dermatoses occurring on the inner surfaces of the thighs are modified by the distinctive environment of this location. Heat, moisture, and rubbing of clothing produce characteristic eruptions.

IN THIS CHAPTER

- Tinea cruris *vs* inverse psoriasis *vs* candidiasis *vs* intertrigo *vs* lichen simplex chronicus
- Condyloma acuminata *vs* skin tags

Tinea Cruris

Tinea cruris ("jock itch") is a common infection of the upper inner thighs and crural area, most often occurring in postpubertal male patients. It is generally caused by the dermatophyte *Trichophyton rubrum*. In contrast to candidiasis and lichen simplex chronicus, it generally spares the scrotum (see also Chapter 19, Buttocks and Perineal Area).

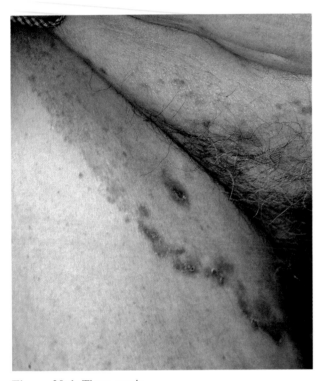

Figure 20-1 Tinea cruris.

DISTINGUISHING FEATURES
- Lesions are usually bilateral, fan-shaped, or annular plaques (plaques with central clearing), with a slightly elevated "active border" (Fig. 20-1)
- Lesions involve the upper thighs, the crural folds, and possibly the pubic area and buttocks (see Fig. 19-1)
- Typically spares the scrotum and penis
- Pruritic, irritating, or asymptomatic

DIAGNOSIS
- The diagnosis is confirmed by a positive potassium hydroxide (KOH) examination or fungal culture
- A positive KOH examination or fungal culture is found most easily by sampling from the border of the lesions. The major diagnostic clue is a scaly or "active" border that can sometimes be pustular or vesicular
- On the basis of clinical manifestations

MANAGEMENT (see Appendix A)
- Topical antifungal creams applied once or twice daily are often effective in controlling, and sometimes curing, uncomplicated, localized infections. Over-the-counter (OTC) preparations of miconazole **(Micatin),** terbinafine **(Lamisil),** and clotrimazole **(Lotrimin),** are available
- For severe inflammation and itching, a mild OTC hydrocortisone 1% preparation or moderate-strength hydrocortisone valerate 0.2% may be used for 4 to 5 days for symptomatic relief
- Systemic antifungal therapy may be necessary in cases that do not respond to topical therapy—chronic recurrent tinea cruris—particularly in immunocompromised patients
- Prevention aims toward decreasing wetness, friction, and maceration by:
  - Using an absorbent powder such as miconazole **(Zeasorb-AF)**
  - Drying the area with a hairdryer after bathing
  - Wearing loose clothing; briefs are less frictional than boxer shorts

Inverse Psoriasis

Psoriasis that is localized in the intertriginous areas such as the axillae (see Chapter 11, Axillae), inframammary, perineal, and inguinal creases, is referred to as *inverse psoriasis* (see also Chapter 19, Buttocks and Perineal Area, Gluteal Cleft). Inverse psoriasis is often difficult to distinguish from atopic dermatitis, seborrheic dermatitis, intertrigo, and candidiasis.

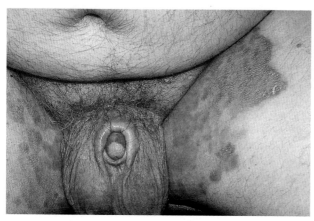

Figure 20-2 Inverse psoriasis. Note involvement of scrotum and glans penis.

DISTINGUISHING FEATURES
- The deep pink to red color and well-defined borders characteristic of psoriasis may be obvious; often involves the penis and scrotum (Fig. 20-2) (see Figs. 18-20 and 18-21)
- May be pruritic
- Fissures may occur

DIAGNOSIS
- Clinical
- Psoriasis may be present elsewhere on the body
- Negative KOH and/or fungal culture

MANAGEMENT (see Appendix A)
- Low-potency, nonfluorinated topical steroids (class 6 or 7) or, if necessary, a higher-potency (class 5) steroid that is used for several days before it is changed to a lower-potency agent
- Tacrolimus (**Protopic**) ointment 1% or pimecrolimus (**Elidel**) cream 1% is applied once or twice daily for longer-term use

☑ **TIP: Inverse psoriasis is commonly misdiagnosed by non-dermatologists as tinea or candidiasis; consequently, it is often incorrectly treated with topical antifungal agents.**

Candidiasis

Cutaneous candidiasis (see also Chapter 16, Breasts and Inframammary Area; Chapter 19, Buttocks and Perineal Area, Gluteal Cleft) is characterized by infection with *Candida* species. *Candida* is a common secondary and sometimes primary cause of intertrigo in elderly, diabetic, and immunocompromised patients. Most cases of cutaneous candidosis occur in skin folds, where occlusion by clothing produces warm, moist conditions. Candidal infection of the skin under the breasts occurs when areas become macerated under pendulous breasts.

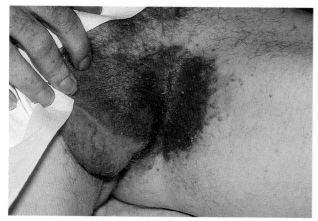

Figure 20-3 Candidiasis. Note beefy red color and "satellite" pustules.

DISTINGUISHING FEATURES
- Beefy red color to the lesions
- Satellite pustules may be seen beyond the border of the plaques (Fig. 20-3)
- Maceration and fissures may be present
- Discomfort and/or pruritus

DIAGNOSIS
- Positive KOH examination for budding yeast or positive culture for *Candida* species

MANAGEMENT (see Appendix A)
- The skin should be patted dry or dried with a hair dryer (no heat)
- Topical nystatin powder, ketoconazole, clotrimazole, or miconazole twice daily
- Patients with extensive infection may require the addition of fluconazole (**Diflucan**) or itraconazole (**Sporanox**) or ketoconazole

INGUINAL AREA

Intertrigo

Intertrigo occurs in places where opposing skin surfaces rub against each other: the axillae, creases of the lips (see Chapter 7, Lips and Perioral Area), inguinal, intragluteal creases, and under the breasts (see Chapter 11, Axillae; Chapter 16, Breasts and Inframammary Area).

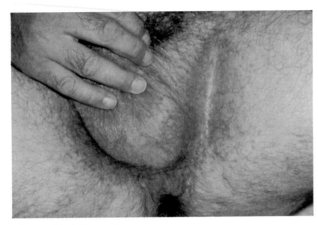

Figure 20-4 Intertrigo.

DISTINGUISHING FEATURES

- It begins as a mild erythema followed by erythematous, well-demarcated patches or plaques that oppose each other on either side of the skin folds (mirror image) (Fig. 20-4)
- Often pruritic; may progress to erosions, oozing, exudation, and painful fissures

DIAGNOSIS

- Clinical
- Exclusion of other diagnoses (e.g., contact dermatitis, psoriasis, seborrheic dermatitis), as well as bacterial or fungal infection (negative potassium hydroxide [KOH] and/or fungal culture), although such infections may be may be secondary phenomena

MANAGEMENT (see Appendix A)

- Low-potency (class 7) OTC hydrocortisone 1% cream or ointment
- Stronger topical steroids (class 6) such as desonide 0.05% or hydrocortisone valerate 0.02% cream (class 5) or ointment (class 4) may be used for very short periods, if necessary
- **ALERT: Potent topical steroids, particularly fluorinated preparations such as contained in** Lotrisone**, are to be avoided in the diaper area.**
- For longer-term use:
- Tacrolimus (**Protopic**) ointment 0.1% once or twice daily
- Pimecrolimus (**Elidel**) cream 1% once or twice daily

Lichen Simplex Chronicus

Lichen simplex chronicus is an often solitary, pruritic eczematous eruption exacerbated and caused by repetitive rubbing and scratching. When it appears in the inguinal or scrotal areas (see Fig. 18-8), it is commonly mistaken for tinea cruris. Lichen simplex chronicus is most often noted in adults, particularly in patients with other atopic manifestations, such as asthma, allergic rhinitis, and atopic dermatitis. The neck, wrists, extensor and flexor forearms, ankles, pretibial areas, or inner thighs are common sites. Lichen simplex chronicus may also involve the vulva, scrotum, intragluteal area, and perianal area (see also Chapter 10, Neck; Chapter 18, Genital Area; Chapter 21, Legs, Lower Legs).

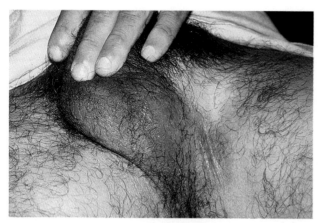

Figure 20-5 Lichen simplex chronicus.

DISTINGUISHING FEATURES
- Atopic history is often present
- Focal lichenified (thickened skin with accentuated skin lines) plaques
- Lesions are confluent (no central clearing)
- Pruritic; crusts and excoriations may be seen
- Lesions are poorly demarcated; they blend gradually into normal surrounding skin (Fig. 20-5)

DIAGNOSIS
- Clinical
- KOH examination and fungal cultures are negative for fungus

MANAGEMENT
- See Intertrigo and Appendix A

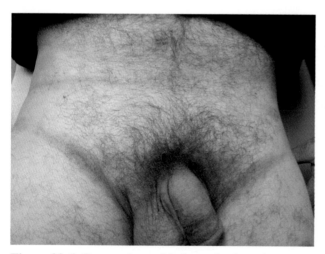

Figure 20-6 Contact dermatitis from elastic underpants.

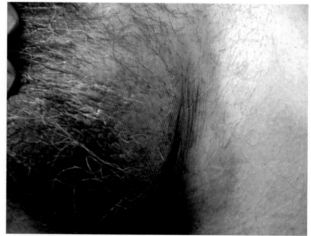

Figure 20-7 Extramammary Paget disease (note similar appearance to Fig. 20-5 above).

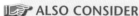 **ALSO CONSIDER**
- Contact dermatitis (Fig. 20-6)
- Intertriginous seborrheic dermatitis

RARELY
- Extramammary Paget disease (Fig. 20-7)

Condyloma Acuminata *vs* Skin Tags

Condyloma Acuminata

Condyloma acuminata warts commonly arise on the scrotum and inguinal creases. They can be easily mistaken for skin tags and common warts (see Figs. 18-23, 18-24, 19-11, and 19-12).

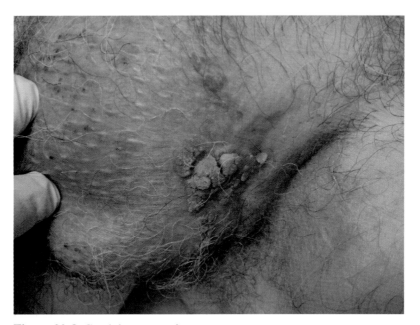

Figure 20-8 Condyloma acuminata.

DISTINGUISHING FEATURES
- May resemble small cauliflowers (Fig. 20-8) or appear as smooth, dome-shaped, or relatively flat papular lesions

DIAGNOSIS (see Appendix B)
- Clinical
- If necessary, snip excisional biopsy or a shave biopsy

MANAGEMENT
- See Appendices A and B
- See Chapter 18, Genital Area; Chapter 19, Buttocks and Perineal Area

Skin Tags

Skin tags (acrochordons) are commonly found in the inguinal crease and medial thighs (see Chapter 10, Neck; Chapter 11, Axillae), as well as in the inframammary area (see Chapter 16, Breasts and Inframammary Area). They are often seen in the body folds, particularly in persons who are obese.

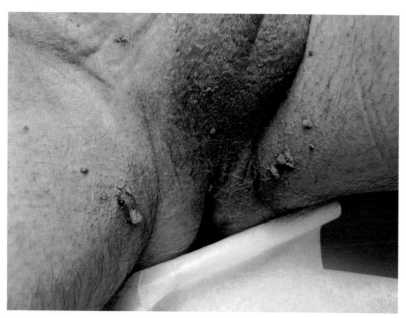

Figure 20-9 Skin tags.

DISTINGUISHING FEATURES

- Small, soft, often pedunculated or sessile papules (Fig. 20-9)
- Skin-colored or darker than the patient's skin
- Most vary in size from 2 to 5 mm in diameter, although larger ones up to 5 cm in diameter (fibroepithelial polyps) are sometimes evident
- Usually asymptomatic unless inflamed or irritated by friction or clothing

DIAGNOSIS

- Clinical
- Easy to recognize; a skin biopsy is rarely, if ever, necessary

MANAGEMENT

- See Appendix B

👉 **ALSO CONSIDER**
- Seborrheic keratosis
- Verruca vulgaris

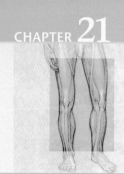

CHAPTER 21

Legs

There are few cutaneous conditions limited to, or particularly characteristic of, the thighs; however, eczema and psoriasis commonly appear in this location. The inner surfaces of the thighs are subject to heat, moisture, and the friction of undergarments. Many of the resultant dermatoses of this region are considered in Chapter 20, Inguinal Area.

In contrast, the lower legs have a unique variety of dermatoses that are influenced by such factors as vascular abnormalities that may result in edema, stasis, purpura, vasculitis, and ulcerations. Atrophic and ulcerative conditions such as necrobiosis lipoidica, diabetic dermopathy, and pyoderma gangrenosum, as well as various panniculitides such as erythema nodosum, also tend to target the lower legs.

Both upper and lower legs are prone to certain benign neoplasms, namely, dermatofibromas, various melanocytic nevi, and seborrheic keratoses, whereas the much more sun-exposed lower legs tend to develop solar keratoses, squamous cell carcinomas, as well as melanomas, in susceptible individuals.

IN THIS CHAPTER

Thighs and Lower Legs
- Nummular eczema *vs* psoriasis
- Dermatofibroma *vs* seborrheic keratosis *vs* melanoma

Knees
- Localized plaque psoriasis *vs* lichen simplex chronicus

Lower Legs
- Xerosis *vs* asteatotic eczema *vs* ichthyosis vulgaris
- Tinea corporis *vs* folliculitis *vs* follicular eczema
- Lichen simplex chronicus *vs* lichen planus *vs* prurigo nodularis
- Pretibial myxedema *vs* elephantiasis nostras
- Erythema nodosum *vs* nodular vasculitis
- Necrobiosis lipoidica *vs* pyoderma gangrenosum *vs* diabetic dermopathy
- Solar keratosis *vs* squamous cell carcinoma *vs* superficial basal cell carcinoma

Lower Legs and Ankles
- Benign pigmented purpura *vs* palpable purpura
- Stasis dermatitis *vs* cellulitis
- Venus ulcers *vs* arterial ulcers

Nummular Eczema *vs* Psoriasis

Nummular Eczema

Nummular eczema may be seen in children who have atopic dermatitis or have an atopic history; thus, it is often a clinical variant of atopic dermatitis. Nummular eczema is also commonly noted in adults, many of whom have an atopic diathesis. The word *nummular* comes from the same root as *numismatic*, meaning "coin-shaped" because lesions are round and have the shape of coins.

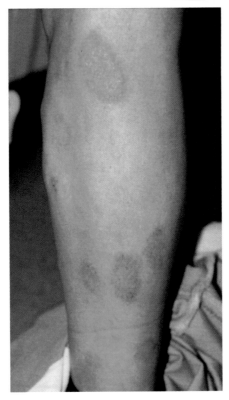

Figure 21-1 Nummular eczema.

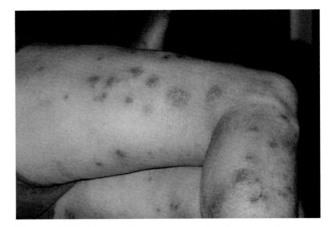

Figure 21-2 Nummular eczema: coin-shaped scaly lesions with postinflammatory hyperpigmentation.

DISTINGUISHING FEATURES
- Lesions are usually coin-shaped, itchy, eczematous patches and plaques that tend to occur in clusters (Fig. 21-1)
- Appear mainly on the legs; less commonly, they occur on the arms and trunk, particularly in children
- The patches or plaques sometimes clear centrally and resemble tinea corporis ("ringworm")
- Healing or resolving lesions often display postinflammatory hyperpigmentation, particularly in dark-skinned individuals (Fig. 21-2)

DIAGNOSIS
- Based on clinical appearance
- If necessary: negative results of a potassium hydroxide (KOH) examination

MANAGEMENT (see Appendices A and B)
- Often can be controlled by an intermediate-strength (class 3 or 4) topical corticosteroid, such as triamcinolone acetonide cream 0.1%, applied sparingly 2 times daily
- If necessary, a high-potency (class 1) topical corticosteroid, such as clobetasol cream 0.05% once or twice daily, may be used
- Recalcitrant cases may require occlusion—provided by a polyethylene wrap or flurandrenolide (**Cordran tape**)—or intralesional corticosteroid injections
- ☑ **TIP: Nummular eczema is frequently misdiagnosed as tinea corporis ("ringworm") and is often inappropriately treated with topical antifungals as well as antifungal–topical steroid combinations (e.g., Lotrisone ointment)**

Psoriasis

Psoriasis can appear anywhere on the body, and the thighs are no exception.

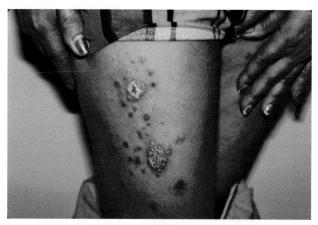

Figure 21-3 Psoriasis. The Koebner phenomenon is evident in this diabetic patient who developed psoriatic plaques at the sites of insulin injections.

DISTINGUISHING FEATURES

- Lesions are typically well-demarcated erythematous plaques with characteristic overlying white or silvery (micaceous) scale
- The Koebner phenomenon (isomorphic response) is seen as a reaction to trauma such as scratching (see lichen planus, below; see Figs. 12-25 and 21-20). The phenomenon in which new psoriatic lesions appear at sites of scratching and rubbing injury or other traumas to the skin (Fig. 21-3)

DIAGNOSIS

- Based on clinical appearance
- Psoriasis elsewhere on the body

MANAGEMENT

- See Appendix A
- See Chapter 12, Arms, Elbows, and Chapter 15, Trunk

🖙 ALSO CONSIDER
- Tinea corporis
- Atopic dermatitis/eczema
- Lichen planus
- Secondary syphilis

RARELY
- Pityriasis rubra pilaris
- Pemphigus foliaceus
- Erythema annulare centrifugum
- Small plaque parapsoriasis or digitate dermatosis
- Subacute cutaneous lupus erythematosus

Dermatofibroma *vs* Seborrheic Keratosis *vs* Melanoma

Dermatofibroma

Dermatofibroma, also known as fibrous histiocytoma and sclerosing hemangioma, is a common lesion that occurs most often on the legs, trunk, and arms, especially in women over 30 years of age. Dermatofibromas are benign growths that are usually brought to medical attention either to rule out skin cancer or because of cosmetic concerns.

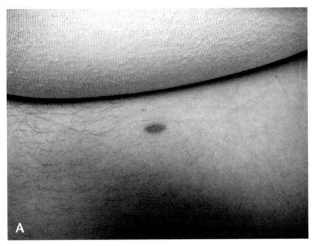 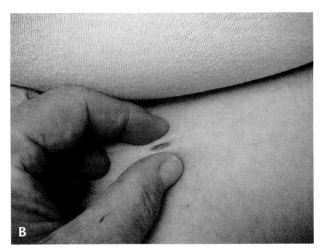

Figure 21-4 A. Dermatofibroma. **B.** Dermatofibroma: "dimple" or "collar button" (retraction) sign is elicited on compression of a lesion when it overlies soft tissue. (From Goodheart HP. *Goodheart's Photoguide to Common Skin Disorders: Diagnosis and Management*. 3rd ed. Philadelphia: Lippincott Williams & Wilkins, 2009, with permission.)

DISTINGUISHING FEATURES
- Lesions are usually freely movable papules or nodules. They may be elevated with a dome shape, flat, or depressed below the plane of the surrounding skin
- The color can vary, even in a single lesion—skin-colored, including chocolate brown, red, or even purple
- The surface may be smooth or scaly, depending on whether the lesion has been modified (e.g., by shaving)

DIAGNOSIS
- Typically, a dermatofibroma feels like a firm pea-sized, buttonlike papule that is fixed to the surrounding dermis (accounting for the "dimple" or "collar button" sign) (Fig. 21-4, A and B)
- If there is any doubt about the diagnosis, a biopsy should be performed

MANAGEMENT
- No treatment is necessary; however, local excision can be performed for biopsy confirmation or cosmetic concerns, or if the lesion is symptomatic
- Deep shave excision is another alternative; however, the lesion may recur
- The patient should be informed that if the lesion is removed, the scar may be more cosmetically objectionable than the original lesion

Seborrheic Keratosis

Seborrheic keratoses (see Chapter 2, Forehead and Temples) are seen in people over the age of 40. Lesions are most often located on the back, chest, arms (see Chapter 12, Arms), and face, particularly along the frontal hairline and scalp (see Chapter 1, Hair and Scalp).

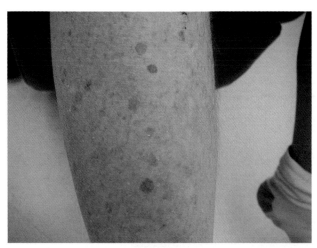

Figure 21-5 Seborrheic keratoses: characteristic flat lesions on shin.

DISTINGUISHING FEATURES
- On the legs, lesions are often flat (Fig. 21-5), freckle-like; fairly uniform in color, varying from brown to dark brown
- Alternatively, lesions may have typical, warty, "stuck-on" appearance with a crumbly, keratotic surface (see Figs. 2-9 and 12-9)

DIAGNOSIS (see Appendix B)
- With experience, seborrheic keratoses are easily recognized
- A biopsy (generally a shave biopsy) is performed if necessary to confirm the diagnosis
- **ALERT: To the untrained eye, however, these lesions may resemble melanomas. An excisional biopsy is unnecessary whenever a melanoma is suspected.**

MANAGEMENT (see Appendix B)
- Shave removal/biopsy; most often for cosmetic purposes
- No treatment at all or:
  - Cryosurgery performed with liquid nitrogen spray or with a cotton swab
  - Electrocautery and curettage

Melanoma

Melanoma (see also Chapter 12, Arms, and Chapter 15, Trunk). In contrast to nonmelanoma skin cancers such as basal cell and squamous cell carcinoma, melanomas are more likely to occur on areas that are less often exposed to the sun, specifically the backs of men and the legs of women. Risk factors include:
- Light complexion, an inability to tan, and a history of sunburns
- Moles that are numerous, changing, or atypical, such as dysplastic nevi
- A personal or family history of melanoma (first-degree relatives)
- A personal or family history of basal or squamous cell carcinoma

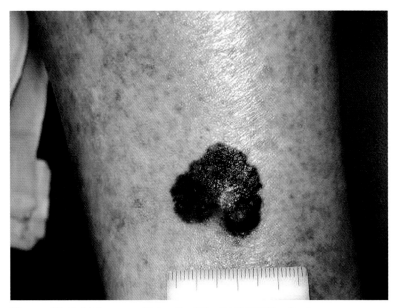

Figure 21-6 Melanoma. Note all of the "ABCDE" criteria.

DISTINGUISHING FEATURES
- Superficial spreading melanoma, by far the most common type, may arise de novo or in a pre-existing nevus
- The lesions of superficial spreading melanoma may conform to some (or all) of the "ABCDE" criteria for melanoma, in which the primary lesion is a macular lesion or an elevated plaque that displays the following (Fig. 21-6):
  - **Asymmetry:** if the lesion "folded" on itself, the halves do not match
  - **Border:** irregular or jagged (like a jigsaw puzzle)
  - **Color:** varied or having different shades (may have brown, black, pink, blue gray, white, or admixtures of these colors)
  - **Diameter:** greater than 6 mm (the size of a pencil eraser); may be smaller when first detected
  - **Evolution** (or change in a pre-existing lesion): change in size, color, elevation, or any new symptom such as bleeding, itching, or crusting (Fig. 21-7)

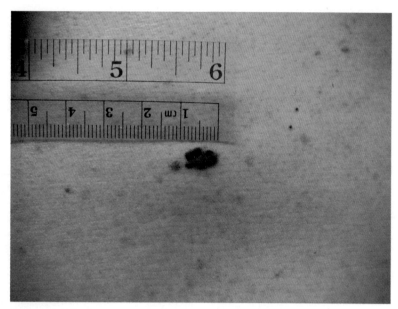

Figure 21-7 Melanoma in situ. This small nevus has evolved (E) into a melanoma.

DIAGNOSIS

- Dermoscopy, also referred to as *dermatoscopy* (see Appendix B), is a noninvasive method that allows the evaluation of colors and microstructures of the epidermis. Diagnostic patterns related to the distribution of colors and dermoscopy structures can better suggest a malignant or benign lesion
- Excisional biopsy that includes as much of the pigmented lesion as possible

MANAGEMENT

- See Appendix B
- See Chapter 12, Arms, and Chapter 15, Trunk

ALSO CONSIDER
- Melanocytic nevi
- Café-au-lait spots
- Solar lentigo

RARELY
- Dermatofibrosarcoma protuberans

Localized Plaque Psoriasis

Localized plaque psoriasis (see also Chapter 12, Arms, Elbows), the most common presentation of psoriasis.

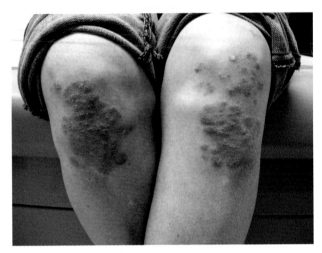

Figure 21-8 Psoriasis.

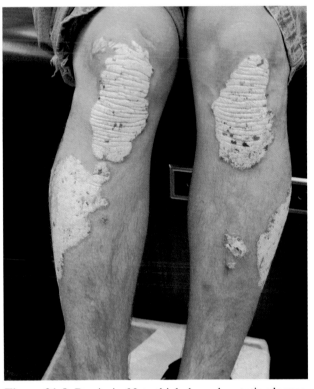

Figure 21-9 Psoriasis. Note thick, hyperkeratotic plaques.

DISTINGUISHING FEATURES
- In its mildest manifestation, psoriasis is an incidental finding and consists of mildly erythematous, well-demarcated, whitish or silvery plaques on the elbows and/or knees (Fig. 21-8). Lesions on the knees tend to be thicker and more verrucous than those on the elbows (Fig. 21-9)
- Usually not pruritic (compare lichen simplex chronicus, discussed later)
- Tends to be symmetric

DIAGNOSIS
- Clinical
- Skin biopsy if the diagnosis is in doubt

MANAGEMENT
- See Appendix A
- See Chapter 12, Arms, Elbows

Lichen Simplex Chronicus

Lichen simplex chronicus is caused by repetitive rubbing and scratching. When this condition appears on the elbows or knees, it is commonly mistaken for psoriasis. It is most often noted in adults, particularly in patients with other atopic manifestations, such as asthma, allergic rhinitis, and atopic dermatitis. The neck, wrists, extensor and flexor forearms, ankles, pretibial areas, or inner thighs are other common sites. Lichen simplex chronicus may also involve the vulvae, scrotum, intragluteal area, and perianal area (see also Chapter 10, Neck; Chapter 18, Genital Area, Scrotum/Vulva).

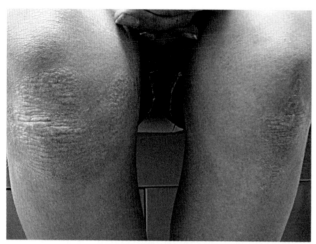

Figure 21-10 Lichen simplex chronicus.

DISTINGUISHING FEATURES
- Atopic history often present
- Focal lichenified (thickened skin with accentuated skin lines) plaques often on both knees (Fig. 21-10)
- Pruritic; crusts and excoriations may be seen
- Lesions are poorly demarcated (they blend gradually into normal surrounding skin)

DIAGNOSIS
- Readily apparent and made on clinical grounds

MANAGEMENT
- See Appendix A
- See Chapter 12, Arms, Elbows

ALSO CONSIDER
- Acquired and congenital hyperkeratosis
- Frictional lichenoid dermatitis in children

Xerosis *vs* Asteatotic Eczema *vs* Ichthyosis Vulgaris

Xerosis

Xerosis, or dry skin, is a common occurrence in winter climates, particularly in conditions of cold air, low relative humidity, and indoor heating. In Western societies, where people tend to overbathe and live in overheated spaces, dry skin is a common complaint. The plethora of moisturizing skin care products are testimony to the prevalence of this condition. Xerosis is believed to be caused by diminished production of sebum (asteatosis), as well as by reduced eccrine sweat activity.

Xerosis becomes especially common in the elderly and tends to be most apparent on the hands and lower legs. The word "dry" is sometimes misapplied. Skin that appears to be dry (i.e., showing a buildup of scale) may not always be suffering from a lack of water but from an overadherence or hyperproliferation of scale, which also occurs in patients with ichthyosis (see following discussion).

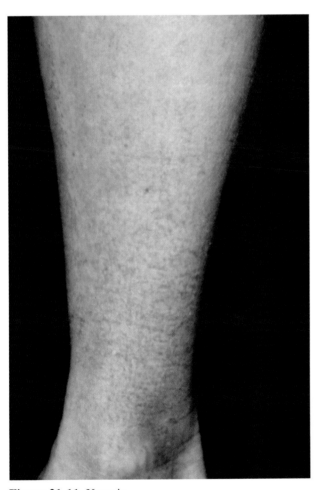

Figure 21-11 Xerosis.

DISTINGUISHING FEATURES
- Whitish scale (Fig. 21-11)

DIAGNOSIS
- Clinical

MANAGEMENT (see Appendix A)
- Less frequent showers and baths
- Soap avoidance (on affected areas) or mild soaps (e.g., **Dove, Basis**) or a soap substitute (e.g., **Cetaphil lotion**) may be used
- Moisturizers help to retain or "lock in" water that is absorbed while bathing; for that reason they should be applied while the skin is still damp
- Ammonium lactate 12% **(Lac-Hydrin)** lotion or cream is a prescription α-hydroxy acid preparation that may be applied after bathing. It is very effective and used for more severe cases of xerosis. It may be purchased as the over-the-counter (OTC) formulation **AmLactin**

Asteatotic Eczema

Asteatotic eczema, also referred to as *winter eczema*, appears exclusively in adults and most commonly arises on the thighs and shins. This form of eczema is a common, sometimes pruritic, low-grade dermatitis. It is caused by a relative loss of water from the skin through evaporation, a lack of normal desquamation, and, possibly, a decline in the production of sebum.

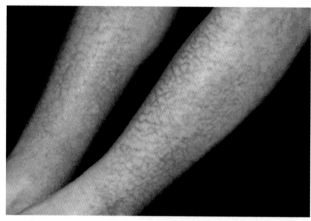

Figure 21-12 Asteatotic eczema.

DISTINGUISHING FEATURES
- Scaly, erythematous eruption
- Early on, the affected skin feels and looks dry; subsequently, an inflammatory dermatitis may evolve
- Seasonal recurrences during dry winter months
- Because the skin often resembles the surface of a cracked porcelain vase, it is often referred to as *erythema craquelé*. It is also likened to the appearance of a dry river bed (Fig. 21-12)

DIAGNOSIS
- Clinical

MANAGEMENT (see Appendix A)
- As with xerosis (see previous discussion), asteatosis is managed with moisturizers
- For itching, low-potency to medium-potency (class 4 to 6) topical corticosteroids are helpful for brief periods, when necessary

Ichthyosis Vulgaris

Ichthyosis vulgaris (hereditary ichthyosis vulgaris), the most common form of ichthyosis, first evident in early childhood, is a common disorder that is associated with atopy. Inheritance is autosomal dominant. The term *ichthyosis* is derived from the Greek root *ichthys*, meaning fish because of the resemblance to fish scales. Typically, shedding of skin occurs unnoticed; however, individuals with ichthyosis produce new skin cells at a rate faster than they can shed them or produce them at a normal rate but shed them too slowly. Either way, there is a buildup of dry, scaly skin. Many patients with hereditary ichthyosis vulgaris have associated atopic manifestations (e.g., asthma, eczema, hay fever). Such atopic conditions can be found in family members, with or without signs of ichthyosis.

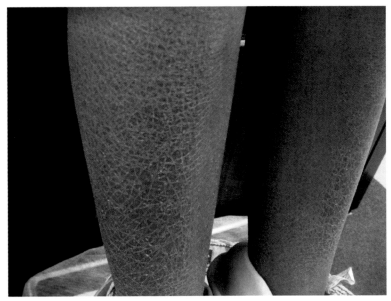

Figure 21-13 Ichthyosis vulgaris.

DISTINGUISHING FEATURES
- Symmetrical scaling of the skin, which varies from barely visible roughness and dryness to thick horny plates
- Lesions are most apparent on the shins; resemble fine fish scales (Fig. 21-13)
- Scales are small, fine, irregular, and polygonal in shape, often curling up at the edges to give the skin a rough feel
- Usually starts in the first year of life, progresses until puberty, then usually improves with age and sun exposure

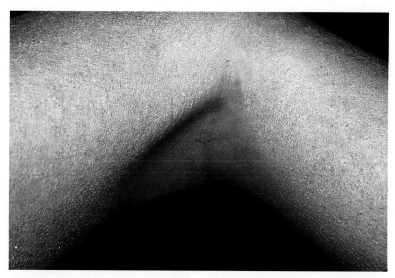

Figure 21-14 Ichthyosis vulgaris. Note flexural sparing.

DIAGNOSIS

- Clinical
- Skin biopsy is rarely necessary
- ☑ **TIP: Sparing of the flexural folds (e.g., antecubital and popliteal fossae) is an important diagnostic feature (Fig. 21-14)**
- ⚠ **ALERT: Later-onset acquired ichthyosis, is extremely rare, usually appearing for the first time in adulthood, is a nonhereditary condition that may be associated with internal disease such as sarcoidosis or as a marker of an underlying malignancy.**

MANAGEMENT (see Appendix A)

- Hydration of the skin and application of an ointment to prevent evaporation
- Ammonium lactate 12% (**Lac-Hydrin**) or OTC **AmLactin** are very effective

ALSO CONSIDER

- Atopic dermatitis (often have xerotic, sensitive, itchy skin)
- Nummular eczema

RARELY

- Acquired ichthyosis

Tinea Corporis *vs* Folliculitis *vs* Follicular Eczema

Tinea Corporis

Tinea corporis ("ringworm") is most often acquired by contact with an infected animal or human. It may also be autoinoculated from other areas of the body that are infected by tinea. Majocchi granuloma, a variant of tinea corporis, is defined as a granulomatous folliculitis due to a cutaneous dermatophyte infection. Majocchi granuloma is most commonly due to *Trichophyton rubrum* infection and less commonly to *Trichophyton mentagrophytes* and *Epidermophyton floccosum*. It tends to occur in women who frequently shave their legs, although it also appears as a result of the use of potent topical steroids on unsuspected tinea (tinea incognito).

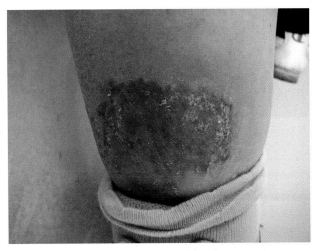

Figure 21-15 Tinea corporis: positive for potassium hydroxide. Note less well-defined (not annular) scaly patches.

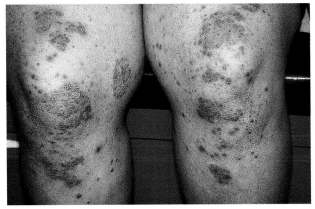

Figure 21-16 Tinea corporis ("incognito"). This patient was initially treated with topical steroids.

DISTINGUISHING FEATURES
- Lesions may be characteristically annular, with peripheral enlargement and central clearing; however, less well-defined patches, papules, or scaly plaques tend to occur on the legs (Fig. 21-15)
- Lesions are single or multiple
- If multiple lesions are present, their distribution is typically asymmetric
- May be pruritic or asymptomatic.
- Majocchi granuloma may result when inappropriate therapy, such as topical steroids, or shaving drives the fungi into hair follicles
- ⚠ **ALERT: Tinea corporis is very often misdiagnosed and treated with topical steroids (tinea incognito) (Fig. 21-16).**

DIAGNOSIS
- Diagnosis is confirmed by a positive KOH examination or fungal culture
- ✔ **TIP: It is especially easy to find hyphae in those patients who have been previously treated with topical steroids**

MANAGEMENT (see Appendix A)
- Topical antifungal agents are useful
- Systemic antifungal agents such as terbinafine (**Lamisil**), itraconazole (**Sporanox**), or griseofulvin are sometimes necessary when multiple lesions are present or in areas that are repeatedly shaved, especially women's legs

Folliculitis

Folliculitis of the legs is seen most often in young adults (see also Chapter 9, Chin and Mandibular Area, and Chapter 10, Neck). Causes include actions such as shaving, as well as irritants such as waxing, depilatories, and electrolysis.

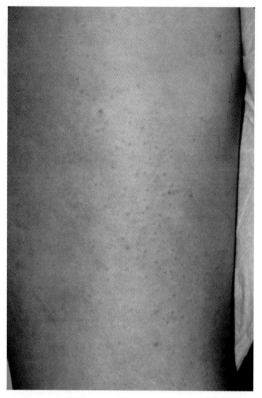

Figure 21-17 Folliculitis. Note superficial, small red papules in a grid-like pattern.

DISTINGUISHING FEATURES
- Superficial, small, red, relatively asymptomatic papules and/or pustules (Fig. 21-17), often in a grid-like pattern

DIAGNOSIS
- Bacterial culture and sensitivity, if necessary

MANAGEMENT (see Appendix A)
Nonbacterial
- Discontinuance or removal of external causes and irritants (e.g., waxing, shaving)

Bacterial
- Mild cases of bacterial folliculitis can sometimes be prevented or controlled with antibacterial soaps (e.g., **Hibiclens**)
- Topical antibiotics, such as clindamycin (**Cleocin**) 1% solution, foam, or gel, may be applied once or twice daily
- If staphylococcal colonization is present, mupirocin 2% (**Bactroban**) ointment should be applied
- If necessary, a systemic antibiotic for coverage of *Staphylococcus aureus*. Dicloxacillin or a cephalosporin are generally the first choice

Follicular Eczema

Follicular eczema is an eczematous eruption that affects the hair follicles. It is most likely to appear on the lower legs, thighs, back, and upper arms, although it can appear anywhere on the body.

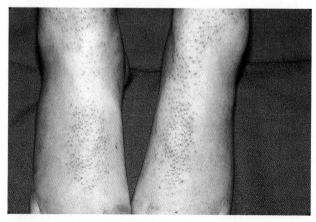

Figure 21-18 Follicular eczema. Note grid-like pattern on feet and lower legs.

DISTINGUISHING FEATURES
- Characterized by the appearance of small, rough, red papules in a grid-like pattern, often with crusting and marked pruritus (Fig. 21-18)

DIAGNOSIS
- Clinical
- Atopic diathesis

MANAGEMENT
- Potent or superpotent topical steroids are often necessary because the inflammatory lesions tend to be deep in the hair follicles
- See Appendix A and Chapter 12, Arms, Elbows

ALSO CONSIDER
- Contact dermatitis
- Insect bite reaction
- Psoriasis

RARELY
- Acquired perforating disease

Lichen Simplex Chronicus *vs* Lichen Planus *vs* Prurigo Nodularis

Lichen Simplex Chronicus

Lichen simplex chronicus (see also Knees, previously discussed) is caused by repetitive rubbing and scratching (see also Chapter 10, Neck, and Chapter 18, Genital Area, Scrotum/Vulva).

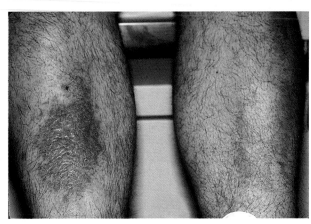

Figure 21-19 Lichen simplex chronicus (compare to stasis dermatitis, Fig. 21-42).

DISTINGUISHING FEATURES
- Atopic history often present
- Focal lichenified (thickened skin with accentuated skin lines) plaques (Fig. 21-19)
- Pruritic; crusts and excoriations may be seen
- Lesions are poorly demarcated

DIAGNOSIS
- Readily apparent and is made on clinical grounds

MANAGEMENT
- See Appendix A
- See Chapter 12, Arms, Elbows

Lichen Planus

Lichen planus (LP) often appears on the shins. Its morphology may be characterized by the typical "seven Ps" (see Chapter 12, Arms). LP often tends to be hypertrophic in this location.

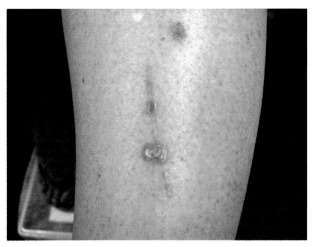

Figure 21-20 Lichen planus. Note the Koebner phenomenon (isomorphic response) due to scratching.

DISTINGUISHING FEATURES
Typical ("Classic") Lichen Planus
- Lesions are flat-topped violaceous flat-topped, polygonal, papules
- The presence of Wickham striae, characteristic white streaks the surface of lesions, and/or the Koebner phenomenon in which new LP lesions appear at sites of scratching (Fig. 21-20) (see also Fig. 12-25)

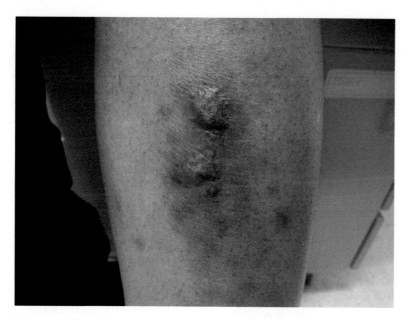

Figure 21-21 Lichen planus (hypertrophic): nodules with dark hyperpigmentation.

Hypertrophic Lichen Planus
- Often pruritic, papules or plaques and nodules
- Become hypertrophic, chronic, and tend to heal with residual very dark hyperpigmentation (Fig. 21-21)

DIAGNOSIS
- Clinical
- Skin biopsy is performed, if necessary
- Characteristic oral lesions are helpful in making the diagnosis
- ⚠ **ALERT: Underlying diseases such as hepatitis C or drugs associated with a LP-like reaction should be ruled out.**

MANAGEMENT (see Appendices A and B)
- High-potency (class 2) or superpotent (class 1) topical steroids may be used alone or with polyethylene occlusion, or with **Cordran Tape**
- Intralesional corticosteroids
- Systemic steroids
- Oral acitretin (**Soriatane**), cyclosporine, psoralen with ultraviolet A (PUVA) therapy, and griseofulvin have been reported to be occasionally helpful

Lichen Simplex Chronicus *vs* Lichen Planus *vs* Prurigo Nodularis (*Continued*)

Prurigo Nodularis

Prurigo nodularis appears most often on the shins and is seen mainly in adults 20 to 60 years of age. The cause is unknown; however, most patients have a personal or family history of atopic dermatitis, asthma, or hay fever. It is seen in the same clinical context as lichen simplex chronicus and may be considered a papular or nodular form of it. Prurigo nodularis tends to be one of the more resistant skin conditions to treat.

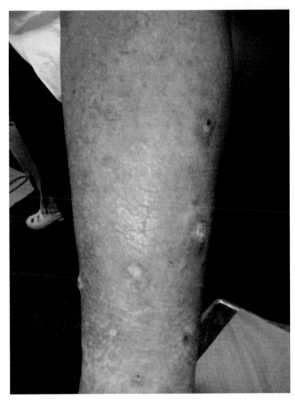

Figure 21-22 Prurigo nodularis.

DISTINGUISHING FEATURES
- Lesions are reddish, brown, or very darkly hyperpigmented, dome-shaped papules or nodules (Fig. 21-22)
- Most commonly appear on the pretibial shafts; less commonly on the extensor areas of the arms
- They are often crusted or excoriated—pruritus may be intense and lead to vigorous scratching and sometimes secondary infection
- Healing results in significant postinflammatory hyperpigmentation (Fig. 21-23)

DIAGNOSIS
- Clinical
- Skin biopsy if the diagnosis is in doubt

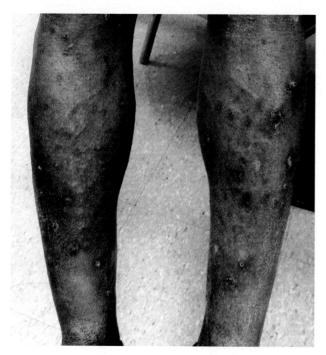

Figure 21-23 Prurigo nodularis. These hyperpigmented nodules are clinically indistinguishable from lichen planus (see Fig. 21-21)

MANAGEMENT (see Appendices A and B)
Local Treatments
- Superpotent (class 1) topical steroid ointments or creams, applied under occlusion (cover with a plastic dressing) to enhance their effect
- **Cordran Tape**
- Intralesional corticosteroids
- Systemic steroids

Systemic Treatments (More Severe Disease)
- Phototherapy (UVB and PUVA)
- Cryotherapy with liquid nitrogen
- Antidepressants such as amitriptyline or doxepin
- Oral corticosteroids
- Systemic retinoids such as acitretin, which may shrink the nodules and reduce the severity of the itch
- Naltrexone, an opiate antagonist, has been reported to reduce itching in some patients
- Thalidomide has been reported as effective in recalcitrant cases.
- ⚠ **ALERT: Thalidomide should not be used in women who are pregnant. In the United States, only physicians who are part of a special registry are permitted to administer this drug**

👁 **ALSO CONSIDER**
- Insect bite reaction
- Pretibial myxedema

RARELY
- Nodular amyloidosis
- Lymphomatoid papulosis

Pretibial Myxedema *vs* Elephantiasis Nostras

Pretibial Myxedema

Pretibial myxoedema (PTM) is a form of diffuse mucinosis that is generally considered a cutaneous manifestation of thyroid disease. It affects 5% of patients with Graves disease. Pretibial myxoedema may appear before, during, or after the thyrotoxic state and is sometimes associated with an underactive thyroid. It is thought to be caused by a circulating autoimmune γ-globulin, which acts as a thyroid-stimulating hormone. Lesions are found most frequently on the lower legs and less commonly, on other parts of the body.

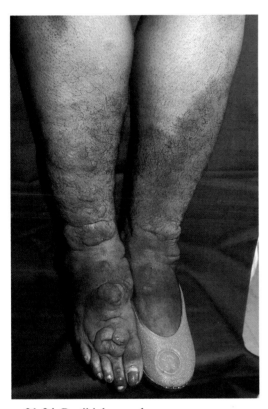

Figure 21-24 Pretibial myxedema.

DISTINGUISHING FEATURES
- Appear on the shins and sometimes the feet (Fig. 21–24)
- Early lesions are flesh-colored, waxy infiltrated translucent plaques that slowly progress to form bilateral, firm, plaques or nodules
- Skin pigmentation becomes erythematous, shiny pink to purple-brown, or violaceous
- Prominent hair follicles impart a "peau d'orange" appearance; alternatively, lesions may coalesce into a verrucous, "elephantiasic" form of PTM
- Enlarging areas of nonpitting edema may develop
- Overlying hyperhidrosis or hypertrichosis may be present

DIAGNOSIS
- Diagnosis of both hyperthyroid and hypothyroid disease is made by specific thyroid function tests
- Long-acting thyroid stimulator levels are elevated in about 50% of patients with PTM
- Skin biopsy reveals characteristic histopathologic features deposition of mucin deposition (glycosaminoglycans) in the dermis

MANAGEMENT
- Treatment of pretibial myxedema lesions can be attempted with high-potency topical steroids and intralesional steroids, although the response generally is poor

Elephantiasis Nostras

Elephantiasis nostras is an unusual progressive cutaneous hypertrophy due to chronic lymphedema, characterized by repeated inflammatory episodes. Long-standing lymphatic obstruction, stasis dermatitis, or low-grade recurrent cellulitis leads eventually to massive enlargement of the lower dependent legs. Obesity is a significant predisposing factor in its pathogenesis.

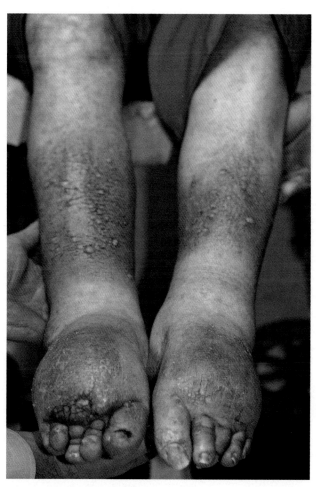

Figure 21-25 Elephantiasis nostras.

DISTINGUISHING FEATURES
- Lichenification, hyperkeratotic papules, nodules, and verrucous, cobblestone-like plaques (Fig. 21-25)
- Nonpitting edema, skin fibrosis, and massive enlargement of the lower legs

DIAGNOSIS
- The diagnosis of elephantiasis nostras can most often be made based on the clinical findings

MANAGEMENT
- Encourage weight loss
- Mainstay of therapy is elevation, use of pressure devices, and administration of antibiotics
- Although medical and surgical treatments are limited in their value, pneumatic pumps are effective in refractory cases
- ⚠ **ALERT: It is important to recognize this rare condition in its initial stages in order to prevent debilitating deformities of the legs.**

ALSO CONSIDER
- Stasis dermatitis
- Cellulitis

RARELY
- Lipodermatosclerosis
- Nodular amyloidosis
- Papillary mucinosis
- Scleredema
- Filariasis

Erythema Nodosum *vs* Nodular Vasculitis

Erythema Nodosum

Erythema nodosum (EN) is a type of panniculitis, an acute inflammatory reaction of the subcutaneous fat. It is considered a delayed hypersensitivity reaction to various antigenic stimuli. Erythema nodosum is 3 times more common in females than in males and has a peak incidence between 20 to 30 years of age.

The most common causes of EN in the United States are sarcoidosis, streptococcal infections, pregnancy, and the use of oral contraceptives. In children, streptococcal pharyngitis is the most likely underlying cause. Approximately 40% of cases are idiopathic. EN is also associated with a variety of other conditions: deep fungal infections (in endemic areas), including coccidioidomycosis, histoplasmosis, and blastomycosis; tuberculosis; *Yersinia enterocolitica* infection; inflammatory bowel disease, including ulcerative colitis and Crohn disease; malignant disease, including lymphoma and leukemia; postradiation therapy; and Behçet syndrome. In addition, drugs such as sulfonamides, penicillin, gold, amiodarone, and opiates have been implicated as causes of EN.

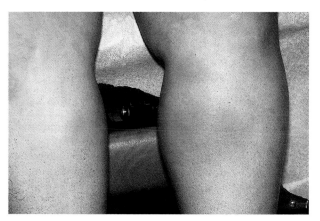

Figure 21-26 Erythema nodosum, acute. (From Goodheart HP. *Goodheart's Photoguide to Common Skin Disorders: Diagnosis and Management.* 3rd ed. Philadelphia: Lippincott Williams & Wilkins, 2009, with permission.)

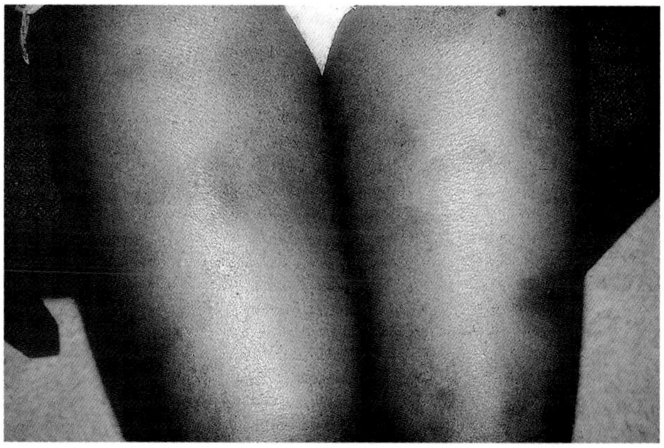

Figure 21-27 Erythema nodosum: healing "contusiform" lesions. (From Goodheart HP. *Goodheart's Photoguide to Common Skin Disorders: Diagnosis and Management.* 3rd ed. Philadelphia: Lippincott Williams & Wilkins, 2009, with permission.)

DISTINGUISHING FEATURES
- Lesions begin as bright red, deep, extremely tender nodules (Fig. 21-26)
- During resolution, lesions become dark brown, violaceous, or bruiselike macules ("contusiform") (Fig. 21-27)
- Tends to occur in a bilateral distribution on the anterior shins, thighs, knees, and arms
- Malaise, fever, arthralgias, and periarticular swelling of the knees and ankles may accompany the panniculitis
- Other symptoms may also be present, depending on the cause of EN
- Spontaneous resolution of lesions occurs in 3 to 6 weeks, regardless of the underlying cause
- ☑ **TIP: Generally, EN indicates a better prognosis in patients who have sarcoidosis.**

DIAGNOSIS
- The diagnosis of EN is usually made on clinical grounds, but a biopsy may be helpful for confirmation
- An excisional skin biopsy shows panniculitis with infiltration of lymphocytes in the septa of the fat

MANAGEMENT (see Appendix A)
- Usually, a complete blood count, erythrocyte sedimentation rate, throat culture, antistreptolysin titer, *Yersinia* titers, purified protein derivative skin test, and chest film are all that are necessary
- Treatment is symptomatic, consisting of bed rest and leg elevation for severe EN
- Firm supportive bandages or stockings should be worn
- Aspirin or nonsteroidal anti-inflammatory drugs (NSAIDs)
- A course of potassium iodide may be effective in clearing it
- Further tests, such as gastrointestinal tract evaluation and serum angiotensin-converting enzyme determination, can be performed if suggested by the review of systems and physical examination
- Systemic corticosteroids, which often bring dramatic improvement, can be used if an infectious cause is excluded
- Ultimately, treatment or avoidance of the underlying cause, if discovered, should be attempted

Nodular Vasculitis

Nodular vasculitis is an idiopathic panniculitis and vasculitis. When associated with *Mycobacterium tuberculosis,* it is known as erythema induratum. Both conditions had been traditionally considered to be the same disease entity but are now separated based on cause. Erythema induratum is due to the tubercle bacillus and is rare in Western countries, whereas, nodular vasculitis refers to the idiopathic type.

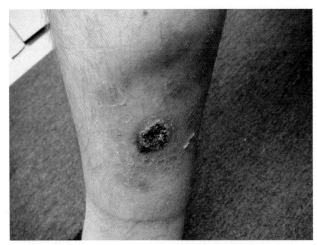

Figure 21-28 Nodular vasculitis: recurrent ulcers and subcutaneous atrophy secondary to panniculitis.

DISTINGUISHING FEATURES
- Crops of small, tender, erythematous nodules may be observed
- Both nodular vasculitis and erythema induratum are most often seen in females
- The lower extremities are the most common sites for lesions to arise—often the calves (Fig. 21-28). However, the shins and ankles are also sometimes involved
- Lesions ulcerate, resulting in permanent atrophy scarring and hyperpigmentation
- The nodules have a chronic, recurrent course

DIAGNOSIS
- Skin biopsy demonstrates vasculitis of the larger vessels and panniculitis
- Patients with erythema induratum have a positive purified protein derivative skin test, suggesting that it is a hypersensitivity reaction to *M. tuberculosis*

MANAGEMENT (see Appendix A)
- Bed rest with systemic steroids may be indicated if an infectious cause is excluded
- Potassium iodide
- Antituberculous therapy, if indicated

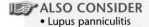**ALSO CONSIDER**
- Lupus panniculitis

RARELY
- Subcutaneous panniculitic T-cell lymphoma
- Erythema nodosum leprosum
- Factitial panniculitis
- Infectious panniculitis due to agents other than *M. tuberculosis*
- α_1-Antitrypsin deficiency panniculitis
- Pancreatic panniculitis

Necrobiosis Lipoidica *vs* Pyoderma Gangrenosum *vs* Diabetic Dermopathy

Necrobiosis Lipoidica

Necrobiosis lipoidica (NL), formerly known as necrobiosis lipoidica diabeticorum, was renamed to exclude diabetes because not all patients with NL have diabetes mellitus. Necrobiosis lipoidica is more common in women than in men. It is seen more frequently in type 1 than in type 2 diabetes and may occur before the onset of clinical diabetes. A minority of patients have no clinical evidence or family history of diabetes.

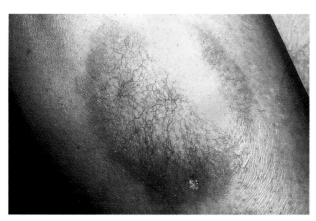

Figure 21-29 Necrobiosis lipoidica. Note the shiny atrophic patch in this diabetic patient.

DISTINGUISHING FEATURES
- Necrobiosis lipoidica appears most commonly on the pretibial areas but may arise on other sites
- It is characterized by yellow-red to brown, translucent shiny patches and plaques that slowly enlarge over months to years, resulting in epidermal atrophy and telangiectasias (Fig. 21-29)
- As lesions progress, the center becomes depressed and yellow
- Ulceration is not uncommon and can occur after minor trauma

DIAGNOSIS
- Clinical findings
- Punch biopsy if diagnosis is in doubt

MANAGEMENT (see Appendix A)
- Because localized trauma can cause ulcerations, protection of the legs with support stockings may be helpful
- Treatment for NL is not very satisfactory; it is typically chronic with progression and scarring
- High-potency topical steroids or intralesional steroid injections are used and can lessen the inflammation of early active lesions and the active borders of enlarging lesions, but have little positive effect on atrophic lesions.
- Antiplatelet aggregation therapy with aspirin and dipyridamole may be of some benefit
- Pentoxifylline **(Trental)** is believed to decrease blood viscosity by increasing fibrinolysis and red blood cell deformity and platelet aggregation
- Other treatments include perilesional heparin injections, topically applied 0.1% topical tacrolimus ointment **(Protopic),** bovine collagen, as well as oral ticlopidine, cyclosporine, nicotinamide, clofazimine, etanercept, and infliximab

Pyoderma Gangrenosum

Pyoderma gangrenosum is a rare ulcerative process of the skin that is seen in association with certain systemic diseases, including ulcerative colitis, regional enteritis, monoclonal gammopathy, hematologic malignancy or paraproteinemia, Behçet disease, Sweet syndrome, hepatitis, human immunodeficiency virus/acquired immunodeficiency syndrome (HIV/AIDS), systemic lupus erythematosus, Sjögren syndrome, Takayasu's arteritis, and rheumatoid arthritis. Pyoderma gangrenosum mainly occurs in the fourth and fifth decades of life. In 50% of patients, no underlying systemic disease is present.

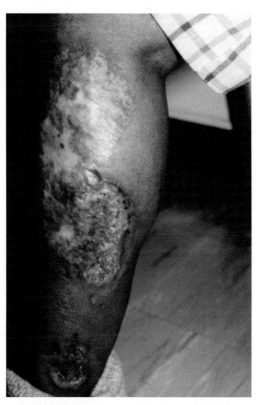

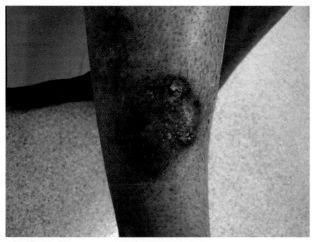

Figure 21-30 Pyoderma gangrenosum. This patient with Crohn disease attributed her nonhealing ulcer to a spider bite.

Figure 21-31 Pyoderma gangrenosum. These ulcerations are starting to heal.

DISTINGUISHING FEATURES

- Often painful ("stabbing") skin ulcers that are 2 to 10 cm in diameter (lesions may also be bullous, pustular, and vegetative)
- ☑ TIP: Often, patients give a history of a spider bite, but they rarely have evidence that a spider actually caused the initial event (Fig. 21-30)
- The classic lesions are deep, rapidly expanding, painful ulcerations with an erythematous to violaceous border that overhangs the ulcer bed (Fig. 21-31)
- The border is often undermined (a probe can be placed under the overhanging edge of the lesion)
- Most commonly found on the lower extremities (shins and ankles) but may also occur on the dorsal surface of the hands and the extensor aspects of the forearms
- Spontaneous healing may occur with scarring
- Ulcerations may occur after trauma or injury to normal or involved skin in some patients; this process is termed *pathergy*
- May occur around stoma sites (peristomal pyoderma gangrenosum)

DIAGNOSIS

- Generally made on a clinical basis and can be difficult. Often made by excluding other causes of similar-appearing cutaneous ulcerations, including infection, stasis ulcers, malignant disease, vasculitis, collagen vascular diseases, diabetes, and trauma
- Workup for systemic disease should include complete blood count with differential, sedimentation rate, antinuclear antibodies, rheumatoid factor, and a chest radiograph

- Serum or urine protein electrophoresis, peripheral smear, and bone marrow aspirate are performed if indicated, to evaluate for hematologic malignant diseases
- A gastrointestinal series for inflammatory bowel disease should be done if clinically indicated
- Skin biopsy of pyoderma gangrenosum is nonspecific. Specimens should be taken from the edge of the ulcer to rule out other causes of skin ulcers, such as infections or malignant disease (e.g., squamous cell carcinoma)

MANAGEMENT

- Effective pain control and local wound care and dressings
- Therapy focused on treating any underlying disease
- Bacterial, fungal, and viral cultures of the ulcer are performed if clinically indicated

Topical and Intralesional Therapy (see Appendix A)

- Application of superpotent topical corticosteroids
- Intralesional steroid injections (triamcinolone acetonide) administered into the edge of the ulcer
- Tacrolimus (**Protopic**) ointment 1% may be of some benefit in certain patients

Systemic Therapy

- Oral steroids for several weeks to months may be given alone or in combination with "steroid-sparing" agents such as dapsone, azathioprine, or chlorambucil
- Oral cyclosporine has been shown to be effective
- The following drugs have also met with some success: mycophenolate mofetil (**CellCept**), tacrolimus (**Prograf**), cyclophosphamide, thalidomide, and nicotine chewing gum
- Intravenous therapy can be administered using pulsed methylprednisolone, pulsed cyclophosphamide, or human immunoglobulin

Surgery

- Surgical grafting and microvascular free flaps are best reserved once the disease is inactive
- ⚠ **ALERT: Surgical débridement of the lesions of pyoderma gangrenosum should be avoided, if possible, because this can result in further wound enlargement (pathergy).**

Other Therapies

- Hyperbaric oxygen
- Biologics such as etanercept (**Enbrel**), adalimumab (**Humira**), and infliximab (**Remicade**)

Diabetic Dermopathy

Diabetic dermopathy is typically a late manifestation of diabetes and is usually asymptomatic. This condition tends to occur in older patients or those who have had diabetes for at least 10 to 20 years. The cause is unknown, but it may be associated with diabetic neuropathic and vascular complications because studies have shown it to occur more frequently in patients who have diabetes as well retinopathy, neuropathy, and nephropathy.

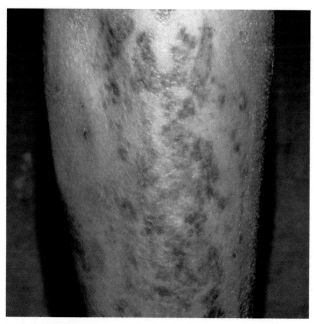

Figure 21-32 Diabetic dermopathy. (From Goodheart HP. *Goodheart's Photoguide to Common Skin Disorders: Diagnosis and Management.* 3rd ed. Philadelphia: Lippincott Williams & Wilkins, 2009, with permission.)

DISTINGUISHING FEATURES

- Characterized by small reddish brown, atrophic, scarred, hyperpigmented plaques (Fig. 21-32)
- Round or oval-shaped
- Commonly occur on both shins

DIAGNOSIS

- Clinical

MANAGEMENT

- Does not require treatment

ALSO CONSIDER

- Morphea (localized scleroderma)
- Sarcoidosis
- Xanthomas
- Granuloma annulare
- Basal cell carcinoma
- Squamous cell carcinoma
- Bacterial infections
- Deep fungal infections
- Herpes simplex virus infections
- Collagen vascular diseases
- Vasculitis

RARELY

- Antiphospholipid antibody syndrome
- Polyarteritis nodosa
- Behçet disease
- Wegener's granulomatosis
- Antiphospholipid antibody syndrome
- Necrobiotic xanthogranuloma

Solar Keratosis *vs* Squamous Cell Carcinoma *vs* Superficial Basal Cell Carcinoma

Traditionally, most nonmelanoma skin cancers occurred almost exclusively in men. Men older than 50 years of age, particularly those of northern European descent with a history of chronic sun exposure (e.g., farmers, athletes, sailors, gardeners), were far more likely to develop solar keratoses, squamous cell carcinomas, and basal cell carcinomas. However, in the past several decades, there has been a marked degree of lifestyle changes for women. Shorter dresses, skirts, and shorts that now expose the legs to the sun, less wearing of broad-brimmed hats, increased participation in outdoor sports-related activities, and the use of tanning parlors has led to an increase in the incidence of nonmelanoma skin cancers.

Solar Keratosis

Solar keratoses (see Chapter 1, Hair and Scalp; Chapter 2, Forehead and Temples; Chapter 4, Ears; Chapter 5, Nose and Perinasal Area; Chapter 6, Cheeks) are extremely common on the sun-exposed legs, extensor forearms, and hands (see Chapter 13, Hands and Fingers, Dorsal Surface) of certain individuals.

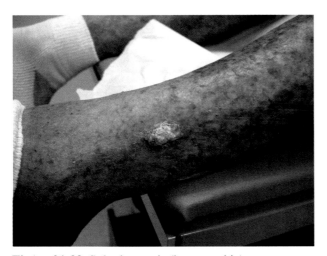

Figure 21-33 Solar keratosis (hypertrophic).

DISTINGUISHING FEATURES
- Males are affected more than females (increasing incidence in women)
- Elderly whites most often affected
- Single or multiple elevated scaly papules with an erythematous base covered by a white, yellowish, or brown scale (hyperkeratosis)
- Palpation reveals a gritty rough-to-the-touch sandpaper-like texture
- May evolve into hypertrophic solar keratosis (Fig. 21-33) or a cutaneous horn (see also Chapter 4, Ears; Chapter 6, Cheeks)
- A small percentage progress to squamous cell carcinoma (see following discussion)

DIAGNOSIS
- Clinical
- A shave biopsy when diagnosis in doubt or to rule out a squamous cell carcinoma

MANAGEMENT
- See Chapter 1, Hair and Scalp
- See Appendix B

Squamous Cell Carcinoma

Most cutaneous **squamous cell carcinomas** (SCCs) arise in solar keratoses, The anterior lower legs are common sites for these lesions. The dramatic escalating incidence in the United States is due to such factors as increasing sun exposure in the general population, the aging of the population, the earlier and more frequent diagnosis of SCC, and the rising number of immunosuppressed patients, who are at greater risk for developing SCC. The incidence is highest in Australia and in the Sun Belt of the United States.

⚠ **ALERT:** Metastases are much more likely to arise from lesions that appear de novo without a preceding solar keratosis. Lesions that are softer, nonkeratinizing, or ulcerated also carry a greater risk. Poorly differentiated, large (>2 cm) lesions are more likely to spread. This is especially a concern in the immunocompromised patient.

DISTINGUISHING FEATURES
- Males are affected more than females (increasing incidence)
- Elderly whites; fair skin
- Scaly papule, plaque, or nodule (Fig. 21-34) with a smooth or thick hyperkeratotic surface

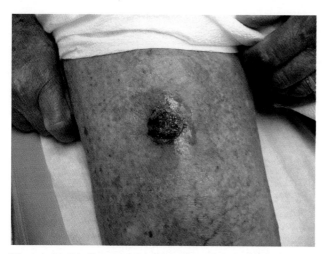

Figure 21-34 Squamous cell carcinoma: poorly differentiated nodule in an immunocompromised patient.

- Ulceration may be the only finding (see Fig. 12-17)
- Clinical variants include SCC in situ (Bowen disease) (see Fig. 12-18)
- As with solar keratoses (see previous discussion), an SCC, as well as an SCC in situ, may also produce a cutaneous horn on its surface
- Often indistinguishable from a hypertrophic solar keratosis (see Fig. 21-33)

DIAGNOSIS
- Shave or excisional biopsy
- ☑ **TIP: An isolated lesion of SCC in situ (Bowen disease) may be clinically indistinguishable from a superficial basal cell carcinoma (see following discussion) or a localized patch/plaque of psoriasis.**

MANAGEMENT
- See Chapter 1, Hair and Scalp
- See Appendix B

Superficial Basal Cell Carcinoma

Superficial basal cell carcinomas (BCCs) most often appear on the trunk and lower legs. They have little tendency to become invasive. In contrast to superficial BCCs that arise on the trunk, lesions on the lower legs are associated with chronic sun exposure. Lesions may mimic psoriasis and SCC in situ.

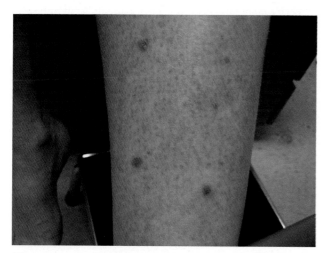

Figure 21-35 Multiple superficial basal cell carcinomas. Note subtle erythematous macules.

DISTINGUISHING FEATURES
- Males are affected more than females
- Arise as very subtle, small, pink to red patch or patches (Fig. 21-35)
- Lesions of superficial BCC tend to be indolent, asymptomatic, and the least aggressive of BCCs
- Often multiple, occurring primarily on the thighs and pretibial area

DIAGNOSIS (see Appendix B)
- A shave biopsy is all that is necessary

MANAGEMENT (Appendix A)
- Electrodesiccation and curettage
- Cryosurgery with liquid nitrogen
- Imiquimod cream (**Aldara**) for multiple lesions

ALSO CONSIDER
- Solitary plaque psoriasis
- Seborrheic keratosis
- Disseminated superficial actinic porokeratosis

RARELY
- Porokeratosis of Mibelli

The lower legs are the most common location for purpura to appear as well as being the primary site of peripheral venous disease such as stasis dermatitis (see following discussion). Purpuric lesions can be a sign or symptom of other vascular disorders such as coagulopathies or vasculitis and may serve as clues to systemic diseases such as systemic lupus erythematosus. Purpuric skin is purple, violaceous, or dark red in color and it does not blanch because blood is present outside the vessel walls. In contrast, erythema that is red in color blanches on compression because blood remains within the vessels.

Red, pinpoint macules (petechiae) or bruises (ecchymoses) are seen most often on dependent areas (i.e., lower legs and ankles and the buttocks in bedridden patients). Older lesions become purple and then brown as hemosiderin forms.

Benign Pigmented Purpura

Benign pigmented purpura, also referred to as *nonpalpable purpura,* is the name given to a number of harmless skin conditions that are caused by capillaritis ("leaky" capillaries), which allows blood to extravasate from small vessels and create petechiae and small ecchymoses. As their name implies, these benign purpuras are not associated with any systemic disease. The cause of capillaritis is most often idiopathic. Occasionally it arises as a reaction to a medication such as aspirin, clopidogrel (**Plavix**), an NSAID, or warfarin (**Coumadin**), agents that increase clotting time. In some instances, minor trauma or a viral infection has been implicated. Also, capillaritis may also develop after exercise (exercise-induced capillaritis). The so-called benign variants of purpura have various names based on their description such as purpura annularis telangiectodes, cayenne pepper purpura, pigmented purpuric lichenoid dermatosis, and lichen aureus.

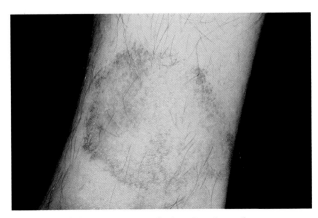

Figure 21-36 Purpura annularis telangiectodes (Majocchi's purpura). (Image courtesy of Art Huntley, MD. From Goodheart HP. *Goodheart's Photoguide to Common Skin Disorders: Diagnosis and Management.* 3rd ed. Philadelphia: Lippincott Williams & Wilkins, 2009, with permission.)

DISTINGUISHING FEATURES

- Lesions are generally asymptomatic, but they may be mildly pruritic
- Benign pigmented purpura may be of cosmetic concern to patients; however, most patients wish to be reassured that purpura is not a sign of a serious disease
- Lesions may persist for months to years or indefinitely
- Variants include:
  - Purpura annularis telangiectodes *(Majocchi's purpura)*
    - Asymptomatic annular lesions may be seen in especially in adolescents and young adults
    - Pigmentation that is annular with central clearing (Fig. 21-36). The purple, yellow, or brown patches consist of telangiectases and hemosiderin deposition
  - Cayenne pepper purpura *(Schamberg disease)*
    - Occurs primarily in adults, especially in the elderly
    - Characterized by tiny red dots, lesions are described as cayenne pepper spots (Fig. 21-37 and 21-38). Over time, they become brown and then slowly fade over weeks to months

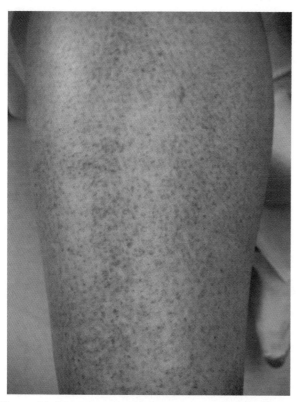

Figure 21-37 Cayenne pepper purpura (Schamberg disease).

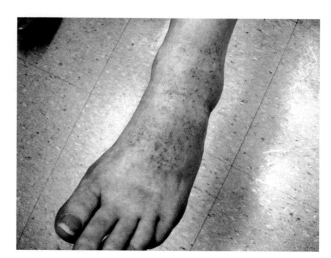

Figure 21-38 Cayenne pepper purpura. These lesions resolved spontaneously.

DIAGNOSIS

- The diagnosis is made on clinical presentation.
- Lesions are not palpable and are nonblanching on diascopy (direct pressure)
- Biopsy may be necessary at times to distinguish benign purpura from leukocytoclastic vasculitis, the histopathologic finding in palpable purpura (see following discussion)
- Lesions can disappear within a few weeks, recur from time to time, or frequently persist for years

MANAGEMENT

- Benign pigmented purpura generally requires no workup
- Possible offending drugs should be evaluated regarding their risk-to-benefit ratio
- A coagulopathy or blood dyscrasia should be ruled out if it is clinically suspected

Palpable Purpura

Palpable purpura is a vasculitis that affects the vessels that lie within the middle to upper dermis. When the vasculitis is more extensive and affects internal organs—most commonly the gastrointestinal tract, kidneys, central nervous system, and joints—it is then referred to as a *systemic* or *hypersensitivity vasculitis*. Common to all forms of vasculitis are the inflammation and destruction of blood vessel walls by inflammatory cells. Palpability of lesions is due to the accumulation of inflammatory cells and the leakage of blood from the vessels. It is believed that the deposition of circulating immune complexes in the postcapillary venules is the cause of vasculitis. The circulating immune complexes may also deposit in organs, causing a vasculitis with resultant gastrointestinal bleeding, hematuria, and arthralgias.

The cutaneous vasculitis may be associated with a hypersensitivity to antigens from drugs (most often antibiotics), NSAIDs, allopurinol, thiazide diuretics, and hydantoins. In some cases, suggested causes include malignancies; infectious diseases; cryoglobulinemias; or other underlying diseases such as systemic lupus erythematosus, Sjögren syndrome, rheumatoid arthritis, and inflammatory bowel diseases also paraproteinemia, ingestants, and infections such as β-hemolytic streptococcal infection; and viral hepatitis, particularly hepatitis C, and HIV infection, may be associated with it. More than 50% of cases are idiopathic and may occur in the absence of any systemic disease.

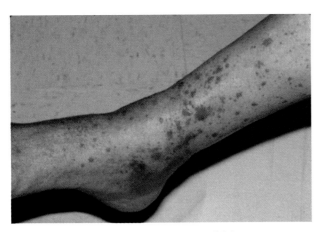

Figure 21-39 Palpable purpura (vasculitis).

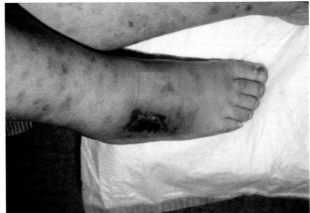

Figure 21-40 Palpable purpura (vasculitis) with ulceration.

DISTINGUISHING FEATURES

- Lesions tend to appear in crops; they are red to violaceous to purple in color and are nonblanching (Fig. 21-39)
- Infrequently, hemorrhagic vesicles or bullae may occur and develop into painful ulcerations (Fig. 21-40)
- Healing takes place within a week or 2 and may result in postinflammatory hyperpigmentation and/or scarring
- Lesions are characteristically symmetrical in distribution and are most often seen in dependent areas such as the lower legs and ankles and on the buttocks in bedridden patients
- In severe forms, lesions can become generalized.
- May be asymptomatic, mildly pruritic, slightly painful, or very painful (ulcers)

- Can be recurrent; however, the majority of patients have only a single episode
- There may be associated malaise and possible fever
- In systemic vasculitis, symptoms are referable to the organ involved
- Henoch-Schönlein purpura is a variant
  - *Henoch-Schönlein purpura* is a term that should be reserved for disease that follows an upper respiratory infection, generally in children
  - It is a type of hypersensitivity vasculitis caused by group A streptococci
  - Clinical and histopathologic findings are similar to those of hypersensitivity vasculitis
  - Abdominal pain, arthralgia, hematuria, and proteinuria may be present
  - In children and in some adults, serologic testing for a possible streptococcal infection should be considered

DIAGNOSIS

- Laboratory investigations that are useful for identifying any underlying disease include complete blood count, a blood chemistry panel, erythrocyte sedimentation rate, urinalysis, and stool examination for occult blood. Further studies (e.g., serum complement, antinuclear antibodies) should be directed by the patient's symptoms. Further laboratory evaluations such as s serum protein electrophoresis, cryoglobulins, and hepatitis C antibody may be indicated
- Biopsy of fresh lesions shows characteristic leukocytoclastic vasculitis ("nuclear dust")

MANAGEMENT

- If known, the precipitating cause (e.g., drug) should be eliminated or the responsible underlying disease (e.g., systemic lupus erythematosus) should be treated
- Elevation of the legs (above the level of the heart) may be useful because the disease often affects dependent areas
- In general, no treatment is necessary for mild, self-limited episodes
- For painful cutaneous lesions or arthralgias, NSAIDs may help
- For severe, extensive, or recalcitrant cases, oral corticosteroids are indicated
- For recurrent or persistent lesions, dapsone and colchicine have also been reported to be effective
- In cases of rapid progression or systemic involvement, immunosuppressants such as cyclophosphamide (**Cytoxan**), azathioprine (**Imuran**), methotrexate, and mycophenolate mofetil (**CellCept**) have been used in conjunction with systemic steroids as steroid-sparing agents
- Rituximab (**Rituxan**) has been reported to be helpful in some cases
- **ALERT: Other rare, life-threatening causes of vasculitis (e.g., Wegener's granulomatosis, polyarteritis nodosa, and Churg-Strauss syndrome) are potentially fatal diseases. Treatment with systemic corticosteroids and/or immunosuppressive/cytotoxic agents are necessary in these instances.**

ALSO CONSIDER

- Arthropod bite reactions
- Erythema multiforme

RARELY

- Septic vasculitis (e.g., meningococcemia, gonococcemia)
- Polyarteritis nodosa
- Pyoderma gangrenosum
- Wegener's granulomatosis
- Churg-Strauss syndrome
- Cholesterol emboli
- Buerger disease
- Thrombotic thrombocytopenic purpura
- Idiopathic thrombocytopenic purpura
- Waldenström's hypergammaglobulinemia
- Other causes of decreased platelets

Stasis Dermatitis *vs* Cellulitis

Stasis Dermatitis

Stasis dermatitis (gravitational dermatitis) often appears on the medial ankles of middle-aged and elderly patients and rarely occurs before the fifth decade of life. The dermatitis is a consequence of chronic venous insufficiency ("leaky valves") and is seen more often in women, particularly those with a genetic predisposition to develop varicosities. Venous insufficiency refers to improper functioning of the one-way valves in the veins and results in back pressure and edema that collects in the tissues. Stasis dermatitis may also occur in patients with acquired venous insufficiency resulting from surgery (e.g., vein stripping or harvesting of saphenous veins for coronary bypass), deep venous thrombosis, or other types of traumatic injury to the lower venous system.

The pathogenesis of stasis dermatitis may be explained by the following sequence of events: varicose veins allow for a reversed blood flow through incompetent valves, the diminished venous return and increased hydrostatic capillary pressure contribute to peripheral edema and relative tissue hypoxia. The preceding process may account for the pruritic, eczematous eruption seen in the early stages.

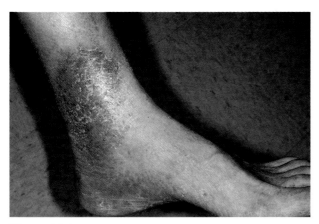

Figure 21-41 Acute stasis dermatitis.

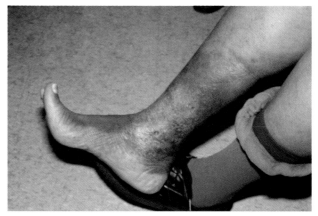

Figure 21-42 Chronic stasis dermatitis. Note ulceration.

DISTINGUISHING FEATURES

- Most cases of stasis dermatitis and resultant ulcers are located on the medial malleolus
- Often associated with varicose veins
- The affected ankle is usually swollen, particularly after prolonged standing
- Lesions begin with pruritic erythema and scale (eczematous dermatitis) (Fig. 21-41)
- Ultimately, the rash may become more erythematous and edematous; erosions, crusts, and may become secondarily infected (impetiginized) and ulcerate (Fig. 21-42)

- May spread to the foot or calf and may progressively lead to the chronic stages of stasis dermatitis, in which pigmentary changes occur and possibly affect the leg circumferentially
- Ultimately, the skin may thicken and become less supple, nonpitting, and feels permanently bound down and fibrotic ("woody") on palpation

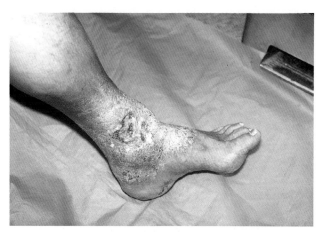

Figure 21-43 Chronic stasis dermatitis with venous stasis ulcer, nonpitting edema ("woody" fibrosis) surrounding the ulcer (lipodermosclerosis). (From Goodheart HP. *Goodheart's Photoguide to Common Skin Disorders: Diagnosis and Management.* 3rd ed. Philadelphia: Lippincott Williams & Wilkins, 2009, with permission.)

- Possible complications include the following:
  - Lipodermatosclerosis: induration may progress to lipodermatosclerosis, which has a classic "inverted water bottle" appearance (Fig. 21-43)
  - Autoeczematization (id reaction); this widespread, often explosive, acute eczematous eruption is presumably triggered by secondary bacterial infection (impetiginization) of eczema, with resultant circulating immune complexes released from the site of the stasis dermatitis lesions. It is hypothesized that patients become sensitized to their own tissue-breakdown products

- Venous stasis ulcers (Fig. 21-43) (see following discussion): the ulcers may be exacerbated by trauma (e.g., scratching), bacterial infection, or improper care of the eczematous rash. Generally painless, such ulcers sometimes produce a dull pain

DIAGNOSIS
- Clinical
- **ALERT: Stasis dermatitis is frequently misdiagnosed as cellulitis.**

MANAGEMENT (see Appendix A)
- Compression is the mainstay of therapy for venous insufficiency and venous leg ulceration
- Support hose, elastic bandages and specialized compression (**Jobst**-type) stockings
- Sitting in a reclining chair
- Discourage smoking
- Venous return can be increased by engaging in regular exercise, such as brisk walking and bicycling, which augments the "calf pump," the mainstay of therapy for venous insufficiency
- **TIP: Furthermore, the affected leg should be elevated above the level of the heart (sitting with the leg elevated by a stool is inadequate).**
- At night, leg elevation can be accomplished by propping up the foot end of the bed by 1 to 2 inches of plywood or a bedding fabric such as sheets
- **ALERT: In the presence of arterial insufficiency, compression therapy is contraindicated.**
- Topical therapy includes:
  - A mild-to-moderate strength (class 4, 5, or 6) topical corticosteroid ointment (such as desonide 0.05%, hydrocortisone valerate 0.2%, or, if necessary, triamcinolone 0.1%) applied twice daily is usually sufficient to treat the eczematous rash and to alleviate any itching

⚠ **ALERT: OTC preparations that contain benzocaine, lanolin, or neomycin should also be avoided. (Patients with stasis dermatitis tend to develop contact dermatitis quite easily.)**
  • **Burow solution** soaks to help dry oozing or infected areas
• Obvious superficial infections (impetiginization) should be treated with systemic antibiotics that have activity against *S. aureus* and *Streptococcus* species (e.g., dicloxacillin, cephalexin, or a fluoroquinolone)

• A widespread autoeczematized eruption may require treatment with both systemic corticosteroids and oral antibiotics
✔ **TIP: Often the "soak and smear" technique with a superpotent topical steroid can be used initially and the use of systemic steroids can be avoided (see Appendix B).**

Cellulitis

The term ***cellulitis*** is used to indicate a nonnecrotizing inflammation of the dermis and hypodermis. In immunocompetent individuals, cellulitis is usually due to Gram-positive aerobic cocci (e.g., *S. aureus, Staphylococcus pyogenes*); however, the isolation of methicillin-resistant *S. aureus* is steadily increasing. Cellulitis may follow a break in the skin, such as a fissure, cut, laceration, insect bite, or puncture wound. Patients with toe web intertrigo and/or tinea pedis and those with lymphatic obstruction, venous insufficiency, pressure ulcers, and obesity are particularly vulnerable to recurrent episodes of cellulitis (see earlier discussion of Elephantiasis Nostras). Recurrent cellulitis due to streptococci may be observed in patients with chronic lymphedema (e.g., from lymph node dissection, irradiation, and Milroy disease).

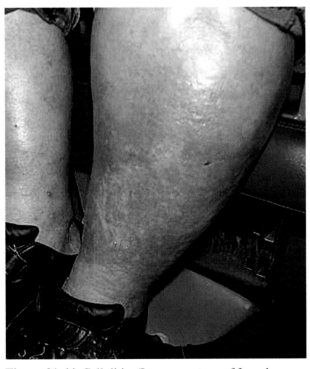

Figure 21-44 Cellulitis. (Image courtesy of Joseph Eastern, MD.)

DISTINGUISHING FEATURES
• Characterized by localized pain, swelling, tenderness, erythema, and warmth
• Legs are red, hot, swollen, and tender (Fig. 21-44)
• Lymphangitis, regional lymphadenopathy, or both, may be present.
• Fever and malaise are common
• Overlying skin may develop areas of necrosis

DIAGNOSIS

- The diagnosis is based on the clinical features
- A complete blood count is likely to show leukocytosis

MANAGEMENT

☑ **TIP: As with stasis dermatitis (see previous discussion), the leg should be elevated above the level of the heart.**

- At night, leg elevation can be accomplished by propping up the foot end of the bed by 1 to 2 inches of plywood, bedding such as sheets or a pillow
- Oral antibiotics are given for mild infections; intravenous antibiotics are indicated for more severe cases and for patients who are immunocompromised

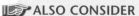**ALSO CONSIDER**
- Contact dermatitis
- Atopic dermatitis
- Dermatophytosis (tinea)
- Arterial disease (see following discussion)

Venous Ulcers *vs* Arterial Ulcers

Venous Ulcers

Venous ulcers are generally a consequence of stasis dermatitis (see previous discussion). The ulcers presumably result from the increased venous pressure that causes fibrin deposits around the capillaries, which in turn act as a barrier to the flow of oxygen and nutrients to muscle and skin tissue. The death of tissue cells leads to the ulceration.

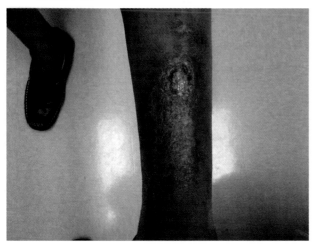

Figure 21-45 Venous ulceration. This ulceration and chronic surrounding lichen simplex chronicus developed from trauma (knife wound) that resulted in a varicosity proximal to the affected area.

DISTINGUISHING FEATURES
- Most cases ulcers are located on the medial malleolus (see Figs. 21-42 and 21-43)
- Some ulcers may be due to trauma to veins (e.g. surgery) (see Fig. 21-45)
- Relatively painless unless infected
- Associated with end of day aching and swollen lower legs that feel more comfortable when elevated

DIAGNOSIS
- Clinical

MANAGEMENT (see Appendix A)
- Stasis ulcers are managed by treating the underlying eczematous dermatitis, controlling weight, preventing infection, and using compression dressings
- Pain is generally relieved by elevation
- **Unna boot** is a commercially available bandage **(Dome-Paste bandage, Gelocast bandage)** that is impregnated with zinc oxide paste. It is best applied in the morning before edema progresses. After application, the bandage hardens into a cast. The boot decreases edema, promotes healing, and serves as a barrier from trauma (e.g., from scratching). It should be changed weekly until the ulcer heals
- If feasible, corrective surgery, such as skin grafts or vascular procedures, may be another option
- The ulcer can be treated with moist wound healing methods, high-compression therapy, fibrinolytic agents, and newer modalities, such as growth factors, matrix materials, and biologically engineered tissue. (These methods are beyond the scope of this chapter)

⚠ **ALERT: Patients should be advised not to apply topical corticosteroid preparations directly into the ulcers, because the preparations may interfere with healing.**

⚠ **ALERT: Compression must not be used if there is significant arterial disease because it will aggravate an inadequate blood supply.**

Arterial Ulcers

Arterial ulcers are most often due to atherosclerosis and are aggravated by smoking and hypertension that result in tissue breakdown. Other factors and conditions that have been linked with the development of arterial leg ulcers include renal failure, sickle cell anemia, obesity, rheumatoid arthritis, clotting and circulation disorders, a history of heart disease, cerebrovascular disease, collagen vascular disease, and peripheral vascular disease.

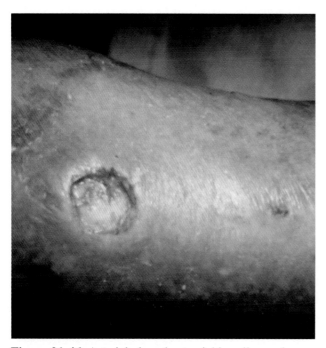

Figure 21-46 Arterial ulcer due to sickle cell anemia. Note punched-out appearance.

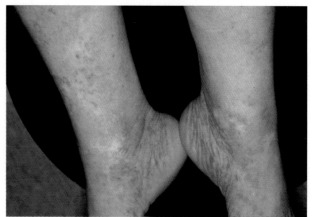

Figure 21-47 Atrophie blanche. Note characteristic porcelain-white stellate (star-shaped) scars arising around the ankles.

DISTINGUISHING FEATURES
- Usually found distally (lower shins, feet, heels, or toes)
- The borders of the ulcer appear as though they have been punched out (Fig. 21-46)
- Frequently painful, particularly when the legs are at rest and elevated; also intermittent claudication
- Associated with cold white or cyanotic, shiny feet

DIAGNOSIS
- Clinical

MANAGEMENT
- It is important to treat underlying diseases such as diabetes, and to discontinue smoking
- Meticulous skin care, debridement, and cleansing of the wound are essential.

- Treating tissue infection
- Antibiotics are not necessary unless there is tissue infection
- Specialized wound dressings
- Dressings are usually occlusive as ulcers heal better in a moist environment
- Surgery may be considered if the ulcer fails to heal with conservative measures
- The ulcer (s) can be treated with moist wound healing methods, high-compression therapy, fibrinolytic agents, and newer modalities, such as growth factors, matrix materials, and biologically engineered tissue. (These methods are beyond the scope of this chapter)

ALSO CONSIDER
- Atrophie blanche (Fig. 21-47)
- Cryoglobulinemia
- Antiphospholipid syndrome
- Protein C deficiency
- Skin cancer
- Pyoderma gangrenosum
- α_1-antitrypsin deficiency panniculitis
- Pancreatic panniculitis
- Lupus panniculitis

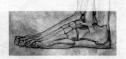

CHAPTER 22

Feet

The dermatologic conditions of the feet are similar to those of the hands. Inflammatory conditions such as psoriasis and eczema often mirror palmar disorders. Similarly, bacterial, viral (e.g., warts), and fungal infections are also prone to appear in this location. As with fingernails, toenails are constantly in contact with, and exposed regularly to harsh contactants, trauma, and irritants. Toenails protect the vulnerable tips of the toes by shielding them from the impact of footwear and external trauma. Toenails also are important contributors to the aesthetic appearance of the feet (see Chapter 13, Hands and Fingers; Chapter 14, Fingernails). Inflammatory disorders that involve the nail matrix, such as psoriasis and eczema, can result in distinctive deformities of the nails.

Melanocytic nevi, plantar warts, and other benign lesions must be distinguished from the rare, but potentially fatal, acral lentiginous melanoma.

IN THIS CHAPTER

Dorsal Feet and Toe Webs
- Tinea pedis *vs* granuloma annulare
- Contact dermatitis *vs* atopic dermatitis

Plantar Feet and Toes
- Acute and chronic tinea pedis *vs* atopic dermatitis *vs* plantar psoriasis
- Plantar warts *vs* corns
- Raynaud phenomenon *vs* perniosis

Toenails
- Onychomycosis *vs* psoriatic nail dystrophy
- Subungual hematoma *vs* junctional melanocytic nevus *vs* acral lentiginous melanoma

Tinea Pedis

Tinea pedis (TP) (athlete's foot) is an extremely common problem. TP thrives in warm, humid conditions and is most commonly seen in young adult men. Ubiquitous media advertisements for athlete's foot sprays and creams are testimony to the commonplace occurrence of this annoying dermatosis. Most cases are caused by *Trichophyton rubrum*, which evokes a minimal inflammatory response, and less often by *Trichophyton mentagrophytes*, which may produce vesicles and bullae. In addition, *Epidermophyton floccosum* may be responsible less frequently. Interdigital TP is the most common type of tinea pedis. It is seen predominantly in men between 18 and 40 years of age. There are various presentations such as acute vesicular TP (see following discussion) and chronic plantar TP (see Plantar Feet and Toes, later).

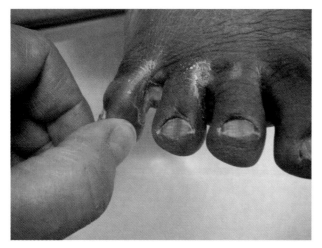

Figure 22-1 Tinea pedis.

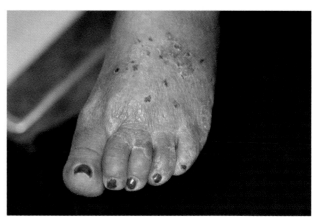

Figure 22-2 Tinea pedis.

DISTINGUISHING FEATURES: Interdigital Tinea Pedis

- Scale, maceration, and fissures of toe webs are characteristic, especially between the fourth and fifth toes (Fig. 22-1); however, any web space, as well as the dorsal foot (Fig. 22-2) may be involved
- Tinea pedis is often asymptomatic; however, it may itch intensely
- Marked inflammation and fissures suggest bacterial superinfection

DIAGNOSIS: Interdigital Tinea Pedis

- A positive potassium hydroxide (KOH) examination or fungal culture is diagnostic

MANAGEMENT: Interdigital Tinea Pedis (see Appendix A)

- For acute oozing and maceration, **Burow** solution is helpful
- Broad-spectrum topical antifungal agents such as ketoconazole **(Nizoral),** ciclopirox **(Loprox),** or clotrimazole **(Lotrimin)** are applied twice daily
- Prevention consists of maintaining dryness in the area by:
  - Using a hairdryer after bathing
  - Applying powders such as **Zeasorb-AF** that contains miconazole as an active antifungal ingredient

Granuloma Annulare

Granuloma annulare is an idiopathic, generally asymptomatic, ring-shaped grouping of dermal papules (see also Chapter 13, Hands and Fingers; Chapter 12, Arms, Elbows). The papules are composed of focal granulomas that coalesce to form circles or semicircular plaques, which are often misdiagnosed as tinea ("ringworm").

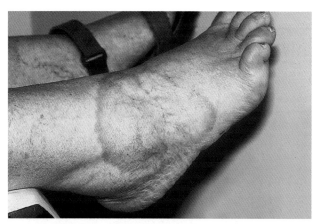

Figure 22-3 Granuloma annulare. (From Goodheart HP. *Goodheart's Photoguide to Common Skin Disorders: Diagnosis and Management.* 3rd ed. Philadelphia: Lippincott Williams & Wilkins, 2009, with permission.)

DISTINGUISHING FEATURES

- Lesions are generally asymptomatic, red or skin-colored, firm dermal papules that most often arise on the dorsal surfaces of hands, fingers, and feet
- May be individual, isolated papules or joined in annular (Fig. 22-3) or semiannular (arciform) plaques with central clearing (see also Fig. 13-1)
- Lesions have no epidermal change (i.e., scale)
- Centers of lesions may be slightly hyperpigmented and depressed relative to their borders

DIAGNOSIS

- Most often made on clinical grounds
- Skin biopsy, if the diagnosis is in doubt

MANAGEMENT (see Appendices A and B)

- The patient should be reassured of the benign nature of the condition
- Localized lesions in very young children are often best left untreated
- Potent topical steroids, if desired, used may be used alone or under polyethylene occlusion
- Intralesional triamcinolone acetonide **(Kenalog)** may be injected directly into the elevated border of the lesions

ALSO CONSIDER
- Atopic dermatitis
- Bacterial pyoderma
- Candidiasis
- Contact dermatitis
- Xerosis

RARELY
- Sarcoidosis
- Necrobiosis lipoidica

Contact Dermatitis

Contact dermatitis frequently occurs more often on the dorsa of the feet. It is far less common on the plantar surface. Ingredients in the rubber used in a shoe's construction cause most cases of allergic contact dermatitis from footwear. Footwear adhesives, both rubber and nonrubber, can also cause problems. Even leather shoes may contain these agents.

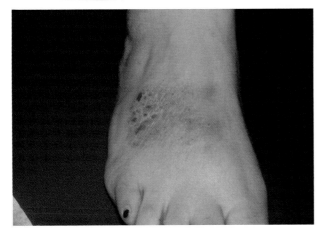

Figure 22-4 Contact dermatitis. This eczematous eruption was caused by leather sandals.

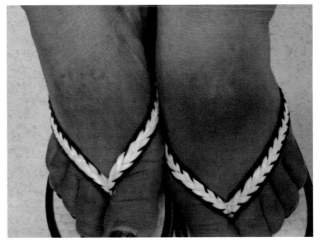

Figure 22-5 Contact dermatitis. The postinflammatory hyperpigmentation is due to chronic irritation from this patient's shoes.

DISTINGUISHING FEATURES

Acute
- Pruritic erythematous papules, "juicy" vesicles, and/or blisters

Subacute and Chronic
- Crusted, pruritic, eczematous plaques (Fig. 22-4)
- Lichenified plaques are generally prominent and tend to blend into surrounding normal skin (see also Fig. 12-20)
- Postinflammatory hyperpigmentation (see Fig. 22-5)

DIAGNOSIS
- Clinical
- Historical evidence of occupational and/or daily habitual exposure may be clues to the specific irritant or allergen
- Consider patch testing to identify relevant allergens (see Appendix B)

MANAGEMENT (see also Chapter 12, Arms; Chapter 13, Hands and Fingers)
- Topical steroids (class 1-3) are applied once or twice daily (see Appendix A)
- After identification, contact with the causative agent must be avoided

Atopic Dermatitis

Atopic dermatitis is often clinically indistinguishable from acute and chronic contact dermatitis. However, atopic dermatitis occurs in association with a personal or family history of hay fever, asthma, allergic rhinitis, sinusitis, or atopic dermatitis itself. Also, a history of allergies to pollen, dust, house dust mites, ragweed, dogs, or cats may be uncovered (see also Chapter 3, Eyelids and Periorbital Area; Chapter 12, Arms; Chapter 13, Hands and Fingers; Chapter 15, Trunk; Chapter 21, Legs).

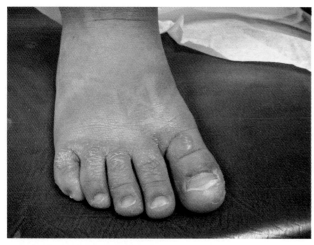

Figure 22-6 Atopic dermatitis.

DISTINGUISHING FEATURES (May be Identical to those of Contact Dermatitis, Previously Discussed)

Acute
- Pruritic erythematous papules, "juicy" dyshidrotic vesicles, and/or blisters

Subacute and Chronic
- Crusted, pruritic, eczematous plaques (Fig. 22-6)
- Lichenified plaques are generally prominent and tend to blend into surrounding normal skin (see Fig. 13-13)

DIAGNOSIS
- Clinical
- Atopic history
- Lack of history of contactant

MANAGEMENT (see Appendix A)
- Topical steroids (class 1-3) are applied once or twice daily
- Frequent application of moisturizers and barrier creams

☞ ALSO CONSIDER
- Stasis dermatitis
- Tinea pedis/corporis

On the soles of the feet, TP, atopic dermatitis, and plantar psoriasis can look very much alike. However, they are managed quite differently (see also Chapter 13, Hands and Fingers).

Acute and Chronic Tinea Pedis

Acute vesicular TP, most often caused by *T. mentagrophytes*, is the least common clinical variant of TP. In contrast, **chronic plantar TP,** usually caused by *T. rubrum*, commonly is seen in its characteristic "moccasin" presentation and sometimes in the "two feet, one hand" distribution.

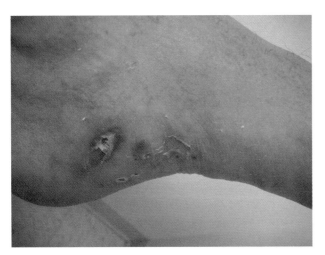

Figure 22-7 Acute tinea pedis.

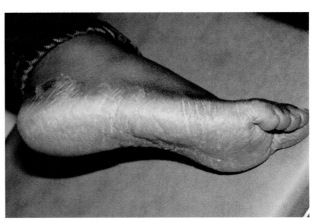

Figure 22-8 Chronic tinea pedis: chronic scaly infection of the plantar surface of the foot in a "moccasin" distribution.

DISTINGUISHING FEATURES
Acute Vesicular Tinea Pedis
- Clusters of pruritic vesicles, bullae, or pustules on the sides of the feet, insteps, or soles (Fig. 22-7)

Chronic Plantar Tinea Pedis
- "Moccasin" tinea is hyperkeratotic, in which the skin of the entire sole, heel, and sides of the foot is "dry" and hyperkeratotic, but not inflamed (Fig. 22-8)
- Borders are distinct along the sides of the feet and may extend to the Achilles area (Fig. 22-9)
- There is often nail involvement (onychomycosis)
- Symptoms are minimal unless painful fissures occur
- "Two feet, one hand" (palmar/plantar): Tinea can present on one or both palms (tinea manuum). This is pathognomic for tinea (see Fig. 13-11)

DIAGNOSIS
Acute Vesicular Tinea Pedis
- A specimen should be obtained from the inner part of the roof of the blister for KOH examination or fungal culture

Chronic Plantar Tinea Pedis
- The KOH examination from the "active border" or fungal culture is positive

MANAGEMENT (see Appendix A)
Acute Vesicular Tinea Pedis
- For acute oozing and maceration, **Burow solution** compresses are used
- Broad-spectrum topical antifungal agents such as ketoconazole **(Nizoral),** ciclopirox **(Loprox),** or clotrimazole **(Lotrimin)** are applied once or twice daily
- Oral antifungal agents such as terbinafine **(Lamisil),** itraconazole **(Sporanox),** fluconazole **(Diflucan),** or griseofulvin may be necessary if topical therapy is unsuccessful

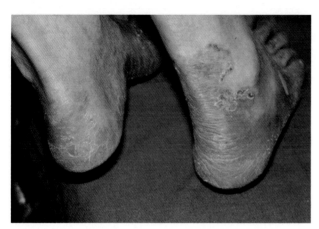

Figure 22-9 Chronic tinea pedis extending to the Achilles area in this patient.

Chronic Plantar Tinea Pedis

This is the most difficult type of tinea pedis to cure because topical agents do not effectively penetrate the thickened epidermis. Consequently:

- Systemic, as well as topical antifungals are often necessary
- Oral antifungal agents such as the following may be prescribed:
    - Terbinafine (**Lamisil**) 250 mg once daily for 14 days or longer, if necessary
    - Itraconazole (**Sporanox**) 200 mg once daily for 14 days or longer, if necessary
    - Fluconazole (**Diflucan**) 150 to 200 mg once daily for 4 to 6 weeks, if necessary
- Nail involvement may require longer treatment because nails may serve as reservoirs for reinfection (see Chapter 14, Fingernails)
- Prevention involves decreasing wetness, friction, and maceration. Absorbent powders, such as miconazole (**Zeasorb-AF**) powder, should be applied after the eruption clears to prevent recurrence

✔ **TIP: Not all rashes of the feet are fungal. In fact, if a child younger than 12 years has what appears to be tinea pedis, it is probably another skin condition, such as atopic dermatitis.**

FEET

Atopic Dermatitis

Atopic dermatitis of the soles is analogous to that of hand eczema (see Chapter 13, Hands and Fingers). More often than not, it occurs in association with an atopic diathesis. Often chronic, it runs a relapsing and remitting course.

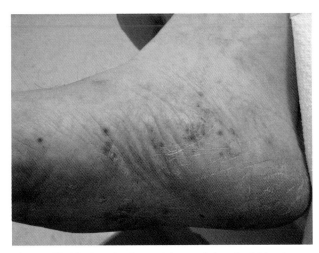

Figure 22-10 Atopic dermatitis resolving dyshidrotic vesicles (potassium hydroxide negative). Note similarity to acute (see Fig. 22-7) and chronic tinea pedis (see Fig. 22-8).

DISTINGUISHING FEATURES
- Lesions may appear as itchy, clear, dyshidrotic vesicles ("wet" type) (Fig. 22-10) or as the nondyshidrotic ("dry" type) characterized by scale, erythema, and sometimes painful fissures (see also Figs. 13-7 and 13-8)

DIAGNOSIS
- Atopic history often elicited
- A negative KOH examination or fungal culture

MANAGEMENT (SEE APPENDIX A)
- The regular use of emollients and avoidance of frequent contact with irritants
- For oozing lesions, compresses with **Burow solution**
- Class 1-3 topical corticosteroids are the mainstay of treatment; used under occlusion or "soak and smear" therapy (see Appendix B)
- For severe or refractory cases, the short-term use of systemic corticosteroids, acitretin **(Soriatane),** psoralen and ultraviolet A phototherapy (PUVA), broadband and narrow band UVB, excimer laser therapy, oral cyclosporine, azathioprine, mycophenolate mofetil **(CellCept),** and low-dose methotrexate may be tried

Plantar Psoriasis

Psoriasis may involve the palms and soles (palmoplantar psoriasis), or these areas may be a part of more extensive psoriasis that is also present elsewhere on the body. The location of these lesions often presents additional problems to the patients such as pain, impairment of function, and fissuring. This condition runs a chronic course and is often very difficult to manage.

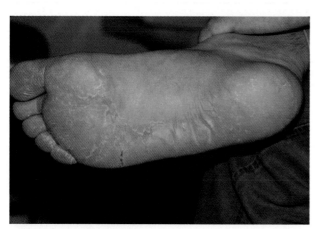

Figure 22-11 Plantar psoriasis. Note well-demarcated plaque.

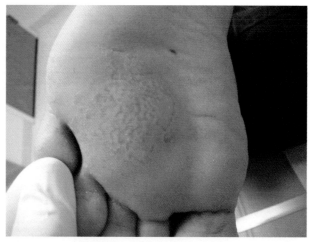

Figure 22-12 Pitted keratolysis. Note pits in stratum corneum caused by prolonged occlusion, hyperhidrosis, and bacterial proliferation.

DISTINGUISHING FEATURES
- Psoriasis has sharply demarcated plaques, often with thick scales (Fig. 22-11) (see also Fig. 13-9)
- Pustular variant is much less common
- Positive family history of psoriasis (50%)
- Less likely to itch than eczema
- Nails may show characteristic changes (see Chapter 14, Fingernails, and Toenails, later in this chapter)

DIAGNOSIS
- Clinical
- A negative KOH examination or fungal culture
- Psoriasis may be seen elsewhere on body

MANAGEMENT
- See Chapter 13, Hands and Fingers
- See Appendix A

ALSO CONSIDER
- Pitted keratolysis (Fig. 22-12)

RARELY
- Pityriasis rubra pilaris
- Various hereditary keratodermas

Plantar Warts

Plantar warts commonly appear on the soles of the feet in children and young adults. They usually arise on the metatarsal area, heels, insteps, and toes in an asymmetric distribution.

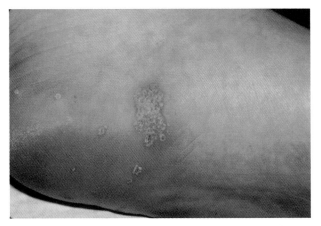

Figure 22-13 Plantar warts. Note loss of normal skin markings and "black dots," or thrombosed capillaries.

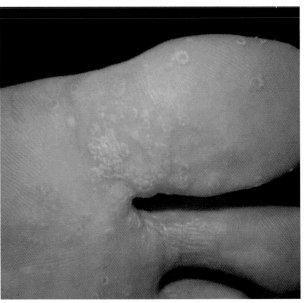

Figure 22-14 Mosaic plantar warts. Note the clustering, "kissing lesions."

DISTINGUISHING FEATURES
- A loss of normal skin markings (dermatoglyphics) such as finger, foot, and hand prints (Fig. 22-13)
- Lesions may be solitary or multiple, or they may appear in clusters (*mosaic warts*) (Fig. 22-14)
- Can be tender and painful
- Extensive involvement on the sole of the foot may impair ambulation, particularly when present on a weight-bearing surface

DIAGNOSIS
- Clinical

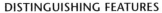 **TIP: Often, there are pathognomonic "black dots" (thrombosed dermal capillaries) and punctate bleeding that become evident after paring with a no. 15 blade (Fig. 22-15).**

⚠ **ALERT: Verrucous carcinoma, a slow-growing, locally invasive, well-differentiated squamous cell carcinoma, may also be easily mistaken for a plantar wart.**

MANAGEMENT (see Chapter 13, Hands and Fingers, as well as Appendix A)
- Paring with a no. 15 blade parallel to the skin surface often immediately relieves pain on walking
- The patient should be instructed to apply salicylic acid preparations between visits, as well as to perform "sanding" with an emery board, foot file such as **Dr. Scholl's Callous Removers,** or pumice stone, which keeps the wart flat and thus painless. This is followed by the application of an over-the-counter salicylic acid solution or **Mediplast,** a 40% salicylic acid plaster cut to the size of the wart

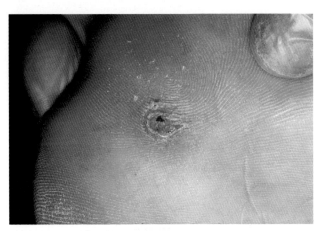

Figure 22-15 Plantar wart. Characteristic punctate bleeding is present after paring. (From Goodheart HP. *Goodheart's Photoguide to Common Skin Disorders: Diagnosis and Management.* 3rd ed. Philadelphia: Lippincott Williams & Wilkins, 2009, with permission.)

- Liquid nitrogen, blunt dissection, electrodesiccation, and curettage are reserved for more recalcitrant warts or when patients insist on aggressive therapy
- **Aldara cream** 5% (imiquimod), a local inducer of interferon that stimulates immune upregulation, may be applied at home by the patient. It is only approved for the treatment of genital warts (condyloma acuminatum)
- ✔ **TIP: No single therapy for warts is uniformly effective or superior; thus treatment involves a certain amount of trial and error. Thus, conservative, nonscarring treatments are preferred. A "cure" is achieved when the skin lines are restored to a normal pattern and there is no recurrence.**

Corns

Corns (clavi) and calluses are localized areas of thickened skin that are caused by response to friction and pressure. Wearing high-heeled shoes—particularly shoes that shift the body weight into a narrow, tapering toe box—can produce corns or calluses. Corns are sometimes difficult to distinguish from warts. A callus (tyloma) is an area of painless thickened, indurated skin.

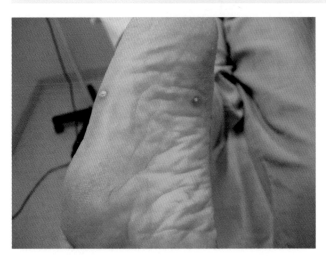

Figure 22-16 Corn (clavus). After paring, the circular central translucent core resembles a kernel of corn.

DISTINGUISHING FEATURES
- Lesions are usually hard and circular-shaped, with a polished or central translucent core, like the kernel of corn from which they take their name

- Can be tender and painful
- Extensive involvement on the sole of the foot may impair ambulation, particularly when present on a weight-bearing surface
- Corns most commonly develop on the tops and the tips of toes, the metatarsal area, heels, and along the sides of the feet; also are typically seen between the fourth and fifth toes ("kissing corns")
- Corns do not have "black dots," and skin markings are retained, except for the area of the central core (Fig. 22-16)

DIAGNOSIS
- Clinical

MANAGEMENT
- Separate toes using cotton or moleskin to relieve pressure
- Adhesive corn plasters
- Orthotic devices
- Foot file such as **Dr. Scholl's Callous Removers** or a pumice stone
- Keratolytic creams containing urea, salicylic acid or lactic acid
- Podiatric referral

ALSO CONSIDER
- Interdigital neuroma

RARELY
- Keratosis punctata
- Porokeratosis plantaris

Raynaud Phenomenon

Raynaud phenomenon is an episodic reduction in the blood supply to the fingers and/or toes occurring mainly in response to cold (vasospasm). The condition most commonly affects the hands but sometimes involves the feet and toes. Primary Raynaud phenomenon, also known as *Raynaud disease*, is not associated with any other conditions; in fact, it can be regarded as an exaggeration of the normal response of the circulation to cold. It affects many women. Secondary Raynaud phenomenon is associated with identifiable conditions such as the connective tissue diseases systemic sclerosis (scleroderma) and CREST syndrome (see Chapter 13, Hands and Fingers). It also occurs in systemic lupus erythematosus, dermatomyositis, Sjögren syndrome, and Wegener's granulomatosis. Furthermore, certain occupations are known to be associated with Raynaud phenomenon, such as use of vibrating tools (e.g., pneumatic drill operators) and industrial exposure to vinyl chloride polymerization processes.

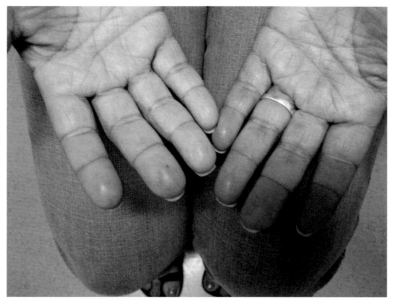

Figure 22-17 Secondary Raynaud phenomenon of the fingers. This patient has systemic lupus erythematosus.

DISTINGUISHING FEATURES
- Characteristically one or more toes or fingers turn white and, on rewarming, violaceous (Fig. 22-17) because of a sluggish blood flow
- This is then sometimes followed by a bright red color due to a compensatory increased blood flow before the skin becomes a normal color
- Episodes may be painful and can last from minutes to hours

DIAGNOSIS
- Clinical

MANAGEMENT
- Warm gloves, thick socks, and slippers
- Discontinue smoking
- Calcium channel blockers, such as nifedipine
- Antiadrenergic drugs
- Pentoxifylline (**Trental**)
- Sildenafil (**Viagra**), which has been reported to be of benefit

Perniosis

Perniosis, also known as *pernio* and "chilblains," is considered to be a localized form of vasculitis that occurs as a reaction to mild nonfreezing cold and humidity. It is most frequently seen in young and middle-aged women and in children. Rarely, a chronic presentation of pernio may be secondary to various systemic diseases such as dysproteinemia, macroglobulinemia, cryoglobulinemia, cryofibrinogenemia, cold agglutinins, and the antiphospholipid antibody syndrome.

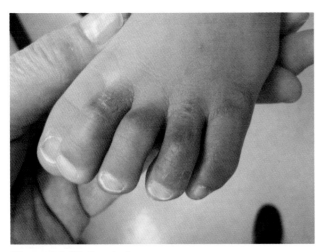

Figure 22-18 Perniosis.

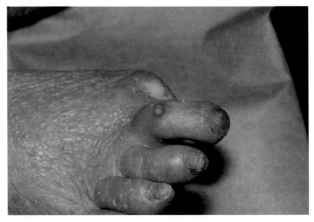

Figure 22-19 Vasculitis. Note amputated toe as a result of cholesterol emboli.

DISTINGUISHING FEATURES
- Most often involves the toes and fingers; also the thighs, especially in horseback riders
- Pernio lesions present 12 to 24 hours after cold exposure as red or violaceous macules (Fig. 22-18), papules, nodules, or plaques, which may form vesicles or ulcerate
- Patient may experience pain or pruritus lasting 1 to 3 weeks

DIAGNOSIS
- Clinical

MANAGEMENT
- Warm clothing, thick woolen socks, comfortable protective footwear, and gloves; avoidance of nicotine and caffeine
- Most cases resolve without any adverse reactions
- Vasodilator medications such as nifedipine **(Procardia)**
- ⚠ **ALERT: In severe cases, ulceration can occur.**

☞ ALSO CONSIDER
- Vasculitis
- Hypertensive ulcer
- Sarcoidosis
- Arterial emboli

RARELY
- Erythromelalgia
- Acrocyanosis
- Purple toe syndrome
- Septic or cholesterol emboli (Fig. 22-19)
- Dysproteinemias
- Macroglobulinemia
- Cryoglobulinemia, cryofibrinogenemia, cold agglutinins
- Antiphospholipid antibody syndrome

Onychomycosis

Onychomycosis refers to an infection of the fingernails or toenails caused by various fungi, yeasts, and molds. Uncommon in children, the prevalence of onychomycosis increases with advancing age, with rates as high as 30% in those 70 years of age and older. The major causes of onychomycosis are dermatophytes, and the resulting condition is referred to as *tinea unguium. Candida* infection of the nail plate generally results from paronychia that becomes established around the proximal the nail fold (see Chapter 13, Hands and Fingers).

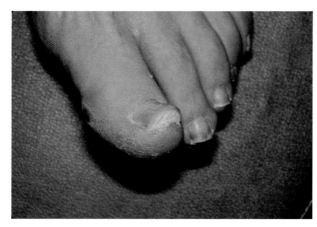

Figure 22-20 Onychomycosis.

DISTINGUISHING FEATURES

- May affect one or more toenails, most often the great toenail (Fig. 22-20) or the little toenail
- Nail thickening, dystrophy, and subungual hyperkeratosis (see Fig. 14-3)
- Nail discoloration (yellow, yellow-green, white, or brown)
- Onycholysis
- Generally asymptomatic, aside from footwear causing occasional physical discomfort and the psychosocial liability of unsightly nails

✔ **TIP: Toenail infections are cured less quickly and effectively than those of the fingernails.**

DIAGNOSIS

- Positive KOH examination and/or growth of dermatophyte. Clippings should be taken from crumbling tissue at the end of the infected nail

MANAGEMENT

- See Appendix A
- See Chapter 14, Fingernails

Psoriatic Nail Dystrophy

Psoriatic nail dystrophy is a chronic, primarily cosmetic condition. Involvement of nails is very common in patients with psoriasis (see Chapter 14, Fingernails). In some instances, thickened psoriatic toenails can become painful and deformed, and this may interfere with function.

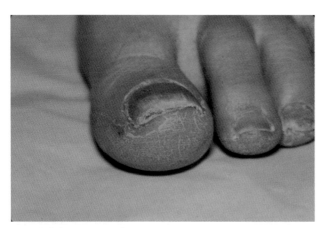

Figure 22-21 Psoriatic nail dystrophy: subungual hyperkeratosis and "oil spots."

DISTINGUISHING FEATURES
- Any of the following may be noted: pitting (see Fig. 14-4), onycholysis, "oil spots" (see Fig. 14-5), and subungual hyperkeratosis (Fig. 22-21) similar to onychomycosis (also see previous discussion) (see Fig. 14-6)

DIAGNOSIS
- Clinical
- Patients usually have psoriasis elsewhere on the body
- ☑ TIP: Psoriasis of the toenails may be indistinguishable from, or coexist with, onychomycosis.

MANAGEMENT
- See Appendix A
- See Chapter 14, Fingernails

☞ **ALSO CONSIDER**
- Ingrown toenail
- Acute paronychia and chronic paronychia (see Chapter 13, Hands and Fingers)
- *Candida* paronychia
- Saprophytic mold infections
- Nail dystrophy secondary to eczematous dermatitis
- Lichen planus
- Onychogryphosis (seen in the elderly)

RARELY
- Pachyonychia congenita
- Darier disease
- Yellow nail syndrome

By far, trauma is the most common cause of nail disorders. However, an injury that results in a collection of blood under the nail can be quite unsettling because a neoplasm often is not easy to rule out (see also Chapter 14, Fingernails).

Subungual Hematoma

Subungual hematomas result from trauma to the nail matrix or nail bed, such as repeated minor injuries (e.g., tight shoes, sports injuries). An acute subungual hematoma that results from rapid accumulation of blood under the nail plate can be very painful and is readily diagnosed (see Fig. 14.11), whereas small asymptomatic lesions may be painless and may go unnoticed for some time.

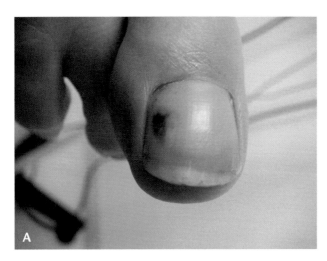

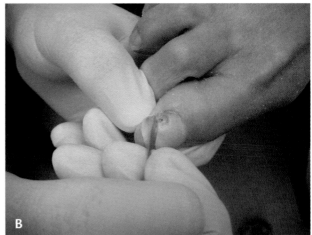

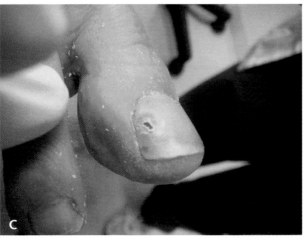

Figure 22-22 A. Subungual hematoma. **B.** Subungual hematoma: the nail plate is pared down with no. 15 scalpel blade. **C.** After paring, the coagulated blood is seen.

DISTINGUISHING FEATURES
• Darkly pigmented spot under toenail (usually the great toenail) (Fig. 22-22)

DIAGNOSIS
• Clinical

⚠ ALERT: Chronic, painless, subungual hematomas that are clearly not the result of trauma may appear similar to a neoplasm, such as an acral lentiginous melanoma (see later discussion). A coagulated bloodstain often remains until the nail grows out (8-12 months for toenails); thus, the diagnosis can be in doubt for some time.

☑ TIP: A rapid method to substantiate the presence of a hematoma is to pare the nail plate gently with a no. 15 scalpel blade or to file it down until the coagulated blood can be visualized (Fig. 22-22, A through C).

MANAGEMENT
• No therapy is necessary for chronic subungual hematomas

Junctional Melanocytic Nevus

Junctional melanocytic nevi are quite common in African-Americans and may be multiple. They are much less common in caucasian.

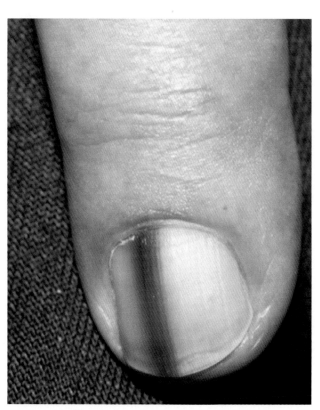

Figure 22-23 Junctional nevus: a brown linear band of longitudinal melanonychia. (From Goodheart HP. *Goodheart's Photoguide to Common Skin Disorders: Diagnosis and Management.* 3rd ed. Philadelphia, Lippincott Williams & Wilkins, 2009, with permission.)

DISTINGUISHING FEATURES
- An evenly pigmented linear nevus that emanates from nests of nevus cells in the nail matrix (Fig. 22-23; see also Fig. 14-12)

DIAGNOSIS
- Clinical
- Dermoscopy (see Appendix B)

MANAGEMENT
- No treatment is necessary
- Biopsy of nail bed or nail matrix if there is any doubt about the diagnosis

Acral Lentiginous Melanoma

Acral lentiginous melanoma (ALM), the least common subtype of melanoma, is relatively rare. However, it accounts for 29% to 72% of melanoma cases in dark-skinned individuals (i.e, African-American, Asian, and Hispanic persons).

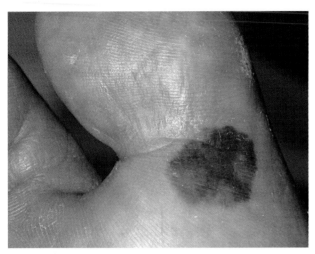

Figure 22-24 Acral lentiginous melanoma. (Courtesy of Charles Miller, MD. From Goodheart HP. *Goodheart's Photoguide to Common Skin Disorders: Diagnosis and Management.* 3rd ed. Philadelphia: Lippincott Williams & Wilkins, 2009, with permission.)

DISTINGUISHING FEATURES

- ALM lesions appear on areas that do not bear hair, such as periungual skin, and beneath the nail plate (see Chapter 14, Fingernails), especially on the thumb or great toe, as well as on the palms and soles (Fig. 22-24)
- A subungual melanoma may manifest as diffuse nail discoloration or a longitudinal pigmented band within the nail plate
- Pigment spread to the proximal or lateral nail folds is termed the *Hutchinson sign*, which is a hallmark for ALM (Fig. 22-25; see also Fig. 14-13)

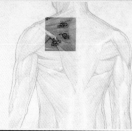

CHAPTER 23

Generalized Eruptions

Previous chapters have discussed drug eruptions and viral exanthems, both of which can become life-threatening. Whether caused by drugs or not, erythema multiforme major (Stevens-Johnson syndrome), toxic epidermal necrolysis, and exfoliative dermatitis (erythroderma) may produce widespread eruptions and present as medical emergencies. Staphylococcal scalded skin syndrome, however, has a generally benign outcome with a very low mortality.

IN THIS CHAPTER

- Exfoliative dermatitis *vs* toxic epidermal necrolysis *vs* staphylococcal scalded skin syndrome

Exfoliative Dermatitis

Exfoliative dermatitis (ED), also referred to as *erythroderma*, is a generalized scaling eruption with a marked loss of exfoliated epidermis due to an increased mitotic rate. It may involve more than 90% of the cutaneous surface. Exfoliative dermatitis may arise idiopathically or secondary to an underlying cutaneous or systemic disease or as a reaction to drugs. When fulminant, this reaction can be fatal. Exfoliative dermatitis is a rare disorder that may appear suddenly or gradually, occasionally accompanied by fever, chills, and lymphadenopathy. Most patients are older than 40 years of age and are mostly males. In young children, ED is most often secondary to severe atopic dermatitis, and in infants, to seborrheic dermatitis. Psoriasis and drug reactions are the most frequent determined causes of ED; it is idiopathic in up to 20% to 30% of cases. Reported causal agents include captopril, codeine, cefoxitin, cimetidine, dapsone, gold salts, hydantoins, isoniazid, lithium, nonsteroidal anti-inflammatory drugs (NSAIDs), omeprazole, para-aminosalicylic acid, penicillins, phenylbutazone, phenothiazines, St. John's wort, sulfonamides, sulfonylureas, thalidomide, vancomycin, and erlotinib (**Tarceva**).

Less commonly, ED has been noted as a finding in the following skin disorders:
* Allergic contact dermatitis
* Stasis dermatitis with secondary autoeczematization
* Pityriasis rubra pilaris
* Graft-versus-host disease
* Ichthyosiform dermatoses
* Pemphigus foliaceus
* Papulosquamous dermatitis of acquired immunodeficiency syndrome (AIDS)

Other rare reported associations include:
* Sézary syndrome (leukemic variant of mycosis fungoides)
* Reiter syndrome
* Hodgkin and non-Hodgkin lymphoma and leukemia

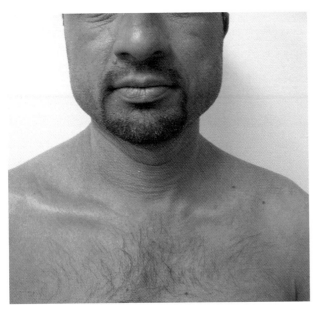

Figure 23-1 Exfoliative dermatitis: erythrodermic type (*l'homme rouge*).

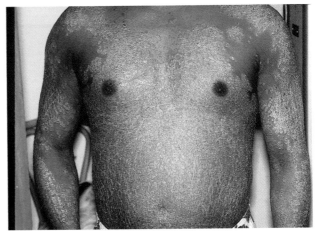

Figure 23-2 Exfoliative dermatitis: secondary to psoriasis.

DISTINGUISHING FEATURES
* Cutaneous involvement consists of generalized erythema (l'homme rouge) (Fig. 23-1) followed by extensive scaling (Fig. 23-2)

* Other findings may include:
  * Pruritus, fever, chills
  * Malaise/weakness
  * Pedal or pretibial edema
  * Lymphadenopathy, usually a reactive type (*dermatopathic lymphadenopathy*)

- Other possible findings include:
  - Eosinophilia, hepatomegaly, splenomegaly (when underlying lymphoma/leukemia is present)
  - Alopecia
  - Nail dystrophy
  - Hypoproteinemia, anemia
  - Dehydration
  - High-output cardiac failure
  - Tachycardia

DIAGNOSIS

- Diagnosis of ED is made on a clinical basis. Determination of the underlying cause is often elusive
- Eliciting a history of drug ingestion or a pre-existing dermatosis or disease is often valuable
- A skin biopsy may have characteristics of an underlying cutaneous disease; however, findings are most often nonspecific
- Infrequently, repeated or multiple biopsies sometimes provide a specific underlying diagnosis
- There are no specific diagnostic laboratory tests for ED. A chest radiograph, lymph node biopsy, and/or bone marrow biopsy may be indicated

MANAGEMENT (see Appendix A)

- Discontinuance of any implicated medications or treatment of any identified underlying infection/disease
- Because acute ED can evolve rapidly, with complications of secondary infection, hypothermia, dehydration, or heart failure, a patient may require hospitalization, where fluid replacement, adequate nutrition with sufficient protein intake, temperature control, and expert topical skin care are available.

- Bed rest, cool compresses, lubrication with emollients, antipruritic therapy with oral antihistamines, and low-to-intermediate strength topical steroids are applied
- Local bland, moisturizing ointments/lotions
- Systemic antibiotics, if signs of secondary infection are observed
- **ALERT: Systemic steroids may be helpful in some cases but should be avoided in suspected cases of psoriasis.**
- When psoriasis is determined to be the underlying cause, oral retinoids, cyclosporine, methotrexate, etretinate, phototherapy, photopheresis, photochemotherapy, as well as monoclonal antibodies such as infliximab and alemtuzumab, may be effective
- Photochemotherapy may also be useful therapy for treating exfoliative dermatitis associated with mycosis fungoides
- Isotretinoin has been used when pityriasis rubra pilaris is the underlying cause
- Certain antimetabolites/cytotoxic drugs
- The prognosis of ED depends largely on underlying etiology
- In patients with an identified underlying cause, the course and prognosis generally parallel the primary disease
- Exfoliative dermatitis due to a drug eruption usually clears when the drug is stopped
- The prognosis in acute, severe episodes, particularly in elderly persons or in persons with pre-existing heart disease, is more guarded
- In patients with idiopathic ED, the prognosis is poor and recurrences are not uncommon

Toxic Epidermal Necrolysis

Toxic epidermal necrolysis (TEN) is a rare, life-threatening mucocutaneous condition that is most often induced by an unusually severe adverse reaction to certain drugs. Toxic epidermal necrolysis involves a prodrome of painful skin, followed by rapid, widespread, skin detachment. It is the result of massive keratinocyte cell death and has a mortality rate of 30% to 50%. Infection is more commonly implicated as a cause in children, whereas medication exposure is a more common etiology in adults. Some authors consider TEN to be a severe form of Stevens-Johnson syndrome (erythema multiforme major) (see Chapter 8, Oral Cavity and Tongue; Chapter 15, Trunk).

The drugs most often implicated in TEN are antibiotics such as sulfonamides, NSAIDs, allopurinol, antiretroviral drugs, corticosteroids, and anticonvulsants such as phenobarbital, phenytoin, carbamazepine, and valproic acid. Also, immunizations, transplants of bone marrow or organs, and infections from agents such as *Mycoplasma pneumoniae* or herpesvirus have been implicated. Septicemia, pneumonia, or multisystem organ failure are the primary causes of death.

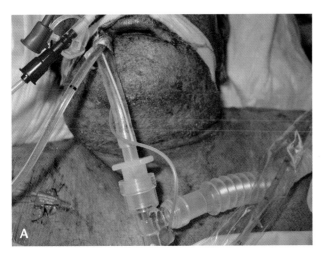

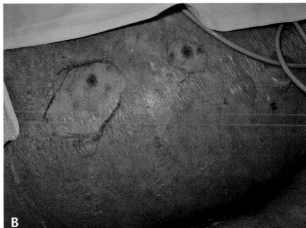

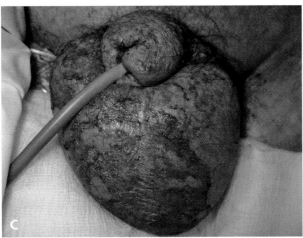

Figure 23-3 A–C. Toxic epidermal necrolysis. Severe, extensive, generalized eruption with epidermal necrosis and denuded erosive areas. (Courtesy of Benjamin Barankin, MD.)

DISTINGUISHING FEATURES

- The cutaneous eruption begins as poorly defined, erythematous macules with purpuric centers. Over a period of hours to days, the rash coalesces to form flaccid blisters and sheetlike epidermal detachment
- Lesions predominate on the torso and face, sparing the scalp
- Often preceded by a prodrome of high fever, cough, sore throat, and malaise
- Mucous membrane involvement of the mouth, eyes, penis, and vagina can result in gastrointestinal hemorrhage, ocular abnormalities, and genitourinary complications
- The rapid evolution of painful, widespread erythema, necrosis, and coalescing blisters result in detachment of the skin similar to that seen in burns (Fig. 23-3, A through C)
- Flaccid bullae tend to separate with slight pressure (Nikolsky sign)

DIAGNOSIS

- Often, the diagnosis can be made clinically
- Sometimes, however, examination of affected tissue under the microscope may be needed to distinguish it between TEN and other entities such as staphylococcal scalded skin syndrome (see following discussion)

MANAGEMENT

- Withdrawal of responsible drug(s), early referral and management in burn units or intensive care units, supportive management, and nutritional support
- The second line is intravenous immunoglobulin
- The third line is cyclosporine, cyclophosphamide, plasmapheresis, pentoxifylline, *N*-acetylcysteine, ulinastatin, infliximab, and/or granulocyte colony-stimulating factors (if TEN-associated leukopenia exists)

✔ **TIP: Systemic steroids are unlikely to offer any benefit.**

⚠ **ALERT: Loss of the skin leaves patients vulnerable to infections from fungi and bacteria, and this can result in sepsis, the leading cause of death from the disease.**

Staphylococcal Scalded Skin Syndrome

Staphylococcal scalded skin syndrome (SSSS) is primarily a disease of children and neonates. Also known as *Ritter disease,* SSSS includes a spectrum of superficial blistering skin disorders caused by the hematogenous spread of exfoliative toxins type A or B of *Staphylococcus aureus.* It is a syndrome of acute exfoliation of the skin. Severity varies from a few blisters localized to the site of infection to a severe exfoliation affecting almost the entire body. Staphylococcal scalded skin syndrome is characterized by red blistering skin that looks like a burn or scald, hence its name. Children are believed to be more at risk because of lack of immunity and immature renal clearance capability (exfoliative toxins are renally excreted). Maternal antibodies transferred to infants in breast milk are thought to be partially protective, but neonatal disease can still occur, possibly as a result of inadequate immunity or immature renal clearance of exotoxin.

The exotoxins from *S. aureus* produce a red rash and separation of the epidermis beneath the granular cell layer, which differs from the more severe TEN; the cleavage site in SSSS is intraepidermal, as opposed to TEN, which involves necrosis of the full epidermal layer (at the level of the basement membrane). Bullae form, and diffuse sheet-like desquamation occurs. Outbreaks are usually due to infection picked up from asymptomatic carriers in neonatal and newborn nurseries. Reports implicating methicillin-resistant *S. aureus* (MRSA) and community-acquired MRSA as a cause of SSSS are increasing.

The decrease in frequency of SSSS in adults is thought to be explained by the presence of antibodies specific for exotoxins and also improved renal clearance of toxins that are produced. The mortality rate from SSSS in children is very low (1%–5%), unless associated sepsis or an underlying serious medical condition exists. The mortality rate in adults is higher (as high as 50%–60%), although this may be a reflection of another underlying disorder.

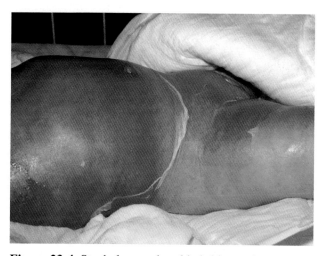

Figure 23-4 Staphylococcal scalded skin syndrome. (From Burkhart C, Morell D, Goldsmith LA, et al. *VisualDx: Essential Pediatric Dermatology.* Philadelphia: Lippincott Williams & Wilkins, 2009, with permission.)

DISTINGUISHING FEATURES

- Presents as an erythematous rash followed by diffuse epidermal exfoliation characterized by the appearance of large fluid-filled flaccid bullae that rupture easily, leaving an area that looks like a burn (Fig. 23-4)
- Fever, although patients may be afebrile; in fact, most patients do not appear severely ill
- Tenderness and warmth on palpation
- Nikolsky sign (gentle stroking of the skin causes the skin to separate at the epidermis)
- Exfoliation may be patchy or sheetlike in nature
- Facial edema
- Perioral crusting
- Dehydration may be present and significant

DIAGNOSIS

- Suspected from the characteristic history and physical examination
- May be confirmed with a biopsy and bacterial culture

MANAGEMENT

- Treatment usually requires hospitalization, as intravenous antibiotics are generally necessary to eradicate the staphylococcal infection
- Maintenance of fluid and electrolyte balance
- Strict handwashing with antibacterial soap

ALSO CONSIDER
- Extensive acute eczematous dermatitis
- Viral or bacterial exanthems

RARELY
- Pemphigus vulgaris
- Paraneoplastic pemphigus
- Toxic shock syndrome
- Phototoxic skin reactions
- Disseminated herpes zoster
- Sézary syndrome (erythrodermic of mycosis fungoides)
- Hypersensitivity syndrome

Formulary

This appendix includes many of the topical and systemic medications and treatments that are discussed in this book (see Appendix C for the formulary for acne and rosacea). The management sections of the book give additional instructions about the various medications and present more information about their complete use. This discussion is not intended to be a complete listing of all the pharmaceutical preparations available for dermatologic conditions.

TOPICAL STEROIDS

- Topical therapy, which is generally safer than systemic therapy, is the mainstay in the treatment of most inflammatory dermatologic conditions

General Principles It is necessary to become familiar with only one or two agents from each potency group to manage the majority of dermatoses:
- Creams are less greasy than ointments
- Ointments are more potent, more lubricating, and less likely to be irritating or sensitizing
- Lotions, solutions, and foam preparations spread more easily on the skin
- Lotions, gels, aerosols, and solutions are useful on hairy areas
- When possible, the lowest-potency steroid should be used for the shortest possible time. On the other hand, one should avoid using a preparation that is not potent enough to treat an intended condition
- Occlusion (discussed later) increases hydration, and hydration increases penetration, which, in turn, increases efficacy
- To help minimize tachyphylaxis, dosing may be cycled (pulse dosing). A preparation is applied until the dermatosis clears and then is resumed on recurrence
- Only nonfluorinated, mild topical steroids should be applied to the face and intertriginous areas, and, ideally only for short periods of time, to avoid atrophy and steroid rosacea

✔ **TIP: This rule can be broken, however. For example, for the treatment of a severe acute contact dermatitis of the face, a superpotent topical steroid used briefly may be preferable to a mild ineffective topical agent or systemic drugs.**

- Thin eyelid skin requires the least potent topical steroid preparations for the shortest periods of time. The intertriginous (skin touching skin) areas such as the axillae, perineum, inframammary, and groin areas similarly respond to lower potencies because the apposition of skin surfaces acts like an occlusive dressing and thus increase the ability of the medication to penetrate the skin
- For severe dermatoses, a very potent steroid may be used to initiate therapy and a less-potent preparation may be used afterward for maintenance ("downward titration") ("*strong, but not long*")

Percutaneous Penetration
- Topical steroids are ineffective unless they are absorbed into the skin
- The barrier to cutaneous penetration lies in the stratum corneum. The thicker the stratum corneum—as on the palms, soles, elbows, and knees—the harder it is for a topical agent to penetrate the skin
- Percutaneous penetration varies among individual patients, and it can be manipulated by changing the drug, the vehicle, and the length of exposure. It also depends on the anatomic surface area to which the drug is applied and whether the skin is inflamed and therefore, is less of a barrier to penetration (e.g., as in eczematous skin)
- Penetration also varies with the presence or absence of occlusive dressings
- Percutaneous penetration is enhanced by:
  - Soaking or bathing an affected area before the application of a topical steroid; "soak and smear" (see Appendix B)
  - Occlusion: a "nonbreathing" polyethylene wrap such as **Saran Wrap** or **Handi-Wrap,** held in place by tape, a bandage, a sock, or an **Ace bandage,** can provide occlusion to an area where topical steroids have been applied
  - Similarly, a plastic shower cap can be used after steroid application to the scalp
  - **Cordran tape,** which is impregnated with the steroid flurandrenolide, is helpful for occlusive therapy when treating relatively small areas
  - Rubber or vinyl gloves or finger cots may be used for the hands and finger tips
  - Small plastic bags such as **Baggies** may be used for the feet
  - Occlusive garments (sauna suits) can be worn when extensive areas are involved

✔ **TIP: Many topical steroids can be just as effective when they are applied only once per day.**

A vast array of topical steroids are available (Table A-1). Those in the same group have roughly the same potency. They differ primarily in vehicle and price. It is necessary to become familiar with only one or two agents from each potency group to manage the majority of dermatoses.

Table A-1   TOPICAL STEROID FORMULARY

Generic Name	Brand Name
Class 1 Superpotent	
Clobetasol propionate cream/ointment, 0.05%	**Temovate**
Clobetasol propionate lotion/foam	**Clobex, Olux**
Diflorasone diacetate ointment, 0.05%	**Psorcon-E, ApexiCon**
Halobetasol propionate cream/ointment, 0.05%	**Ultravate**
Flurandrenolide, 24 and 80 inch rolls	**Cordran Tape 4 mcg/cm^2**
Fluocinonide cream, 0.1%	**Vanos**
Betamethasone dipropionate gel, ointment 0.05%	**Diprolene**
Class 2: Very High Potency	
Desoximetasone cream/ointment, 0.25%/gel 0.05%	**Topicort**
Fluocinonide cream/ointment/solution/gel, 0.05%	**Lidex**
Amcinonide ointment, 0.1%	**Cyclocort**
Diflorasone diacetate ointment, 0.05%	**Florone, Maxiflor**
Halcinonide, 0.1% cream	**Halog**
Betamethasone dipropionate cream, 0.05%	**Diprolene AF**
Class 3: High Potency	
Triamcinolone acetate ointment, 0.1%	**Aristocort A**
Amcinonide cream, lotion, 0.1%	**Cyclocort**
Fluticasone propionate ointment, 0.005%	**Cutivate**
Fluocinonide cream, 0.05%	**Lidex E cream**
Class 4: Upper Mid-Strength	
Hydrocortisone valerate ointment, 0.2%	**Westcort**
Betamethasone valerate lotion, 0.1%	**Valisone**
Desoximetasone cream, 0.05%	**Topicort-LP**
Fluocinolone acetonide ointment, 0.025%	**Synalar**
Flurandrenolide ointment, 0.05%	**Cordran**
Triamcinolone acetonide cream, 0.1%	**Kenalog**
Class 5 Lower Mid-Strength	
Betamethasone valerate foam, 0.12%	**Luxiq**
Fluocinolone acetonide cream, 0.025%	**Synalar**
Fluticasone propionate cream, 0.05%	**Cutivate**
Hydrocortisone butyrate cream, 0.1%	**Locoid**
Hydrocortisone valerate cream, 0.2%	**Westcort**
Prednicarbate cream, 0.1%	**Dermatop E**
Class 6 Low Potency	
Alclometasone dipropionate cream/ointment, 0.05%	**Aclovate**
Desonide cream/ ointment/lotion, 0.05%	**DesOwen, Tridesilon**
Class 7 Least Potent	
Hydrocortisone cream/ointment/lotion, 1%	**Cortaid, Cortizone-10** (over the counter)
Dexamethasone cream, 0.1%	**Decadron Phosphate**
Hydrocortisone, 0.5%, 1%, 2.5%	Generic (**Hytone,** others)
Methylprednisolone, 1%	**Medrol**

Table A-2   ANTIFUNGAL DRUG FORMULARY

Generic Name	Brand Name	Form(s)
TOPICAL AGENTS		
OVER-THE-COUNTER		
Terbinafine, 1%	**Lamisil**	Cream, solution, spray; applied 1 to 4 weeks, twice daily
Clotrimazole, 1%	**Lotrimin**	Cream lotion, solution; applied twice daily
Miconazole 2%	**Micatin**	Cream, lotion, spray; applied twice daily
Tolnaftate 1%	**Tinactin**	Cream; applied twice daily
Miconazole 2%	**Zeasorb-AF** powder	Powder; applied as needed
PRESCRIPTION		
Ketoconazole 2%	**Nizoral**	Cream; applied once daily
Econazole 1%	**Spectazole**	Cream; applied once daily for 4 weeks
Ciclopirox 0.77%	**Loprox**	Cream, lotion, shampoo; applied as needed for 4 weeks
Naftifine 1%	**Naftin**	Cream, gel; applied once daily
Sulconazole	**Exelderm**	Cream, solution; applied twice daily for 4 weeks
Miconazole	**Monistat-Derm**	Cream; applied twice daily for 4 weeks
Oxiconazole 1%	**Oxistat**	Cream, lotion; applied once to twice daily for 4 weeks
SYSTEMIC AGENTS		
Griseofulvin	**Fulvicin P/G, Grisactin, Gris-PEG**	Microsized: 250-, 500-mg tablets; ultramicrosized: 125-, 250-, 333-mg tablets Pediatric: microsized: 125 mg/tsp pediatric suspension
Terbinafine	**Lamisil** tablets and **Lamisil Oral Granules**	250-mg tablets 125 mg and 187.5 mg
Itraconazole	**Sporanox**	100-mg capsules Oral solution (10 mg/mL)
Fluconazole	**Diflucan**	50-, 100-, 150-, 200-mg tablets; oral solution 10 mg/mL, 40 mg/mL

Table A-3 SEBORRHEIC DERMATITIS FORMULARY

General Type	Specific Agent
SCALP	
Shampoos/gels/lotions	
Antiseborrheics	Pyrithione zinc (**Head & Shoulders**[a]) shampoo Coal tar (**Neutrogena T/Gel**[a]) shampoo Coal tar (**Zetar**[a]) shampoo and emulsion Tar plus salicylic acid (**Neutrogena T/Sal**[a]) shampoo 2.5% selenium sulfide shampoo 1% ketoconazole shampoo (**Nizoral**[a])
Antifungals	2% ketoconazole shampoo (**Nizoral**), ciclopirox 0.77% (**Loprox** shampoo and gel).
Keratolytics (agents that remove excessive scale)	Sulfur 2%, salicylic acid 2% (**Sebulex**[a]) shampoo, or **Salex** cream or lotion, or **Keralyt** gel
Topical corticosteroids	
Medium potency (class 4)	Betamethasone valerate 0.1% (**Valisone**) Desoximetasone (**Topicort**) gel 0.05%, betamethasone valerate 0.12% (**Luxiq Foam**)
High potency (class 2)	Fluocinonide (**Lidex**) gel or solution 0.05%
Superpotency (class 1)	Clobetasol gel, foam, or scalp application 0.05%
FACE AND INTERTRIGINOUS AREAS	
Topical steroids	
Very low potency (class 7)	Hydrocortisone cream or ointment 1%
Low potency (class 6)	Desonide (**DesOwen**) cream, lotion 0.05%, desonide 0.05% foam (**Verdeso**)
Medium potency (classes 4 and 5)	Hydrocortisone valerate (**Westcort**) cream, ointment 0.2%
Topical creams/ointments	
Antifungals	Ketoconazole (**Nizoral**[a]) 1% cream, ciclopirox 0.77% (**Loprox** gel), and econazole cream 1% (**Spectazole**[a]) Ketoconazole (**Nizoral**) 2% cream, gel (**Xolegel**)
Immunomodulators	Tacrolimus 0.03% and 0.1% (**Protopic**) ointment Ketoconazole (**Nizoral**) 2% cream, gel (**Xolegel**)
Nonspecific anti-inflammatory	**Promiseb**

[a]Available over the counter.

Table A.4 PSORIASIS FORMULARY

Generic Name	Brand Name
TOPICAL AGENTS	
Keratolytics	
Salicylic acid 6%	**Keralyt Gel** (1 oz)
Salicylic acid 6%	**Salex** cream (400 g) and lotion (441 mL)
Topical vitamin D₃	
Calcipotriene 0.005% solution	**Dovonex** cream/ointment, scalp
Topical vitamin D₃–topical steroid combination	
Calcipotriene–betamethasone dipropionate 0.064%	**Taclonex** ointment
Topical immunomodulators	
Tacrolimus ointment 0.03%, 0.1%	**Protopic**
Pimecrolimus 1% cream	**Elidel**

Generic Name (Brand Name)	Comments
SYSTEMIC AGENTS	
Acitretin (**Soriatane**)	Synthetic derivative of vitamin A that is effective in treating the pustular and erythrodermic forms of psoriasis ⚠ **ALERT: Teratogen; contraindicated during pregnancy**
Methotrexate (**Rheumatrex**)	Antimetabolite that hinders DNA synthesis and cell reproduction in tissues with high rates of turnover, such as those found in psoriatic plaques. Often prescribed in a low-dose weekly regimen
Cyclosporine (**Neoral, Sandimmune**)	Suppresses humoral and cell-mediated immune reactions; inhibits production of interleukin 2, the cytokine responsible for inducing T-cell proliferation
"Biologics" Etanercept (**Enbrel**) Infliximab (**Remicade**) Adalimumab (**Humira**) Alefacept (**Amevive**) Ustekinumab (**Stelara**)	Act as immunologically directed inhibition in the pathogenesis of psoriasis; interact with specific targets in T-cell–mediated inflammatory processes and have anti-inflammatory effects

Table A-5 WART AND MOLLUSCUM CONTAGIOSUM FORMULARY

Brand and Generic Name	Comments
COMMON WARTS	
DuoFilm Salicylic Acid (17% W/W*)	Keratolytic
Occlusal-HP*	Keratolytic
Compound W*	Keratolytic
Plasters 15%, 40%: 40% salicylic acid plasters **(Dr. Scholl's, Mediplast)**	Keratolytic; available over the counter
Imiquimod **(Aldara)**	Effective as an immune response modifier
MOLLUSCUM CONTAGIOSUM	
Cantharone	Blistering agent (vesicant) solution, cantharidin 0.7%
Cantharone Plus	Podophyllin 5%, cantharidin 1%, salicylic acid 30%
Imiquimod **(Aldara)** 5% cream	Effective as an immune response modifier
GENITAL WARTS	
Podophyllum resin (podophyllin) is applied as a 25% suspension in compound tincture of benzoin or in alcohol	After application to the warts the resin is then washed off after 4 to 6 hours or longer ⚠ **ALERT: Contraindicated in pregnancy**
Condylox (0.5% podofilox)	Antimitotic drug; applied twice daily for 3 consecutive days, then discontinued for 4 consecutive days. This 1-week cycle of treatment may be repeated until there is no visible wart tissue or for a maximum of four cycles
Imiquimod **(Aldara)** 5% cream:	Applied once a day for 3 days a week. Treatment should continue until the warts are completely gone, or for up to 16 weeks

*Over-the-counter (ITAL)

Table A-6 TOPICAL THERAPY FOR SOLAR KERATOSES AND SUPERFICIAL BASAL CELL CARCINOMA

In addition to liquid nitrogen and electrosurgery (see Appendix B), therapy of multiple solar keratoses and superficial basal cell carcinomas can be treated topically with the immunomodulator imiquimod **(Aldara)**. Imiquimod is also used experimentally for other skin disorders such as Bowen disease and lentigo maligna melanoma. Alternatively, fluorouracil, a fluorinated pyrimidine antagonist that acts as an antimetabolite by interfering with DNA synthesis, is used topically for the treatment of multiple solar keratoses, superficial basal cell carcinomas, and Bowen disease.

Generic Name (Brand Name)	Comments
Imiquimod **(Aldara)**, 5% cream	Single-dose packets (box of 24); usually used once a day for 3 days a week
Imiquimod **(Zyclara)**, 3.75% cream	Single-dose packets (28 sachets); once-daily application 2 weeks on, 2 weeks off
Fluorouracil **(Efudex)** 5% topical cream	Fluorouracil preparation indicated for the topical treatment of multiple solar keratoses and superficial basal cell carcinomas
Fluorouracil **(Carac)** 0.5% topical cream	Fluorouracil preparation indicated for the topical treatment of multiple solar keratoses and superficial basal cell carcinomas
Diclofenac sodium 3% **(Solaraze Gel)**	Fluorouracil preparation indicated only for the topical treatment of multiple solar keratoses

Table A-7 ANTIHISTAMINE FORMULARY

Antihistamines are used for acute and chronic urticaria as well as other histamine-induced dermatoses.

Generic Name	Brand Name
FIRST-GENERATION HISTAMINE H1 BLOCKERS	
Diphenhydramine	**Benadryl**[a]
Hydroxyzine	**Atarax**
Cyproheptadine	**Periactin**
NONSEDATING H1 ANTIHISTAMINES	
Fexofenadine HCl	**Allegra**
Loratadine	**Claritin**[a] and **Clarinex**[a]
Cetirizine HCl	**Zyrtec**[a]
COMBINED H1 AND H2 RECEPTOR ANTAGONIST	
Doxepin	**Sinequan**

[a]Available over the counter.

Table A-8 STEROID–FREE BARRIER CREAMS

Barrier creams are steroid-free creams for the management of mild to moderate eczema (atopic dermatitis) and contact dermatitis. They enhance the skin's ability to attract, hold, and distribute moisture and help restore the balance of lipids to increase effective skin barrier function.

Brand Name	Comments
Mimyx, Atopiclair, EpiCeram Emulsion	Prescription required
CeraVe Moisturizing Cream	Available over the counter

Table A-9   TOPICAL ANTIBIOTIC FORMULARY

Generic (Brand) Name	Comments
2% Mupirocin (**Bactroban, Centany**)	Topical antibiotic activity, mostly against gram-positive aerobic bacteria (including *Staphylococcus* and methicillin-resistant *Staphylococcus*) and many strains of *Streptococcus*
Bacitracin ointment[a]	Bactericidal against many gram-positive organisms such as streptococci, staphylococci, and pneumococci but is inactive against most gram-negative organisms
Neomycin[a]	Effective against most aerobic gram-negative organisms. Group A streptococci are relatively resistant.
Polymyxin B	Effective against *Pseudomonas*, *Escherichia coli*, and other gram-negative bacteria. It has little effect on gram-positive organisms.
Polymyxin/neomycin/ bacitracin(**Neosporin**)[a]	Combination of topical antibiotics

[a]ALERT: Frequent contact allergens, particularly in patients with leg ulcers.

Table A-10   Androgenetic Alopecia Formulary

Generic Name	Brand Name
TOPICAL AGENTS	
Minoxidil 5%	**Rogaine** foam
Minoxidil 2% solution	Generic only
ORAL AGENT	
Finasteride	**Propecia,** which acts as a specific competitive inhibitor of 5-alpha-reductase

Table A-11   AGENTS THAT CAUSE HYPOPIGMENTATION ("BLEACHING CREAMS") FORMULARY

Hydroquinone products act to inhibit the enzymatic oxidation of tyrosine, thereby inhibiting melanin formation.

TIP: Use of daily sunscreen and sun avoidance is paramount in the prevention of pigment recurrence. Effects are seen between 2 and 6 months. If there is no improvement after 2 months of treatment, use of the product should be discontinued.

Generic Name	Brand Name	Comments
Hydroquinone, 2%	**Ambi, Esotérica**	Available over the counter as cream, gel, or solution
Hydroquinone, 4%	**Tri-Luma**	Available by prescription only
		A combination topical. corticosteroid, depigmentation agent (hydroquinone), and keratolytic (retinoid)
	Lustra and **Lustra-AF**	Furthermore, also contains a broad-spectrum sunblock including avobenzone that helps minimize ultraviolet induced hyperpigmentation and sun damage
Hydroquinone, 3%	**Melanex**	Topical solution
Azelaic acid	**Azelex** 20% cream	Safe even in pregnancy
Monobenzone	**Benoquin**	Monobenzyl ether of hydroquinone.
		Prevents melanin production and may cause destruction of melanocytes and permanent depigmentation; used to irreversibly depigment normal skin surrounding vitiliginous lesions in patients with disseminated vitiligo vulgaris.
		ALERT: This agent should be used only when permanent depigmentation is desired.

Table A-12   SCABICIDAL AND PEDICULICIDAL FORMULARY

Generic Name	Brand Name	Comments
SCABICIDAL AGENTS		
Topical		
Permethrin cream 5%	**Elimite, Acticin**	Currently considered the treatment of choice for scabies; has not been proven to be safe in infants younger than 2 months or in pregnant and nursing women
Gamma benzene hexachloride (Lindane)	**Kwell** lotion and cream	**ALERT: There have been several reports of neurotoxicity in infants**
Precipitated sulfur ointment (6%)		Used in pregnant or lactating women and in infants younger than 2 months
Oral		
Ivermectin	**Stromectol**	An antihelmintic that can be administered (off-label) in a single oral dose. **Dosage:** 0.2 mg/kg in a single oral dose that is repeated in 10 days. For 6-mg tablets the dose is given below:

Weight (kg)	No. of Tablets
15–24	1/2
25–35	1
36–50	1 1/2
51–65	2
66–79	2 1/2
>80	3 to 4

Generic Name	Brand Name	Comments
PEDICULICIDAL AGENT		
Malathion	**Ovide**	Currently considered the treatment of choice for head lice

SELECTED DRUGS AND THEIR INDICATIONS

The following is a brief description of systemic medications mentioned in the book:

- Acitretin **(Soriatane):** a systemic retinoid with anti-inflammatory and antiproliferative properties
- Azathioprine **(Imuran):** an immunosuppressant used in organ transplantation and autoimmune diseases such as pemphigus, bullous pemphigoid, leukocytoclastic vasculitis, acute lupus erythematosus, and pyoderma gangrenosum.
- Chlorambucil **(Leukeran):** a nitrogen mustard alkylating agent chemotherapy drug mainly used in the treatment of chronic lymphocytic leukemia. It is used in dermatology as an immunosuppressive drug for various autoimmune and inflammatory conditions
- Colchicine: an anti-inflammatory drug that is sometimes used to treat aphthous stomatitis, acute neutrophilic dermatoses (e.g., Sweet syndrome), Behçet disease, dermatomyositis, leukocytoclastic vasculitis, and urticarial vasculitis
- Cyclophosphamide: an alkylating agent used to treat various types of cancer and some autoimmune disorders such as systemic lupus erythematosus and Wegener granulomatosis
- Cyclosporine **(Neoral):** an immunosuppressant drug widely used to reduce the activity of the patient's immune system and, thus, the risk of organ rejection. Cyclosporine is also used in psoriasis, severe atopic dermatitis pyoderma gangrenosum, chronic autoimmune urticaria, and, infrequently, in rheumatoid arthritis and related diseases
- Cyclosporine ophthalmic emulsion: 0.05% **(Restasis)** is prescribed for increasing tear production due to ocular inflammation associated with keratoconjunctivitis sicca
- Dapsone: a primary treatment for dermatitis herpetiformis and acute neutrophilic dermatoses such as erythema elevatum diutinum and granuloma faciale; also an antibacterial drug with potent anti-inflammatory effects for susceptible cases of leprosy
- D-penicillamine: a form of immunosuppression to treat rheumatoid arthritis. It works by reducing numbers of T lymphocytes, inhibiting macrophage function, decreasing interleukin-1, decreasing rheumatoid factor, and preventing collagen from cross-linking
- Hydroxychloroquine **(Plaquenil):** an antimalarial drug used in the treatment of lupus erythematosus, polymorphous light eruption, and sarcoidosis
- Intravenous immune globulin (IVIG): when administered intravenously, contains the pooled immunoglobulin [antibody] G (IgG) extracted from the plasma of more than 1000 blood donors; mainly used as treatment of primary and secondary immune deficiencies, as well as inflammatory and autoimmune diseases
- Mycophenolate mofetil **(CellCept):** indicated for the prevention of organ transplant rejection; increasingly used as a steroid-sparing treatment in immune-mediated disorders such as small vessel vasculitides, pemphigus vulgaris, and psoriasis
- Pentoxifylline **(Trental):** improves flow through the blood vessels. It is used to treat intermittent claudication and in such conditions as atrophie blanche and other types of vasculitis
- Thalidomide: also inhibits angiogenesis, which may help AIDS patients with Kaposi sarcoma, aphthous ulcer, Behçet syndrome, and graft-versus-host disease.

⚠ **ALERT: This drug is a known teratogen.**

TREATMENTS FOR SELECTED SKIN DISORDERS

For proper dosages and contraindications, refer to other current books on therapy. The author is indebted to the following excellent references: Lebwohl MG, Heymann WR, et al. *Treatment of Skin Disease: Comprehensive Therapeutic Strategies.* St. Louis: Mosby, 2002, and Levine N, Levine CC. *Dermatology Therapy: A to Z Essentials.* New York: Springer, 2004.

- Atrophie blanche vasculitis: pentoxifylline **(Trental),** aspirin, clopidogrel **(Plavix);** less commonly, warfarin
- Behçet syndrome: systemic steroids, azathioprine, cyclosporine, colchicine
- Bowenoid papulosis: local excision, electrodesiccation and curettage, cryosurgery, CO_2 laser ablation, 5-fluorouracil cream
- Bullous pemphigoid: systemic and/or superpotent topical steroids, tetracycline in combination with niacinamide, dapsone, methotrexate, azathioprine, intravenous immune globulin (IVIG), other immunosuppressives
- Dermatitis herpetiformis: dapsone, sulfapyridine, gluten-free diet, systemic steroids
- Dermatofibrosarcoma protuberans: wide local excision or Mohs micrographic surgery
- Dermatomyositis: topical steroids, systemic steroids for muscle disease; antimalarials, methotrexate, azathioprine, mycophenolate mofetil, etanercept, infliximab, and IVIG
- Epidermolysis bullosa acquisita: systemic steroids, azathioprine, dapsone, colchicine, IVIG, cyclosporine, extracorporeal photochemotherapy
- Erythromelalgia: elevation of extremity, aspirin, prostaglandins, gabapentin, sodium nitroprusside, calcium channel blockers, nonsteroidal anti-inflammatory agents, treatment of underlying disease (e.g., myeloproliferative disorder) if present
- Fox Fordyce disease: topical and intralesional steroids, topical clindamycin, oral contraceptives, topical retinoids and UVB; also oral retinoids, electrocautery, excision
- Hailey-Hailey disease (familial benign pemphigus): topical steroid preparations (class 5 or 6), topical tacrolimus ointment, topical calcitriol, topical antibiotics (clindamycin or erythromycin), systemic antibiotics. Dapsone, systemic steroids, methotrexate, oral retinoids and other immunosuppressive agents; photodynamic therapy, as well as low-dose botulinum toxin have been reported to be of value; surgical excision and CO_2 laser therapy may be effective
- Kawasaki syndrome: current recommended therapy in the acute phase includes a single infusion of intravenously administered gamma globulin and

high-dose aspirin. Clopidogrel **(Plavix)** may be briefly substituted for aspirin in patients allergic to aspirin. An alternative treatment is infliximab **(Remicade);** other alternative therapies for resistant cases include cyclophosphamide and methotrexate

- Keratosis follicularis (Darier disease): sunscreens, low- or mid-potency topical steroids, and **Burow solution** may be helpful, along with topical retinoids and topical 5-fluorouracil. Systemic medications such as oral retinoids (e.g., acitretin, isotretinoin) and oral antibiotics are used to clear secondary bacterial superinfection

- Pemphigus vulgaris: systemic steroids, cyclosporine, mycophenolate mofetil, azathioprine, IVIG, other immunosuppressives

- Pityriasis rubra pilaris: topical steroids; oral retinoids (e.g., **Soriatane**); methotrexate cyclosporine, azathioprine, and extracorporeal photochemotherapy

- Polyarteritis nodosa: systemic therapies such as corticosteroids, IVIG, pentoxifylline, including immunosuppressive agents such as azathioprine and methotrexate; also tamoxifen and infliximab

- Porokeratosis of Mibelli and disseminated superficial actinic porokeratosis: cryotherapy, topical 5-fluorouracil, oral retinoids, CO_2 laser, imiquimod, topical retinoids, dermabrasion

- Pyoderma gangrenosum: topical superpotent steroids, tacrolimus and pimecrolimus; cromolyn sodium 2% solution, nitrogen mustard, and 5-aminosalicylic acid. Systemic therapies include corticosteroids, cyclosporine, mycophenolate mofetil, azathioprine, dapsone, tacrolimus, cyclophosphamide, chlorambucil, thalidomide, tumor necrosis factor-alpha inhibitors, and nicotine. Intravenous therapies include pulsed methylprednisolone, pulsed cyclophosphamide, infliximab, and IVIG. Hyperbaric oxygen is also used

- Sarcoidosis: topical, intralesional and systemic steroids; antimalarials, and methotrexate. Also isotretinoin, laser, excision, thalidomide, methotrexate, chlorambucil, clofazimine, minocycline, quinacrine, as well as etanercept, have been used in certain cases

- Systemic scleroderma: D-penicillamine, interferon-gamma, mycophenolate mofetil, cyclophosphamide, photopheresis, thalidomide, methotrexate, losartan, etanercept, allogeneic bone marrow transplantation, UVA, UVB-1 (used with varying degrees of qualified success)

Diagnostic and Therapeutic Techniques

DIAGNOSTIC TECHNIQUES

Potassium Hydroxide Examination

The potassium hydroxide examination has the advantage of providing an immediate diagnosis of a superficial fungal infection rather than waiting weeks for the results of a fungal culture. It is performed by gently scraping the "active border" with a no. 15 scalpel blade (Fig. B-1). A thin layer of scale is gathered on a slide and is then covered with a coverslip. A single drop of a potassium hydroxide solution such as **Swartz-Lamkins fungal stain** is used with an eyedropper. The undersurface of the slide is heated gently with a lighter or a match until bubbling begins. Identification is best begun with a low-power scan to identify scale and possibly hyphae. High power (×40) is used to confirm the presence of hyphae and/or spores (Figs. B-2 and B-3).

Wood Lamp Examination

A Wood lamp is a handheld black light that makes hypopigmented areas appear lighter, and depigmented areas (e.g., those produced by vitiligo) appear as a pure "milk-white" fluorescence (Fig. B-4). It is also used to help in the diagnosis of tinea versicolor and erythrasma, as well as in the delineation of certain hyperpigmentation disorders (e.g., melasma).

Tzanck Preparation

A Tzanck preparation is used to aid in the diagnosis of herpes simplex virus (HSV) and herpes zoster virus (HZV); however, it does not enable one to distinguish HSV from HZV. For best results, a fresh, intact vesicle or bulla usually present for less than 24 hours is preferred. The specimen is then air-dried and stained with a supravital stain such as Giemsa, Wright, or methylene blue, which is left on for one minute. Examination under oil immersion (×100) helps identify the characteristic multinucleated giant cells (Fig. B-5).

Patch Testing

Patch testing is used as an aid to identify specific allergens in patients with histories suggestive of allergic contact dermatitis. The allergens most commonly responsible for allergic contact dermatitis are standardized and impregnated on tape. The tape is placed, against the skin of the patient's back for 48 hours, and then removed. A final reading is performed in 96 hours. The presence of erythema, papules, or vesicles (i.e., an acute eczematous reaction) is strongly positive. Interpretation of results and correlation with clinical findings require experience and is generally performed by dermatologists.

Dermoscopy

Dermoscopy, performed with a handheld dermoscope, is a noninvasive in vivo method that allows the evaluation of skin morphology that is not visible to the naked eye. The identification of specific diagnostic patterns and colors can suggest various diagnoses as well as differentiate a malignant pigmented lesion, such as melanoma (Figs. B-6 and

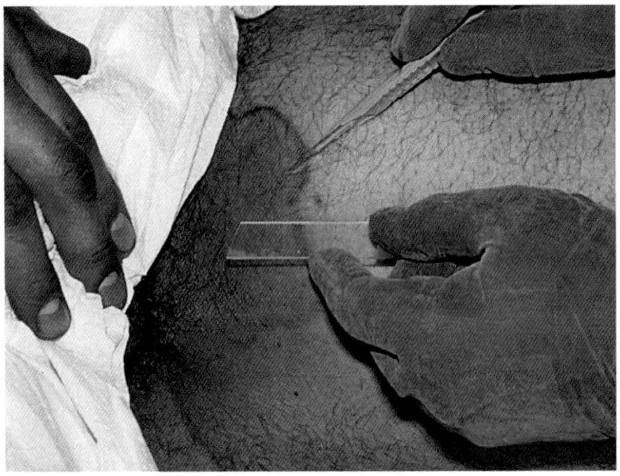

Figure B-1 Potassium hydroxide examination. Collection of scale from the "active" border of a lesion. (From Goodheart HP. *Goodheart's Photoguide to Common Skin Disorders: Diagnosis and Management.* 3rd ed. Philadelphia: Lippincott Williams & Wilkins; 2009, with permission.)

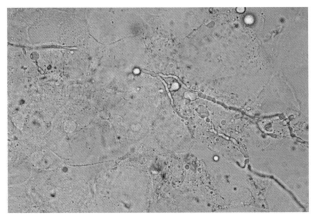

Figure B-2 Potassium hydroxide examination. Dermatophyte. Note the wavy-branched hyphae with uniform widths coursing over cell borders. (From Goodheart HP. *Goodheart's Photoguide to Common Skin Disorders: Diagnosis and Management.* 3rd ed. Philadelphia: Lippincott Williams & Wilkins; 2009, with permission.)

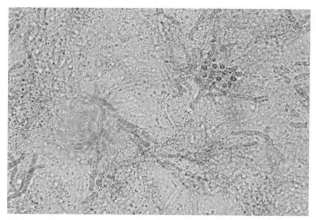

Figure B-3 Potassium hydroxide examination. Tinea versicolor. Note the short, stubby hyphae ("spaghetti") and the clusters of spores ("meatballs"). (From Goodheart HP. *Goodheart's Photoguide to Common Skin Disorders: Diagnosis and Management.* 3rd ed. Philadelphia: Lippincott Williams & Wilkins; 2009, with permission.)

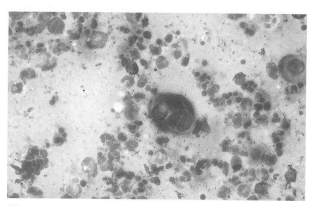

Figure B-5 Positive Tzanck preparations. Note the multinucleated giant cells with large nuclei. Compare to nuclei of normal-sized keratinocytes, which are the size of neutrophils. (From Goodheart HP. *Goodheart's Photoguide to Common Skin Disorders: Diagnosis and Management.* 3rd ed. Philadelphia: Lippincott Williams & Wilkins: 2009, with permission.)

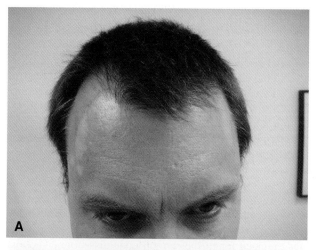

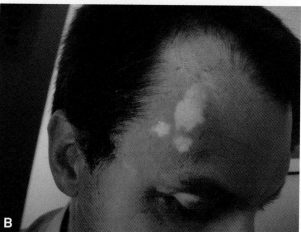

Figure B-4 A: Vitiligo. **B:** Vitiligo: Wood light examination.

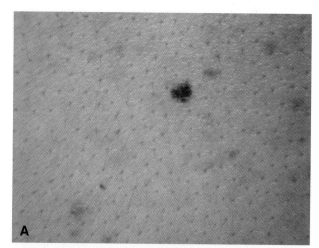

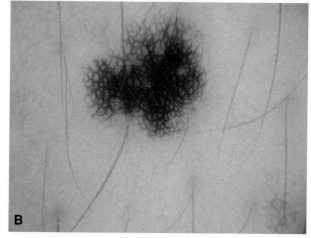

Figure B-6 A: Dermoscopy. Pigmented lesion. **B:** Dermoscopy. Same lesion as B-6A under dermoscopy with a benign network pattern of a melanocytic nevus.

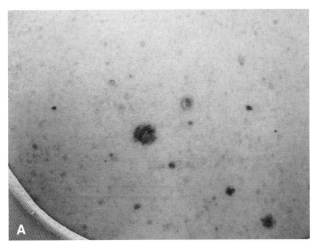
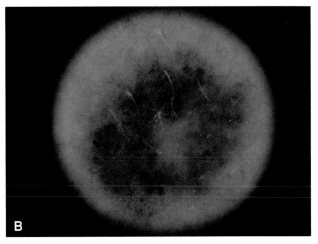

Figure B-7 A: Dermoscopy. Pigmented lesion. **B:** Dermoscopy. Same lesion as B-7A under dermoscopy with an asymmetric pattern, variegation of colors. Biopsy proved this lesion to be a melanoma in situ.

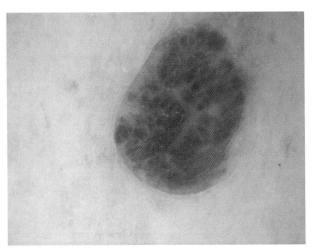

Figure B-8 Dermoscopy. Cherry angioma.

B-7), from a benign melanocytic nevus. It also helps to distinguish a pigmented lesion from a vascular lesion (Fig. B-8).

Sentinel Lymph Node Biopsy

Sentinel lymph node biopsy is used to detect the first lymph node draining from the site of a melanoma. A technetium 99-labeled colloid and a vital blue dye are injected around the area of a primary melanoma or biopsy scar (at the time of wide local excision/re-excision). The sentinel node is thus identified and excised for detection of possible micrometastases.

Sentinel lymph node biopsy is generally indicated for the staging of the regional nodal basin(s) for primary tumors one mm or greater in depth and when certain high-risk histologic features (e.g., ulceration, extensive regression) are present in thinner melanomas. If results are positive, an elective lymph node dissection is usually performed at a later date. A negative sentinel node obviates the need for further lymph node dissection. There is conflicting data and controversy about the improved survival value of sentinel lymph node biopsy for melanoma patients.

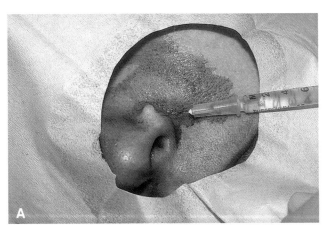
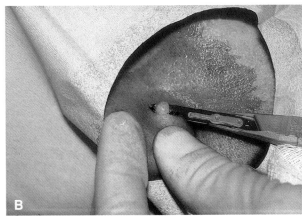

Figure B-9 A: Shave biopsy. **B:** Shave biopsy. (From Goodheart HP. *Goodheart's Photoguide to Common Skin Disorders: Diagnosis and Management.* 3rd ed. Philadelphia: Lippincott Williams & Wilkins; 2009, with permission.)

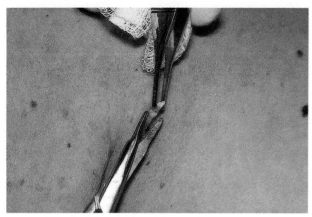

Figure B-10 Snip excision. (From Goodheart HP. *Goodheart's Photoguide to Common Skin Disorders: Diagnosis and Management.* 3rd ed. Philadelphia: Lippincott Williams & Wilkins; 2009, with permission.)

Shave Biopsy And Shave Removal

Shave biopsy and shave removal is used for the diagnosis and therapeutic removal of superficial skin lesions, such as melanocytic nevi, warts, seborrheic and solar keratoses, pyogenic granulomas, and skin tags, as well as other benign and malignant skin tumors (Fig. B-9).

Scissor (Snip) Biopsy And Snip Excision

Scissor biopsy and snip excision is a fast method to remove a single lesion or many lesions in one visit. Certain elevated or pedunculated lesions such as warts, nevi, seborrheic keratoses, and skin tags are ideally suited for removal with scissors and can be precisely removed level to the skin (Fig. B-10).

Punch Biopsy

A punch biopsy is performed by using a 3- to 5-mm cylindric cutting instrument ("punch") to remove all or part of a lesion. This method is most useful for biopsy of relatively flat, inflammatory lesions such as those seen in psoriasis, lichen planus, and vasculitis (Fig. B-11).

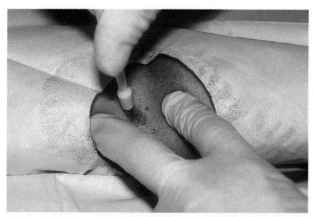

Figure B-11 Punch biopsy. (From Goodheart HP. *Goodheart's Photoguide to Common Skin Disorders: Diagnosis and Management.* 3rd ed. Philadelphia: Lippincott Williams & Wilkins; 2009, with permission.)

⚠ **ALERT: Areas to be avoided are the digits, locations around the facial nerve, or in any region where the operator is unfamiliar with the underlying anatomy.**

Simple Elliptical Excision

Excisional biopsies provide more extensive tissue samples. They may be performed on discrete lesions, such as cysts, basal or squamous cell carcinoma, malignant melanoma, or other solitary tumors and nevi.

THERAPEUTIC TECHNIQUES

Soaking And Smearing

✔ **TIP: The "soak and smear" technique (B, Illustration) is a rapid way to treat various severe inflammatory dermatoses, especially eczema, poison ivy, psoriasis, and lichen planus. The "soaking" hydrates the skin, which increases its permeability to topical steroids and allows the patient to treat precise areas that are involved. It may often obviate the need to prescribe systemic steroids.**

The patient simply soaks in a bathtub, with the entire body or affected body part immersed in plain lukewarm water for 20 minutes. Then, *without* drying the skin, he or she should *immediately* smear the skin with a *thin* film of a potent (class 2-3) or superpotent (class 1) steroid *ointment*. The following day, the patient may be advised to apply a less greasy potent (class 2-3) steroid *cream* once

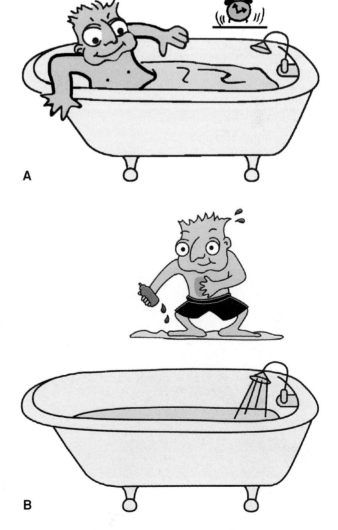

A

B

in the morning and during the day to the most troublesome or itchy areas, if needed.

This routine can lead to fast improvement, even in a day or 2. The ointment is greasy; therefore, the patient is instructed to wear old pajamas after treatment. The number of nights of soaking and smearing depends on how severe the skin condition is and how long it takes to get it under control (generally 2 to 3 days).

If the patient has no bathtub or is unable to use one, he or she should be instructed to take a long, lukewarm shower followed by the application the steroid ointment to the wet skin, which is then covered with a cool water-soaked towel and left on the skin for 20 minutes.

Bleach Baths

For infected, impetiginized skin, the addition of a 1/2 cup (1/4 cup or less for infants) of bleach (**Clorox**) for 2 to 3 days can be mixed in with the bath water. "Bleach bath," which is similar to chlorination in swimming pools, helps control bacteria on the skin. This simple, inexpensive approach often serves as an alternative to systemic antibiotics.

⚠ ALERT: The patient should be instructed to mix the bleach-water solution well and not pour the Clorox directly on the skin.

Burow Solution

Burow solution is a topical antibacterial astringent preparation that helps "dry up" and control weeping, oozing, and infected skin. Burow solution (**Domeboro**, **Bluboro**, **Boropak**) can be obtained in most pharmacies without a prescription. It is available as a powder in packets or tablets that are dissolved in water. The solution is applied using a wet cotton, cloth, or gauze compress moistened by the solution and placed over the affected skin area for 15 to 20 minutes. This is performed 3 to 4 times each day until all areas are no longer oozing.

Intralesional Steroids

Intralesional triamcinolone acetonide (Kenalog, 2.5, 5, 10, 40 mg/mL) is injected using a 30-gauge needle. It may be necessary to repeat the procedure at 4- to 6-week intervals. This medication is useful for the treatment of various skin lesions such as acne cysts, hypertrophic scars and keloids, localized psoriatic plaques (Fig. B-12), lichen planus, and prurigo nodularis.

⚠ ALERT: Possible local atrophy and telangiectasias may result.

Scale Removal For Scalp Psoriasis

When it is necessary to remove thick hyperkeratotic scale, a 6% salicylic acid preparation such as **Keralyt gel** or **Salex cream** or **lotion** is applied to the scaly areas while the hair is wet. After application, the patient is instructed to cover the head with a shower cap, which is left on overnight or at least for several hours. The area then is shampooed again. This is repeated if the scale builds up again. Similarly, the salicylic acid preparation can be used on other hyperkeratotic lesions elsewhere on the body.

Electrodesiccation And Curettage

Electrodesiccation and curettage is a method to remove or destroy many types of benign superficial skin lesions such as warts, seborrheic keratoses, skin tags, molluscum contagiosum, and condylomata acuminatum. Electrodesiccation and curettage is also used as a method to treat skin cancers such as small basal cell and squamous cell carcinomas.

Curettage is a scraping or scooping technique performed with a dermal curette, which has a round or oval sharp ring. Electrodesiccation, without or without curettage, is often used to eliminate warts, skin tags, and spider angiomas and to flatten lesions (e.g., melanocytic nevi). Conversely, curettage without electrodesiccation may also be used to remove many of these epidermal lesions.

Cryosurgery

In cryosurgery, liquid nitrogen is applied with a cotton swab or a cryospray gun. It is most commonly used on warts and solar keratoses (Fig. B-13). Tissue destruction results from intercellular and extracellular ice formation, denaturing liquid protein complexes, and cell dehydration.

✔ TIP: Treatment of filiform warts may be performed with a mosquito hemostat that has been immersed for 10 seconds in liquid nitrogen. The wart is then gently grasped for about 4 to 5 seconds. This simple, relatively painless procedure causes very little collateral damage to the surrounding skin (Fig. B-14).

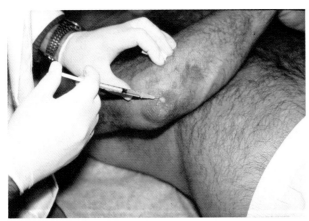

Figure B-12 Intralesional triamcinolone. Given here for the treatment of a psoriatic plaque.

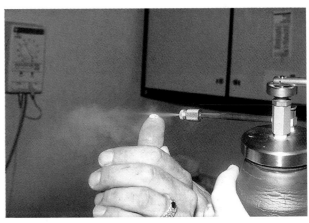

Figure B-13 Cryosurgery. Application with a cryogun apparatus.

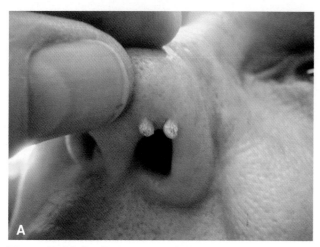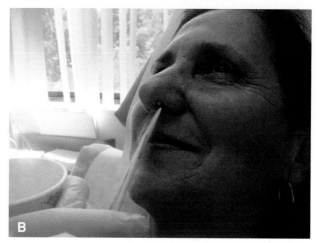

Figure B-14 A: Cryosurgery of filiform warts. **B:** Cryosurgery of filiform warts. Treatment of filiform warts with a mosquito hemostat that has been immersed in liquid nitrogen.

Mohs Micrographic Surgery

Mohs micrographic surgery is a microscopically controlled method of removing skin cancers that allows for controlled excision and maximum preservation of normal tissue. It has the highest cure rate of all surgical treatments. Mohs surgery is most suited for morpheaform basal cell carcinomas and squamous cell carcinomas, recurrent tumors lesions larger than 2 cm in size, as well as tumors situated on the ears, lips, nose, and nasolabial folds.

Phototherapy And Lasers

Many phototherapy and laser modalities are useful in the treatment of various skin disorders. Ultraviolet (UVB, narrowband UVB, psoralen with UVA [PUVA]) treatment is used for extensive and widespread moderate-to-severe plaque psoriasis that is not responding to topical therapy. It is also for conditions such as severe, recalcitrant atopic dermatitis, cutaneous T-cell lymphoma, and vitiligo.

The excimer laser may be effective in treating recalcitrant plaque and palmoplantar psoriasis. The pulsed dye laser is used to treat solar keratoses, actinic cheilitis, sebaceous hyperplasia, acne vulgaris, and warts.

Radiotherapy

Although it is currently used less often than other procedures, radiotherapy is best suited for patients of advanced age and poor general health. Radiation therapy can be used to treat many types of basal cell carcinoma, even those overlying bone and cartilage.

Management of Acne and Rosacea

ACNE

As with rosacea (see later discussion), long-term control of acne should be attempted with topical therapy alone, and oral antibiotics should be reserved for initial control and for breakthrough flares.

Topical Therapies

Benzoyl Peroxide

- Benzoyl peroxide is found in many brand name over-the-counter products such as **Clearasil, Oxy 5,** and **Oxy10** (Table C-1). It is available in both water-based and alcohol-based vehicles, soaps, medicated pads, and washes.
- It can be used alone for mild acne
- There have been no reports of bacterial resistance to this agent
- It can be used in conjunction with topical retinoids as well as topical or systemic antibiotics for moderate to severe acne

Topical Retinoids

- The topical retinoids (Table C-2) are primarily comedolytic (i.e., they treat blackheads and whiteheads)
- They also have potent anti-inflammatory effects

Topical Antibiotics

- Topical antibiotics (Table C-3) can be used alone; however, drug resistance has been reported with these antibiotics. The combination of these agents with benzoyl peroxide (see later discussion) has obviated this problem
- Furthermore, the combination of an antibiotic with benzoyl peroxide appears to add a synergistic effect

Combination of Topical Antibiotic and Benzoyl Peroxide

- **Benzamycin, BenzaClin,** and **Duac** gels are the commonly prescribed combination formulations (Table C-4)

Alternative Topical Prescription Drugs

- Azelaic acid (**Azelex** 20%), as well as preparations that contain sulfur and sodium sulfacetamide such as **Sulfacet-R lotion, Novacet lotion,** and **Klaron lotion,** are alternative topical prescription agents for treating acne

Newer Combinations

- The antibiotic clindamycin combined with a retinoid (**Ziana**) as well a benzoyl peroxide combined with a retinoid (**Epiduo gel**) (Table C-5) are newer combination drugs

Systemic Therapies

- Patients who have moderate-to-severe acne that is unresponsive to topical treatment alone or acne that tends to scar generally receive systemic treatment in addition to topical therapy. Less commonly, alternative antibiotics are used. These include erythromycin, amoxicillin, and azithromycin (**Zithromax**). Other agents are listed in Table C-6

Oral Antibiotics

- The oral antibiotics that are the tetracycline derivatives such as plain tetracycline, minocycline, doxycycline, and the extended-release **Solodyn** are prescribed most often
- Less commonly, alternative antibiotics are used. These include erythromycin, amoxicillin, azithromycin (**Zithromax**), as well as cephalosporins and trimethoprim-sulfasoxazole

Hormonal Treatment

- In female patients, hormonal treatment is an option when conventional topical and systemic therapies are ineffective or when an endocrine abnormality is discovered
- Oral contraceptives and antiandrogenic drugs such as spironolactone (**Aldactone**) may be prescribed in carefully selected situations
- Oral contraceptives such as **Yasmin** and **YAZ, Ortho Tri-Cyclen, Ortho-Cyclen, Ortho-Cyclen Lo, Estrostep, Ortho-Cept, Alesse, Mircette,** and **Desogen** are relatively low in androgenic activity

Oral Retinoids

- The oral retinoid 13-*cis*-retinoic acid (**Accutane**) a synthetic derivative of vitamin A, is reserved for

Table C-1 BENZOYL PEROXIDE–CONTAINING PREPARATIONS FOR ACNE

Preparation	Strength(s)
Over-the-Counter	
Oxy 5, Oxy 10	5%, 10% benzoyl peroxide
Clear y Design	2.5% benzoyl peroxide gel
Clearasil 10%	10% benzoyl peroxide lotion
Prescription	
Desquam-X 5, Desquam-X 10	5%, 10% benzoyl peroxide gel (water-based)
Desquam-E	2.5%, 5%, 10% benzoyl peroxide gel (water-based)
Bevoxyl-4, Bevoxyl-8	4%, 8% benzoyl peroxide gel (water-based)
Triaz pads	3%, 6%, 10% benzoyl peroxide gel (water-based)

Table C-2 TOPICAL RETINOIDS FOR ACNE

Generic Name	Brand Name	Strength	Sizes
Tretinoin	**Retin-A** cream, gel	Creams: 0.025%, 0.05%, 0.1% Gels: 0.01%, 0.025%	20 g, 45 g
Tretinoin	**Retin-A Micro** topical gel	0.04%, 0.1%	20 g, 45 g, 50-g pump dispenser
Tretinoin	**Avita** cream, gel	0.025%	20 g, 45 g
Adapalene	**Differin** cream, gel, solution, pledgets	0.1%, 0.3%	15 g, 45 g 30 mL, No. 60
Tazarotene	**Tazorac** cream, gel	0.05%, 0.1%	30 g, 100 g

Table C-3 TOPICAL ANTIBIOTICS FOR ACNE

Generic Name	Brand Name	Strength	Sizes
Erythromycin	**A/T/S** solution, gel	2%	60 mL, 30 g
Erythromycin	**Akne-Mycin** ointment	2%	25 g
Clindamycin	**Cleocin T** solution, gel, lotion	1%	30 mL, 60 mL
Clindamycin	Evoclin Foam	1%	50 g, 100 g

Table C-4 COMBINATION TOPICAL ANTIBIOTIC AND BENZOYL PEROXIDE AGENTS FOR ACNE

Generic Name	Brand Name	Size(s)
Erythromycin 3%/benzoyl peroxide 5%	**Benzamycin** gel	23.3 g, 46.6 g
Clindamycin 1%/benzoyl peroxide 5%	**BenzaClin** gel	25 g, 50 g
Clindamycin 1%/benzoyl peroxide 5%	**Duac** gel	45 g
Clindamycin 1.5 %/benzoyl peroxide 2.5%	**Acanya** gel	50 g

Table C-5 NEWER TOPICAL COMBINATIONS FOR ACNE

Generic Name	Brand Name	Size(s)
Clindamycin 1.2%/ tretinoin 0.25% gel	**Ziana**	30, 60 g
Adapalene 0.1%/ benzoyl peroxide 2.5%	**Epiduo Gel**	45 g

Table C-6 SYSTEMIC ANTIBIOTICS FOR ACNE AND/OR ROSACEA[a]

Generic Name	Brand Name	Delivery	Common Starting Dose
Tetracycline	(Generic)	Capsules	250 or 500 mg bid
Doxycycline	(Generic)	Capsules, tablets, liquid	50, 75, 100 mg bid
	Oracea	Capsules	40 mg qd
	Adoxa	Tablets	75 or 100 mg bid
Minocycline	(Generic)		50, 75, or 100 mg bid
	Solodyn	Tablets Extended-release tablets	45, 65, 90, 115, or 135 mg once daily (1 mg/kg per day)
	Minocin	Capsules, oral suspension	50 or 100 mg bid
	Dynacin	Capsules, tablets	50 or 100 mg bid

[a]bid, twice daily; qd, every day.

Table C-7 TOPICAL AGENTS FOR ROSACEA

Generic Name	Brand Name	Sizes
Metronidazole 1%	**Noritate** cream	30 g
Metronidazole 1%	**MetroGel, MetroCream**	60 g
Metronidazole 0.75%		45 g
Azelaic acid 15%, 20%	**Azelex, Finevin, Skinoren** creams	30 g, 50 g
Azelaic acid 15%	**Finacea** gel	30 g
Sodium sulfacetamide 10%/sulfur 5%	**Rosac** cream	45 g
Sodium sulfacetamide 10%	**Sulfacet-R** lotion	25 g

more severe, recalcitrant disease. This powerful agent promotes long-term remissions in severe acne. It is reserved for patients with severe nodular acne who are unresponsive to conventional therapy

- The original brand names for oral isotretinoin were **Accutane** in the United States and **Roaccutane** in rest of the world. The drug is now sold under several generic brand names in the United States

⚠ **ALERT: Isotretinoin *can cause severe birth defects if taken by a pregnant woman* or a woman who becomes pregnant while taking the drug, even for a short time.**

⚠ **ALERT: If a patient taking isotretinoin is showing signs of moodiness, depression, or psychosis, the drug should be discontinued.**

Surgery

Comedo Extraction

- Removal of comedones is performed with a comedo extractor, an instrument that minimizes skin injury. (This has been performed less commonly since the topical retinoids have become available)

Intralesional Corticosteroid Injection

- Intralesional injections of glucocorticosteroids, introduced with a syringe and a 30-guage needle, can reduce the inflammatory response and decrease the size of nodular inflammatory lesions of acne

Newer Technologies

- Laser and light therapies such as photodynamic therapy, intense pulsed light, and pulsed dye lasers offer promising, noninvasive treatment alternatives to oral medications

ROSACEA

Topical Therapies

- Some of the topical medications used to treat acne are also very effective for rosacea (Table C-7).

However, some precautions must be taken because many people with rosacea have very sensitive skin

- The following topical preparations can be used in combination with oral antibiotics

Metronidazole

- The "metros" are the most frequently prescribed first-line topical therapy for rosacea
- **Noritate** (metronidazole) 1% cream and **MetroGel** 1% gel are applied once daily on rosacea-prone areas. Metronidazole is also available as a generic 0.75 % cream that is applied b.i.d.

Azelaic Acid

- **Azelex** cream and **Finacea** gel are 15% azelaic acid preparations. (**Skinoren** is available in Europe.) They are considered to be as effective as metronidazole

Sodium Sulfacetamide and Sulfur

- Preparations containing sodium sulfacetamide and sulfur are also effective for rosacea **Klaron** and **Sulfacet-R** are preparations containing sodium sulfacetamide 10% and sulfur 5%
- Brand names include **Klaron, Plexion, Rosula, Rosac, Rosanil, Novacet,** and **Ovace.** These agents are available as lotions, creams, and washes

Systemic Therapy

- The same systemic oral antibiotics used to treat acne are also used to treat the papules and pustules of rosacea. See the previous discussion of acne and Table C-6
- Electrocautery with a small needle is used to destroy small telangiectasias

Newer Technologies

- Pulse dye lasers and intense pulsed light are sometimes used to destroy telangiectasias of rosacea

Index

Note: Page numbers followed by f and t indicates figure and table respectively.